SECRETS OF AN ALTERNATIVE DOCTOR

The Ultimate Compendium of Amazing Health Discoveries

By Keith Scott-Mumby
MD, MB ChB, HMD, PhD, FRCP (Colombo)

Introduction to Health Literacy

SECRETS OF AN ALTERNATIVE DOCTOR
By Keith Scott-Mumby MD, MB ChB, HMD, PhD, FRCP (Colombo)

Copyright © 2014 ALL RIGHTS RESERVED

Disclaimer

The information in this report is not meant to replace the attention or advice of licensed physicians or other healthcare professionals. Nothing contained in this report is meant to constitute personal medical advice for any particular individual.

In no event shall Professor Scott-Mumby be liable for any consequential damages arising out of any use of, or reliance on any content or materials contained herein, neither shall Professor Scott-Mumby be liable for any content of any external internet sites listed and services listed. Always consult your own licensed medical practitioner if you are in any way concerned about your health. You must satisfy yourself of the validity of the professional qualifications of any health care provider you contact as a result of this report.

Please be aware: No holistic alternative or mainstream pain treatment can boast a one hundred percent record of success. As with any medical treatment, results of the treatments described in this report will vary from one person to another.

PLEASE DO NOT USE THE INFORMATION FROM THIS REPORT IF YOU ARE NOT WILLING TO ASSUME THE RISK.

All rights reserved. No part of this publication may be reproduced, stored in a retrieval system, or transmitted in any form or by any means, electronic, mechanical, photocopying, recording or otherwise, whether for financial gain or otherwise, without the prior written permission of the copyright owner.

ISBN: 978-0-9884196-5-0

Published by Mother Whale Inc. PO Box 371225, Las Vegas, NV, 89137

Printed in the United States of America

CONTENTS

1. WHAT DOCTORS NEVER TELL YOU ABOUT YOUR BODY
The Science of Elimination Can Rejuvenate Your Health 3
Do Genes Determine Your Death? 4
The Myth of Evidence-Based Science 5
Understanding the Mid-Life Crisis 8
Back Pain Is a Common Agony….But You Can Beat It 11
Testosterone: Good for the Heart and Blood Pressure 14
Alzheimer's Disease…Something You Don't Want 21
The Body Matrix - Can You Create a Whole New You? 22
Could Stardust Fight Aging and Obesity? 26
How to Avoid a Fatal Blood Clot:
Eye-Opening Study Explains Why Lowering Your Blood Viscosity Is Crucial 29
A Novel Technique for Cleaning Your Teeth 32
How to Fight Candida and Painful Yeast Infections 33
The Brain and Gut Connection – Linked to Alzheimer's Disease 34
Why Antibiotics Make You Fat 35
Why No One Wants to Talk About Parasites 38
Get Tanned, Not Skin Cancer! The Safest Sunscreen 39
The Natural Healing Science of Tissue Cleaning 42
If I Had My Life Over Again… 48

2. TAKING CARE OF YOUR MIND, SOUL, & SPIRIT CAN HELP YOU LIVE LONGER
Quick Tips for Building Self-Confidence 55
Mending the Fragmented Self 56
Finding the Good in Everything, No Matter How Painful 67
True Happiness Is for Life, Not Only Just for the Holidays! 70
Right-Left Brain Myth 72

3. ROMANCE KEEPS YOU HEALTHY: LOVE & SEX
Finding Love in Everything 76
Waves That Thrill (Sex Is Not Intercourse) 78
What Does Love Mean? 79
Does Vigorous Sex Cause Memory Loss? 81
20+ Ways to Show Love 82
The Cuddle Hormone (Can I Get Shots?!) 84
10 Reasons Men Don't Want Sex and Women Have to Fight to Get It 85
All That Said, Here's a List of the 10 Most Common Reasons Why Men May Not Want Sex 85
Are Orgasms Sexual? 87

4. DEATH CREEPS IN AT THE GUMS – WISE DENTISTRY
What Dentists Don't Tell You! 91
Advanced Gum Disease May Raise Cancer Risk 96
Treating Gum Disease May Save Your Life..97
Brush Your Teeth, Live Longer..97

5. CANCER RESEARCH BREAKTHROUGHS
A Testing Breakthrough For Hidden Cancers 101
One of the Greatest Medicines of All Time Is Coming!..104
Could This Be a Living Drug?..107
Can This Plant Substance Kill Cancer Cells? 109
Does Music Destroy Cancer?..110
What Doctors Don't Tell You…About the War on Cancer 112
This Bioactive Compound Stalls Melanoma 114
When Is a Cancer Diagnosis Really Not Cancer? 115
A Final Word on Cancer… 118

6. UNLOCKING THE FOOD CODE
Let's Talk About Weight Loss!...122
Why We Need Salt 124
It's Not Just Fat; It's Fat AND Stress..125
Food Fraud: What Are You Really Eating? 126
Is Caffeine More Toxic Than Drugs? 129
The Truth About Genetically Modified Organisms (GMO's) 130
The Slippery Science of Fats and Oils..134
A Simple Weight-Loss Mind Strategy 137
Yet Again They Attack "Red Meat" 138
The Blood Fats Story Screwed Up..139
Vinegar May Aid in Fat Loss 142
Cholesterol Is GOOD...142
A Big Bum Protects 143
Beware of Those Bathroom Scales - They Lie! 144
If You Want Lasting Weight Loss Keep A Food Diary 145

7. HIDDEN CAUSES OF ALLERGIES & HOW TO GET ALLERGY RELIEF
Food Allergy: What's All the Fuss? 149
Mechanisms of Allergy – Chemical Sensitivity 161
Total Body Load – The Most Important of All Healing Principles.................................163
Symptoms of Allergy..165
CHEMICAL CLEAN UP - Chemical Intolerance & Hypersensitivity 167
Treatment for Allergies..174

8. ANTI-AGING SECRETS REVEALED

Do Genes Determine Your Death? 184
Harmonious Balance – The Key to Anti-Aging 185
Advances in Anti-Aging 186
Your Brain & Aging 188
Folic Acid for a Better Memory 193
Top 10 Non-Hormonal
Anti-Aging Supplements 194
Live a Younger Life 197
Extend Your Life with Carb Control 204
Human Growth Hormone - Do We Need It? 208
Oxygen & Why We Need Antioxidants 212
The Mother Hormone: PREGNENOLONE 215
No More Wrinkles! 216
The Anti-Aging Vitamin 218
Senility Is Inflammation 219

9. VIRTUAL MEDICINE... WHAT I ALSO CALL MEDICINE BEYOND!

Electrotherapy – Discover the Electric Language of the Body for Ultimate
Healing 224
Personalized Medicine Will Revolutionize Healthcare 227
What Is High-Voltage Syndrome? 230

10. THE FORGOTTEN ANTIBIOTICS THAT CAN SAVE YOUR LIFE

The Forgotten Alternatives to Antibiotics That Saved Millions of Lives 238
The Real Surprise Antibiotic…What is Iodine? 241
Alternatives to Antibiotics - These Friendly Viruses Easily Kill Deadly Bacteria 245
How Plant Oils Are Highly Effective Against Drug-Resistant Bacteria 248

11. VITAMINS, ANTIOXIDANTS & SUPERFOODS

Vitamin C Can Halve Your Chance of a Heart Attack 254
Vitamin D Has More Amazing Properties 255
Cocoa in Chocolate Is Good for the Heart 257
Did You Eat Your Sulfur Today? 257
Flax Seed Oil – Simply Amazing! 258
Herbs Can Really Work For Pain 259
The Number One Antioxidant 260
What Is Chia? Does It Work for Weight Loss? 260
Vitamin E Triumphs Again 261
Who Likes Artichokes? 262
Vitamin B1 Mega-Doses Reverse Early-Stage Kidney Disease 263
Something New For Allergies? 263
Some Of My Websites You Might Like to Visit 265

SOMETHING YOU CANNOT AFFORD TO SKIP!

I'm very grateful to the team who trawled through a huge pile of my writings, to extract for you life-changing health education pieces I've written.

I've published nearly 3 million words over the years, on all matters of health, from topics as wide-ranging as using bee venom injected into acupuncture points to amazing electronic devices that transform body metabolism; from herbs that have more power than modern medicines to very unusual advanced holistic psychology; from shining laser light up the nose to hanging upside down from silk cords; from transplanting sh*t from one person to another to swallowing parasite worms as a cure for colitis! I've seen it all: from very controversial cutting-edge discoveries to tried and tested science, the best there is, with many stops and stages in between.

And I've been proved right time and time again in my visions for the future. In fact, I've enjoyed writing an occasional column for years with the theme: *"I told 'em!",* meaning I said it already, often decades before it was supposed to have been discovered.

You've probably heard of "earthing" or "grounding," for example. Various writers (Clint Ober and Stephen Sinatra, for example) have claimed to discover the efficacy of this. They want the credit. But I published why it's necessary and important in a book of mine in 1988—a full 20 years before this was "discovered" by others—and it's a matter of written documentation.

Of course, some of my findings are already out of date, things move so fast in this field. That's not what we have presented for you here. You've got the best, the latest there is. Some of the things I wrote about more than three decades ago were so far ahead of their time that they are only just becoming "current"; and it will be a long time yet before some of them go out of date.

Take food allergies or the inflammatory foods effect: there was a time (early 1980s) when the idea was laughed at and the whole subject derided as "mumby-jumbo" in my hometown. But now no competent doctor on Earth would avoid this topic or not realize it is of crucial importance to patient health. I was called a quack back then but, by the end of the 1990s, the UK National Health Service (NHS) was buying my allergy formulas for NHS patients.

Quack to respectable in just under 20 years is pretty fast in medicine, where it often takes decades for old dogma to die away. Did you know, for example, that some surgeons went on cutting off limbs without anesthetic for over 20 years after anesthetics had been discovered and proven to render the patient senseless to the agony of an amputation? They weren't interested in what they considered new-fangled ideas but also were not interested, as you see, in patient welfare at all.

WHAT IS HEALTH LITERACY?

Medicine can be very slow. But you cannot afford to be left behind. These days, to survive and have any chance of being healthy, you must know about pollution, detoxing, genetic profiling, EMF dangers, inflammatory foods, the effect of GMO's, the gut microbiome, inflammatory markers, glucose metabolism, and much more. It's up to you.

Then you have to know how to protect your liver, your kidneys, brain, heart, and lungs. While we are at it, let's throw in skin health. You also need to know about hormone balancing, using natural viable hormones, and nutritional supplementation, from the right sources, to help our bodies cope with the tide of chemical excess.

To just leave all of this up to your doctor is the highway to disaster. The idea that there is a pill for everything and your doctor is an expert in the "right" pill for you is nonsense. Doctors mess up all the time. It often takes years for them to admit that a fashionable treatment simply isn't working or, even worse, that it's dangerous. Sometimes, because of financial interests, it seems like doctors and other practitioners will never change, unless new laws force them to adopt better practices that are in the patient's interest, instead of their own.

That's where my writings are good for you: I'm offering nourishing knowledge, not trying to sell you anything. I just share my expertise and when I say something is a fact, or based on true clinical experience, I mean it. It's not an advertising line. I just want to tell the truth, the complete truth, just as it really is. Call me old-fashioned but I just enjoy science as it should be.

I'm really saying that you need to become what I call "health literate." It's something you have to do. Get yourself educated so that you know what your doctor should be doing; or, if or she won't do it, that you know enough to go elsewhere and get the specific treatment that's right for you.

Of course a lot of ailments don't really need any "treatment," as such. All you have to do is make sensible changes in your diet and lifestyle. It's all here, in one form or another. This huge compilation is a great place to start your journey into health literacy. You need to become a "professor of you"… Good luck on that journey!

Keith Scott-Mumby MD, MB ChB, HMD, PhD
The Original "Alternative Doctor"
Las Vegas, June 2014

SECTION 1

WHAT DOCTORS NEVER TELL YOU ABOUT YOUR BODY

- THE MYTH OF EVIDENCE-BASED SCIENCE
- DO GENES DETERMINE YOUR DEATH?
- UNDERSTANDING THE MID-LIFE CRISIS
- BACK PAIN IS A COMMON AGONY….BUT YOU CAN BEAT IT
- TESTOSTERONE: GOOD FOR THE HEART AND BLOOD PRESSURE
- ALZHEIMER'S DISEASE… SOMETHING YOU DON'T WANT
- THE BODY MATRIX - CAN YOU CREATE A WHOLE NEW YOU?
- COULD STARDUST FIGHT AGING AND OBESITY?
- HOW TO AVOID A FATAL BLOOD CLOT
- A NOVEL TECHNIQUE FOR CLEANING YOUR TEETH
- HOW TO FIGHT CANDIDA AND PAINFUL YEAST INFECTIONS
- THE BRAIN AND GUT CONNECTION – LINKED TO ALZHEIMER'S DISEASE
- WHY ANTIBIOTICS MAKE YOU FAT
- WHY NO ONE WANTS TO TALK ABOUT PARASITES
- GET TANNED, NOT SKIN CANCER! THE SAFEST SUNSCREEN
- THE NATURAL SCIENCE OF TISSUE CLEANING
- IF I HAD MY LIFE OVER AGAIN…
- WHAT DOCTORS NEVER TELL YOU ABOUT YOUR BODY – BEWARE OF SHAM HOLISTIC PRACTITIONERS

They want your money, just as sure as money-hungry MDs. Some are good; some are bad; some are downright dangerous.

This recently got me mad…

A friend who lives down the road was not feeling well, so I dropped by. Let's call her Annie. She had been feeling weak and actually fainted at one point, we were told; she had to be picked up off the floor. My wife and I just wanted to make sure she was OK.

We knew Annie's current lifestyle and her work was EXTREMELY emotionally stressful at times (I couldn't endure it for more than a few hours, never mind months). She had been diagnosed as having adrenal exhaustion by a holistic practitioner and prescribed large doses of B12 and folic acid, by injection. This is **NOT** a recognized treatment for adrenal exhaustion.

What's more alarming, the doses were seriously wrong: she was injecting 5 mg of B12 every second day. That's insane! (And probably dangerous). When Annie started fainting, the same practitioner had told her to increase the injections to daily. That's 5,000 mcg 7 times a week: 35 times the MAXIMUM dose I would ever consider.

Fainting and headaches is a recognized side effect of B12 overdose. Yet this practitioner had her double the dose she was taking. It's just drug-doctor mentality, not holism.

This was a dangerous practitioner in my view (remember the near-riot conditions at the Nevada assembly two years ago, when there was a move to license all health practitioners, so some control could be brought in against these crazy fools, who demanded their "rights" to practice?)

Annie was also having a chiropractic "adjustment," having been told the problem was really in her spine (see below).

There's more. Annie was taking *ashwaganda*; she felt nauseated and had almost constant headaches. This brings me to a very important point. Ashwaganda is very badly tolerated and makes many people violently ill, mainly headaches and nausea.

It is not a good herb, for all its reputation.

What Many Holistic Practitioners Don't Know About Herbs

I want to point out the folly of the belief that all "herbs" are good, natural, and healthy.

No herbs are good, natural, and healthy by nature. Some have benefits for some people, some of the time—but all contain strong, potentially toxic ingredients (aren't marijuana, opium, and hemlock just "herbs"?)

Now here's the point. My medical paradigm, which has produced tens of thousands of miracles over the years, is that eliminating things is much more crucial than supplementing. If the body is under overload conditions, as was surely the case for Annie, then STOPPING foods and supplements is the way to go.

I told her to quit the ashwaganda and all injections and, in fact, all supplements. Overnight she felt better. As soon as I walked in the door next day, I could hear the difference in her voice. She was over 90% better; the nausea and headaches were gone; her physical strength was improved to the point where she was now out of her housecoat and dressed; her face, which had been grey and drained of color, was looking pinker.

I won't be sharing the rest of the story (it's ongoing) but here's the take-home: **many holistic practitioners, even with licenses and prescribing rights, do not know what they are doing and are potentially dangerous.**

Yet they try to take the moral high ground, yapping about those nasty rotten MDs. Mike Adams (the "Health Ranger") is part of this mindset: all doctors are bad; all holistic practitioners are good. Neither, of course, is even nearly true.

So beware. Choose carefully and remember they speak B*S* as fluently as MDs!

THE SCIENCE OF ELIMINATION CAN REJUVENATE YOUR HEALTH

Just like Annie, you can easily feel better, get rid of terrible allergies, body overload, and relieve inflammation once and for all. There are trigger foods that will spark allergies, increase overload, weight gain, and other illnesses in your body. The truth is that certain foods can be hostile.

Everyone is different and you need to find out which foods are not safe for YOU and how to eliminate them from your diet, even if they are seemingly "healthy foods."

It's a scientific secret I have used with many patients for over 40 years and it works immediately. I'm so glad you've taken the opportunity to get your very own copy of my alternative medicine discoveries. You'll be able to take charge of your health and create a whole new you starting now.

DO GENES DETERMINE YOUR DEATH?

A common question about aging is whether or not genes have an important role to play; in other words, does it matter who your ancestors are and does that have much bearing on how long you will live?

Obviously, if you inherit a gene for a fatal illness, it does. If you inherit a disorder that makes it difficult for your body to perform at optimum function, that too will play a part in how long you survive. Your family history will tell you this.

But the question remains: given a first-rate set of genes, can you control when you will die, even in part, or is it already pre-programmed? Obviously, it is an important point, because if you can influence the outcome of an inherited health trait or override it altogether, then truly your health and survival is in your own hands. The external or environmental factors that we bring to bear on issues can compensate for any destructive genetic material we have been provided with.

The Question Is: Can It Be Done?

The answer is slightly complicated but interesting. It's fashionable today, of course, to believe that everything is in the genes. But genes don't always show up. The gene for blue eyes, for instance, is subordinate to the gene for brown eyes. So if you get one of each (one from your mother and one from your father), the brown eyes will win. This is called a dominant gene (blue eyes are a recessive gene). But then it is found that sometimes even the dominant gene doesn't show up as it should. So scientists are beginning to talk of gene "expression" (whether it will come into play or not).

Many external factors will influence whether or not a gene expresses itself fully or partially.

So really, all this is saying that environmental factors are very important and genes are not the be-all-and-end-all, though science continues to peddle this silly story. Let us make this clearer by inventing an example: supposing that mother eating a lot of garlic while pregnant will suppress the brown eye gene (this is not true, we made it up to illustrate a point!).

Which then controls the eye color, genes or the garlic-rich diet? The answer is that it doesn't matter; because you can't change the genes, but you have the choice of eating garlic or not. So only the garlic is important. Do you see?

Where does this leave us in anti-aging science? There are many genetic factors that are being studied right now. One is in relation to calorie-restricted diets. We have remarked elsewhere that calorie restriction (CR) is the only known way to increase maximum life span (as opposed to average life expectancy).

Dr. Stephen R. Spindler, professor in the Department of Biochemistry at the University of California, Riverside, has studied the effect of long- and short-term CR diets on the expression of some 11,000 age-related genes in animals. He found something remarkable and published it in the *Proceedings of the National Academy of Sciences* (September 11, 2001).

Not only was the age-benefit effect of CR seen over and over again, but genetically determined age changes could be reversed. Till then, science had assumed that the genes took effect but the resulting damaging changes were blocked by CR. What Dr. Spindler showed, using sophisticated microchip technology, was that the expression of many pro-aging genes was actually reversed.

The good news was that this occurred even in elderly animals. Because the effect was not merely blocking damage but undoing gene expression, they became younger animals, so to speak. Naturally, some genes decrease their expression due to aging; Spindler found 26.

These were genes that protect against cancer and enable proper DNA maintenance and several liver functions. The best news of all was that even short-term calorie restriction could produce significant pro-survival health changes. Of the 46 liver function genes studied in mice, 27 benefited from a year or more of CR dieting, and 19 of this 27 (55%) changed for the better after just four weeks of CR.

It is interesting to note that Dr. Spindler found that 40% of the genes that increased expression with age were associated with inflammatory changes and 25% associated with oxidative stress.

We have pointed out that inflammation is one of the key processes of aging; according to this finding, it's more critical than oxidative damage, which is supposed to head the list of aging causes.

No wonder food restriction helps survival, if it reduces inflammation and other stresses. It would also explain the benefits of Luigi Cornaro's diet and indeed any detox (low-allergy) plan.

MY ADVICE: forget about genes and don't use them as an excuse to be lazy about your health.

You can start reversing the expression of known and as yet unknown age-related genes right away. Find out more about it in my book *Diet Wise* (www.alternative-doctor.com/dietwise) fast, if you haven't already done so, and take your love of life seriously: do what we tell you!

HOT TIP

We can't recommend full calorie restriction dieting for humans; the levels used in the animal experiments were very drastic. But you could consider three immediate actions:

Reduce your calorie intake significantly, even if not to the point of hunger, starting NOW.

Consider a 1-, 2-, or 3-day fast as a substitute for calorie restriction dieting.

A weekly one-day grape/juice or full fast. That's 52 days a year of knocking back gene expression!

Look out for drugs that will mimic calorie restriction diets. None are yet on the market but there is a race to get them to you.

THE MYTH OF EVIDENCE-BASED SCIENCE

I'm giving a talk to the European Parliament MPs (like congressmen and women). I've been invited to lay into the Big Pharma society model and explain how it is enslaving whole countries economically—like in the USA, the healthcare bill is 14% of the gross national product (GNP); in Britain it's 7%, and so on.

Pharmaceutical companies have a clear agenda (I almost wrote "hidden" agenda, but it's so blatantly obvious!) for trapping and controlling governments into having to allocate huge sums for the medical care of its citizens, which goes into their coffers.

It is based on two very vicious traps:

No one shall get well, if we can stop it. We want them to remain UN-cured and permanently in medical care.

As many citizens as possible will be made ill, by preventing access to natural and effective health products.

Governments fall for it so consistently, it's OBVIOUS that politicians are getting payoffs and back-handers.

This is going to be a very hard-hitting talk. I'll make the video available to you later.

In the meantime, I thought I would use some of the shocking data I found that's readily available to any honest journalist (sounds like an oxymoron!). Trouble is, the media are very heavily censored in the USA. People are not allowed the truth.

Let me share a few incriminating facts with you about the myth of what is (laughably) called *"evidence-based medicine"* or EBM. It's a new tool, a silly boast, whatever you want to call it, that orthodox doctors use to attack and berate holistically inclined practitioners.

According to this myth, mainstream doctors are guided by pure scientific wisdom; their story is a proven case; science backs up everything they say and do; they work from real evidence.

Whereas holistic practitioners, so the myth goes, have no science behind there crackpot theories; or they use "junk science" at best.

So what's the truth?

They are condemned from their own published journals!

According to the journal *BMJ Clinical Evidence**, which describes itself as "the international source of the best available evidence for effective health care," the myth is very sorry indeed.

The journal's distinguished team of advisors set out in 2007 to answer a simple question: "What proportion of commonly used treatments are supported by good evidence…?"

Around 2500 treatments were reviewed. The results are either hilarious or sickening, depending on your view!

Results:

- Only 13% of current treatments have been found definitely beneficial (less than one-seventh of medicine is what it's cracked up to be!)
- 23% are rated as likely to be beneficial
- 8% can be classified as a tradeoff between benefits and harms
- 6% are clearly unlikely to be beneficial

- 4% are likely to be ineffective or harmful
- A whopping 46% of all current medical treatments are honestly rated as being of unknown effectiveness

What you get from your doctor is really like the outcome of a lottery: it could be worthless, it could kill you, or it could do the job. Nobody knows… throw the dice. Hey! That's my a** on the line. That's not what you want if you seek medical assistance, is it?

HYPOCRISY AND DOUBLE STANDARDS

Given that very few of conventional medicine's standard treatments have been demonstrated to have any clear benefit and, conversely, that a substantial proportion have been shown to be potentially harmful, it is somewhat ironic to see the term "evidence-based medicine" used as a war cry by those who are virulently opposed to complementary and alternative medicines.

But not all orthodox medical doctors are fascist fools (I keep making this point).

Erich Loewy, MD, a bioethicist and professor of medicine at the University of California, Davis (I wish I'd met with him when I lived in Davis) writes:

To me, as a bioethicist and…a physician who has observed the evolution of EBM, I am impressed with the danger to physicians, patients, the educative process, and, ultimately, to the behavior it encourages. Mindless reliance on EBM does exactly what we do not want our students to do: convert what is a suffering human being, with a unique personal life-history, into a specimen of pathophysiology or a heart murmur (Loewy, 2007).

Dr. Loewy points out that "evidence-based medicine," as practiced in large institutions, can have the highly undesirable effect of stifling thought and constraining good diagnostic and clinical judgment.

Doctors who "think outside the box" and who feel that a particular patient is uniquely suited for a treatment option that is currently not listed as standard "evidence-based medicine," risk being disciplined by their institution. "EBM is basically anti-intellectual,"1 Loewy writes.

Furthermore, says Loewy, "evidence-based medicine" protocols must, like drugs or food, have an expiration date, after which they have to be reexamined in far more than a perfunctory way to make sure they are still legitimate.1

Evidence-based medicine, for all its advantages in caring for the "usual case of X," tends to suppress our curiosity and imagination or it at least tends to channel our curiosity and shape our imagination within narrow limits and, therefore, gets in the way of the sort of speculation necessary for scientific progress.[2]

Refusing to publish a paper, by the way, may be a highly effective form of censorship. We badly need a *Journal of Negative Results* devoted to experiments that proved a reasonable hypothesis to be untrue, he says.

I think that's a great idea.

"A herniorrhaphy patient can go home in one or two days." Is that really true? It is probably true if the patient lives in a middle-class suburb with a spouse and adequate sanitation. But is it true for a 55-year-old man who lives in a rat-infested "project" building on the fifth floor and without a functioning elevator? [3]

We are a strange society, says Loewy: on the one hand, we have made autonomy into the supreme virtue; on the other, we have created instruments that force others (physicians) to act in ways they find suboptimal.

One writer compared the dilemma of doctors who don't want to knuckle under to the EBM hypocrisy to the moral dilemma of Germans under the Nazis, who may not have wanted to harm the Jews. But they were forced to conform.

A "system"—a political, economic, or cultural system—insinuates itself between myself and the other. If the other is excluded, it is the system that is doing the excluding, a system in which I participate because I must survive and against which I do not rebel because it cannot be changed…I start to view horror and my implication in it as normalcy.[4]

Let Me Finish with a Telling Joke
The *British Medical Journal* has run a few scientific jokes over the years. This one is a beauty. They published a tongue-in-cheek article looking into what scientific papers, if any, had been published to provide evidence that parachutes were effective for those who were "gravitationally challenged"!

The findings were: "The authors were unable to identify any randomized controlled trials of parachute intervention for gravitational challenge. They concluded that the effectiveness of parachutes has not been subjected to rigorous evaluation by randomized controlled trials."

The authors of this report suggest that everyone might benefit if the most radical proponents of evidence-based medicine organized and participated in a double blind randomized, placebo-controlled crossover trial of the parachute.[5]

I'd like to support such a trial!

* An offshoot of the BMJ: the British Medical Journal.
1. [Erich Loewy MD, Medscape General Medicine. 2007;9(3):30]
2. [Loewy EH. Curiosity, imagination, compassion, science and ethics: do curiosity and imagination serve a central function? Health Care Anal. 1998;6:286-294]
3. [Erich Loewy MD, Medscape General Medicine. 2007;9(3):30]
4. [Barnett V. Bystanders: Conscience and Complicity During the Holocaust. Westport, Conn: Praeger Publishers; 1999:169.]
5. [Ref: Smith GCS, Pell JP. Parachute use to prevent death and major trauma related to gravitational challenge: systematic review of randomized controlled trials. BMJ. 2003;327:1459-1461

UNDERSTANDING THE MID-LIFE CRISIS

The menopause is a well-known, even celebrated, event for women, though it has been late in coming to the understanding of men -- and male doctors in particular. What is much less known is that men have to endure a similar biological and emotional experience. It is obscured by the usual male inability to come to terms with personal issues and the fact that it is perceived as less than masculine to even admit to such feelings.

Matters are made more complicated by the fact that there are really two phenomena rolled into one and they easily become confused. It is vital that women appreciate what is happening to their loved ones and that doctors come to grips with this important aspect of growing older. Although men like to believe they are tough and immune from care, the truth is that they are often desperately insecure and failing to understand what is happening to oneself can be a major cause of anxiety and suffering.

There is a male hormonal shut-down, akin to the menopause, which is therefore named the "andropause." But this is quite distinct from the mid-life crisis, as we shall see in detail. The trouble is that both happen at a similar time, though the crucial difference is that the mid-life crisis tends to occur somewhat earlier. How can we tell these two apart?

Let us consider first the true andropause.

Characteristics of the Andropause

It starts, usually, in the fifth decade. It is unrelated to life events (though it may happen at the same time as an unrelated disaster). There are true biological changes, which can be measured in the laboratory. Testosterone levels fall. The resulting symptoms are not unlike those experienced by a woman at the menopause:

- fatigue
- depression
- aches and pains
- sweating and flushes
- reduced libido

To which may be added: loss of erectile function. The latter is particularly disturbing to a man and difficulty in talking about this problem is one of the reasons why the male menopause has been little attended to.

The True Mid-Life Crisis

This often falls earlier than the andropause, maybe in the fourth decade. Typically, it occurs in response to some outside challenge in a man's life: a breakdown of the marriage, career failure, bankruptcy, death of a peer or loved parent, redundancy, and so on.

Essentially, it is an emotional crisis and not a hormonal one. Deep introspection often results in the feeling that life is passing by and precious years have been wasted with so little achieved. Dreams that were once so important seem to have faded or gone forever beyond reach. It can be a time of great anguish, despair, inadequacy, and feelings of guilt or futility.

Whereas anyone, sooner or later, will experience a shutdown of hormones, the man who suffers the mid-life crisis is typically one who has been challenged and cannot come to terms with his life. There has been a shock which brings him face to face with himself and he doesn't like what he sees. In trying to rationalize the unhappy feelings, he may begin to see his life partner in negative terms or blame his bosses and work dissatisfaction. Therefore he seeks change: a new partner (times of infidelity and experiment), a new career, new home territory, and so on.

Unfortunately, alcohol and drugs are often seen as the answer. They shut out the pain temporarily but, of course, they solve nothing. This may be the start of a slippery slope to abuse, addiction, and early demise.

Far from the libido shutdown characteristic of the andropause, a man in a mid-life crisis wants to boast of sexual prowess and seeks new thrills and adventure. This is the man likely to start buying younger generation fashion clothes and to run off with a tart or to have an affair with his secretary in her twenties. But it is a kind of denial, an admission that things are not as they were, underscored by a great desire to prove everything is OK, "No problem!"

The andropause man lacks any energy or drive and cannot be bothered with sex or adventure. For him, it already is too late (he thinks).

What Lies Beyond
One can gain a deeper insight by looking far beyond the moment of crisis.

The mid-life crisis is a kind of rite of passage. It comes to an end eventually and good may come of it. A marriage may not always be wrecked but may be strengthened and renewed by surviving the threat. A great deal depends on the response of the life partner in this time of upheaval and change.

A man may be renewed through suffering, discover a vision for the future and come home once again to feelings of family and love. He can learn something of great value, about himself, about others, about the deeper nature of life. If the trigger was a financial collapse, he may recover the determination to work hard and rebuild his empire. In this way, some men will go forward and meet the challenge.

Sadly, many do not do so, but give in to what they see as an overwhelming tide of misfortune. Alcohol or drug addiction takes a lasting grip. These individuals rapidly advance into the inertia of age and decrepitude. For them, the mid-life crisis was a disaster from which they do not recover.

Women
And yes, the mid-life crisis can occur for women. Almost all of what is said here applies equally. Even the search for new loves, thrills, and adventure can lead to women too becoming unfaithful or seeking divorce. Obviously it needs to be distinguished from the onset of the menopause.

What You Can Do
The most important first step is to have blood tests to check up on the men's hormones.

If this reveals that there is a problem, testosterone supplements are needed and will work a satisfying and sometimes dramatic change. The fatigue and depression lifts, life becomes worthwhile, energy levels and zest return to former levels, potency problems recede. What is more, testosterone improves circulation, protects against heart disease, aids weight loss, improves skin condition, increases muscle strength, and works in a host of healthy ways to rejuvenate the man.

It is a tragedy that early experiments (with artificial methyl testosterone), bungled by the greed of drug companies, have led to testosterone supplements having bad press.

Testosterone supplementation does need some care and is discussed elsewhere. Generally, though, one can say that the dangers of NOT supplementing testosterone well into old age are far greater than any theoretical risks to prescribing it. Be clear about it: testosterone saves lives and saves hearts and minds!

On the other hand, what if the tests show that testosterone deficiency is not significant? Clearly supplements will not help. This is an emotional or life-events crisis and needs handling as such, at whatever age it befalls.

The first sensible step towards surviving the mid-life crisis is having the problem identified and understood, as above. Kindness, tact, and sympathy are required, despite outrageous and often destructive behavior by the affected individual, because it is still a medical condition.

Any crisis is a time of great stress and stress, we know, is a killer. It shortens lives.

If the individual is already abusing drugs and drink as a solution, then the danger to health and longevity is even greater. Bitter acrimony and rejection from relatives, even though they are badly affected in turn, are counterproductive and simply make everyone suffer more. At all costs, keep the communication flowing; it's the only hope for a sane future and rebuilding friendships.

The man concerned has to be brought to confronting his situation.

The pretense that there is nothing wrong and everyone else is to blame does not help.

Dr. Malcolm Carruthers, a male hormone and lifestyle specialist and author of *The Testosterone Revolution*, makes the point that the kind of man likely to suffer a mid-life crisis is one with an unhappy childhood, maybe abusive or with cold and unloving parents.

Such early formative experiences often engender a feeling of unworthiness that emerges later in life, at a time of crisis. This is fruitful ground for counseling or other therapy.

Even without a therapist, a man can sit down with pen and paper and start to write down what matters. Nothing changes the meaning of life more than working out what one's values truly are. Often we aspire to false goals, imposed by others, that have little meaning to ourselves.

Society at large, and the media in particular, often impose ridiculous standards of goodness and value. There is a cult of greed, materialism, and celebrity worship in vogue which is very dangerous and tends to create envy, desire, feelings of inadequacy, and misery in those who do not have all the trappings of a luxurious film-star lifestyle.

The irony is, you only have to look at the stories in that same press to realize that the people we are supposed to envy have disastrous, miserable, and often very short sick lives.

BACK PAIN IS A COMMON AGONY....
BUT YOU CAN BEAT IT

I know that back pain is probably the **number one reason people visit the doctor.** Probably something to do with our amazing upright posture.

Neck pain and low back pain constitute the most common musculoskeletal complaints in primary care clinics.

Few of us will go through life without at least one episode of severely incapacitating back pain, whether due to a fall, repetitive strain injury, or excessive lifting. Here's some great information you can share with family and friends, if any of them should suffer with this problem.

Low Back Pain
First a warning: low back pain can be a sign of serious pelvic disease, such as cervical or prostatic cancer. Make sure you are OK in this regard before accepting that the problem is merely back pain.

Real back pain is caused usually by a pulling injury or a displacement. Cricking your back due to tearing muscle fibers is common. But the problem is more serious if a part of your back becomes misaligned (the so-called "slipped disc").

If the sciatic nerve (a long nerve down the back of the leg) is affected, pain is felt from the lower back all the way down to the foot. This is called sciatica and it is very unpleasant. The least unguarded movement causes a jolt of pain that runs down the leg and is close to unbearable.

Unaccustomed effort or bad lifting posture are the chief causes of low back injury. Bad sleeping posture is by far the commonest reason for neck pain, especially if it is present on waking.

Most back pain is transient and, where it persists, the real cause is spasm of the muscles. The initial pain causes the muscles to contract hard and that is sufficient to continue the squeeze on the tender nerves. A vicious circle is set up, where pain causes muscle spasm and muscle spasm causes further pain.

I say this with confidence because I have shown time and again to countless patients that if you can break the muscle spasm, the pain melts away. Here's what I do for it.

Lie on the floor in the anatomically natural position – on your back, arms and legs out straights, palms upwards and neck in line with the rest of the spine. You will probably find this uncomfortable at first.

Then, by gradually wriggling and making small adjustments, you search for a position where you don't feel the pain. It may seem a strange idea but, no matter the pain you are in, you will always find such a posture. Usually it will be somewhere in this anatomically "correct" position - but don't be rigid and force it, as if you were standing upright on parade in the army! Relax!

Once you find the pain-free position, then you hold it for as long as possible: 15 minutes at least, 30 minutes is better. In that time the muscle spasm will gradually soften and release, as it is pain that causes the muscle spasm.

If you are lucky, you may have broken the vicious circle. When you get up (carefully, making sure you do not trigger the hurt), the pain is gone. At the very worst. it will have lessened considerably and this is far better than taking painkillers.

You can resume the anatomically true position any time you like. When you go to bed, get yourself into the correct position and follow the procedure I described above. If you can only sleep on your side, make sure you look "ahead," as if you were lying on the floor looking up. Make sure the pillow is exactly the right thickness to have your head in such a way that the spine is straight.

Do not lie on your front because this will force you to twist your neck. Never, never sleep on your front normally, for this same reason. If you don't have neck damage now, you certainly will have it as you age.

Cervical Spondylosis

When the pain is in the neck area, this is usually labeled "spondylosis" (not to be confused with spondylitis, which is an inflammatory condition). Usually this problem is present on waking with a "crick" in the neck and is caused by a bad sleeping posture trapping a nerve. Carrying heavy shopping bags can also do it, because the nerves of the arm are dragged downwards and pulled across the bony protrusions of the vertebrae.

There is pain with most neck movements. First warning here: don't snap your neck from side to side, just to see how it feels. Every time you aggravate the pain by doing this, it slows down recovery. Look straight ahead and don't turn your neck. If you want to see something to the side, rotate your whole body and shoulders.

That means you should not drive a car, because it requires you to turn your head right back, to see into your blind spot, or to reverse while parking.

This leads to the first rule for beating pain: don't provoke the pain. Pain means damage; damage means delayed recovery! It's logical if you think it through – but most people don't.

Chronic Back Pain

If the pain persists, acupuncture is a good option. I have seen awesome results. A randomized trial of 55 subjects with low back pain demonstrated that acupuncture significantly improved disability scores, and the superior outcomes in the acupuncture group remained significant through four weeks after the cessation of treatment. Participants receiving acupuncture also experienced fewer side effects related to analgesic therapy compared with patients receiving conventional therapy alone.[1]

Exercise Can Play a Part

A Finnish study investigating female office workers with chronic back pain and published in the December 2006 issue of *Medicine & Science in Sports & Exercise* showed that effective exercise was very successful at reducing chronic neck pain. Now you know why: the proper toning of muscle helps prevent spasms.[2] Incidentally, this study excluded prolapsed intervertebral disk.

Another study showed that yoga was moderately effective in reducing chronic back pain of all kinds.

"Yoga was more effective than a self-care book for improving function and reducing chronic low back pain, and the benefits persisted for at least several months," according to the authors. "It is important to note that some styles, such as Bikram and Vinyasa, may be too vigorous for patients with back pain who are unfamiliar with yoga whereas other styles (for example, Iyengar) may need modification from normal practice to be appropriate for patients with back pain."[3]

Finally... The Conventional Approach

Conventional therapy is based on bed rest (if pain is severe, as in sciatica) and painkillers. It is rather passive and not addressing any causal issues. For that reason, it has little to offer.

In cases of severe intractable pain, generally over many years, surgery may be suggested. Reject it fully. Published studies show that surgery produces no better results than conservative management. So why endure the risks and trauma of major surgery?

References

1. *Rheumatology.* 2003;42:1508-1517
2. *Med Sci Sports Exerc.* 2006:38:2068-2074.
3. *Ann Intern Med.* 2005;143:849-856

TESTOSTERONE: GOOD FOR THE HEART AND BLOOD PRESSURE

You might say that the male essence is *testosterone*. But remember that male bodies also carry significant amounts of estrogen. Since we don't really understand why it's there, the boffins have tended to say it's unimportant. But, when I was a medical student, they said that about the thymus gland; we now know it is one of the most important organs in the body and regulates T-cells (T for thymus!).

Similarly, women have traces of testosterone. Amongst other things, it drives their libido, so it's pretty important to us guys.

Testosterone gets a bad press. It's supposed to make us harsh, aggressive, and insensitive. I'm sure it does in excess. But lack of it leads to torpor, depression, and negativity. That's not having a "feminine side"; it's sickness. The fact is, we need testosterone.

Not the least because it **protects us from heart disease**. For years the stupid myth was that since women have fewer heart attacks, testosterone causes cardiovascular disease. Probably it raises blood pressure, because it makes men energetic and goal driven; that's stress, *right*?

Another example of scientific bovine excrement. One day, somebody wondered if this myth is actually true. He studied the testosterone levels of men lying in intensive care units, having suffered strokes or coronary infarctions. What was found was that **men with cardiovascular problems had far lower levels of testosterone than average, not higher**.

It emerged that testosterone actually protects from heart disease; totally the opposite of what "science" had said. Incidentally, that's true also for women. When their testosterone levels drop later in life, they eventually assume a similar risk to males.

Testosterone also generates strength and stamina. It regulates youthful protein synthesis, lowers cholesterol, reduces blood sugar levels, and fortifies bone density.

Dr. Eugene Shippen, MD, author of *The Testosterone Syndrome*, points out that this is not just a "sex hormone." **Testosterone is a whole-body hormone.**

So we need that stuff. Enough to feel good, to protect our arteries and live longer; but not enough to make us road freaks and intolerant bullies, right! Otherwise, lacking it, we slide into a male equivalent of the menopause, which has been dubbed the andropause.

Characteristically. the man begins to lose energy and drive; depression, demotivation, and loss of libido follow. Physical decay is soon part of the picture. It's bad news for the wife or partner. Men are hard to live with even when they feel good about themselves; it's ten times worse when their virility deserts them!

A word of enlightenment: it is important to recognize there are two phenomena that can strike a man at about the same age: the andropause and the so-called mid-life crisis.

They are not the same, though they can become inextricably mixed. The mid-life crisis is more of a psychological slump: it is a time of questioning and a looming sense of failure that might strike a man who hasn't yet achieved the things he dreamed of when younger. Possibly a shattered marriage or relationship and the impending sense of being over the hill career-wise add to the picture of gloom. This too will lead to depression, demotivation, and a sharp fall off in sex drive. So the two effects may look similar.

The important difference is that one is caused by a drop in testosterone and the other is brought on by dissatisfaction with life goals.

They have different causes and therefore different treatment modalities. If there is any real doubt, after consultation with a knowledgeable physician, blood levels of free and bound testosterone will usually settle the matter.

Supplementing testosterone has been around for a surprisingly long time. Pioneer work by Dr. Tiberius Reiter and his followers in the 1950s showed dramatic results. As a result there were queues of men outside his door and scientific orthodoxy, typically, ignored the new breakthrough in healing. The know-alls went on decrying the idea of such a thing as the andropause (the majority still do).

When the drug industry finally got into the act, the result was a disaster. True to form, a synthetic patentable analogue of natural testosterone, called methyl testosterone, was brought onto the market. It worked all right but caused a lot of cancers. As a result, testosterone supplementation was discredited and even today ignorant reactionaries cite this tale with dire prognostications. So not only is there no such thing as an andropause, but apparently treating it will probably kill you anyway!

It's a double whammy of yesterday's pseudo-science. For optimum health, you must move with the times.

The fact is that there are safe ways to supplement testosterone these days; Restandol or testosterone undecoanate is one (curiously, methyl testosterone is still licensed in the US by the FDA).

Capsules, patches, and implants are available, each with relative merits and problems. If you are hesitant, take only the natural testosterone molecule and avoid any modified, patented compounds. At the clinic we supply a gel formulated from pure natural testosterone, just as nature makes it.

A Testosterone Study and Comment...

The study, published in *JAMA*, enrolled 237 healthy men aged 60 to 80. All men had a testosterone level below 13.7 nmol/L (rather low). The men were randomly assigned to be either in a group that received a twice-daily oral 80 mg testosterone supplement or a placebo. The researchers measured hand strength, time to stand/sit, cognitive functioning (how well your brain is working), bone density, body composition, cholesterol, insulin, quality of life, and other factors.

Bone density, metabolic, and quality-of-life measures were no different except for one hormone-related quality-of-life measure that improved.

If you read the skeptics, they say there was no real difference in the groups. Yet there was, definitely! For one thing, the testosterone group had a significant improvement in lean body mass. Also their insulin resistance lessened. These are both factors that we know for sure increase longevity (hundreds of supporting studies).

Paradoxically, 47.8% in the testosterone group vs. 35.5% in the placebo group developed the metabolic syndrome ($P = .07$). Since one of the definitions of metabolic syndrome is insulin resistance and one of its measures is LOSS OF LEAN BODY MASS, one can say the results are paradoxical and therefore the study pretty worthless.

No negative effects on prostate safety were detected, which is good and puts paid to the usual squawking argument that testosterone is DANGEROUS and increases the risk of prostate cancer, etc., etc.[1]

CAUTION: The Aromataze Enzyme

The picture isn't quite as simple as it sounds. This is due to the fact that some testosterone is converted into an unwanted estrogen form, by an enzyme called aromataze. More so in later life. A 59-year-old man has, on average, more estrogen then a 59-year-old woman.

It is this male estrogen or xeno-estrogen (measured as sex hormone binding globulin or SHBG), which leads to prostatic enlargement and NOT testosterone itself, as you may have been led to believe. Male estrogen also adds to the risk of heart disease.

Dosing is therefore not a matter for self-treatment. Blood tests are required to learn the existing levels of SHBG. If it's high, this tricks the pituitary and interferes with the secretion of LH (luteinizing hormone), which then scores low. LH is meant to stimulate the testes to secrete testosterone. If LH is high and testosterone low, the regulation pathway is probably OK but the testes are not responding to the signal.

We also need to block the aromataze pathway, to prevent the conversion into male xeno-estrogen, which is otherwise bad news. Failure to grasp the importance of this side path is the chief reason for ineffective and mismanaged male hormone supplementation. Even if you are not contemplating testosterone supplements, this build up of male estrogen can put you in danger, through heart disease and through prostate cancer. At the very least, you will tend to feminize, as older men do.

Known antagonists of aromataze are saw palmetto and zinc. If you are supplementing testosterone, you MUST take at least 300 mg of saw palmetto and 50 mg of zinc daily. Saw palmetto may also block metabolism of testosterone to androstenedione, another potent androgen which has been implicated in prostate disease. Also good news is that plants in the crucifer family (cabbage, kale, broccoli, and Brussels sprouts) contain large amounts of an estrogen antagonist called indole-3-carbinol, I3C for short. This has been shown to be very helpful against women's hormone-dependent cancers, such as breast and cervical cancers. We men can benefit from the same breakthrough. Eat plenty from this group.

Chrysin (passion flower), available as capsules or cream, also has a definite beneficial effect in this context. *Avena sativa* (oats) is also said by some to increase free testosterone.

If the SHBG cannot be brought down to safe levels, it may be wise to consider a drug called Arimidex (anastrozole). It is prescribed for breast cancer patients in order to eliminate the estrogen problem. For a male using it in this way, the correct dose is no more than 0.5 mg two to three times a week. Obviously, this is a prescription-only matter.

Arimidex is NOT used routinely with testosterone supplements.

Vitamin K and Prostate
This is much more important than most doctors recognize. An EPIC study at Heidelberg (it really was an epic: 11,000 men over an average of 8.6 years) showed conclusively that **vitamin K gives critical protection against prostate cancer**. It showed that K1, the plant derivative, was not helpful but K2 (menaquinone, as it's known) did the job well. K2 lasts far longer in the body.

Moreover, K2 is known to protect our arteries and is helpful in preventing osteoporosis.

The current recommended intake of vitamin K in Japan is 55 mcg for women and 65 mcg per day for men. In the US and Canada it is 120 mcg per day for men and 90 mcg per day for women. These figures are disastrously low (as usual) and need to be at least tripled. I repeat, K1 will just NOT do the job.

Take 300 mcg daily, minimum, if you are a man (or woman) over 55.

CAUTION: Do not use external applications of testosterone if you have physical contact with children: there is a case on record of a male child going into premature puberty through contact with testosterone cream on his father's body. Do not use testosterone if you have a raised PSA or known prostate cancer.

Which Brings Us to Prostate Health
As a medical student, I heard male patients being told, "If you get a cancer, choose the prostate." This tumor is a very slow killer and survival for 20 or more years, even without treatment, is not unusual. Many men die of something else, without ever realizing they had an invader, munching away slowly!

Nevertheless, that's a pretty stupid reason to accept it when cancer of the prostate is among the most preventable of all malignancies. Its appearance is all but confined to later years in life and the cause, apart from the general causes of malignancy (DNA decay, nutritional factors and chemical carcinogens), is the steady build up of male estrogen. This leads first to benign prostatic hypertrophy (BPH) and sometimes then on to cancerous growth.

Prostate-specific antigen (PSA) is the usual screening test but hardly a gold standard. It may be negative in the presence of cancer and may be positive when there is none. Nevertheless, to not have regular PSA checks from middle-age onwards is walking blind. Checks are mandatory as a preliminary to supplementing either growth hormone or testosterone on an anti-aging program.

Where there is clear enlargement of the gland and a problem SHBG level, it is vital to raise free testosterone (as opposed to bound testosterone) as a protection and at the same time block the conversion to estrogen. Saw palmetto and zinc are given, as above. While restoring testosterone levels to a normal healthy level (25 to 40 pg/ml) does not cause prostate cancer, it has been suggested that it may induce faster growth in an existing tumor. However, a study from Santa Barbara in California showed that testosterone actually killed the tumor cells. That's more in keeping with the physiology outlined here.

Skullcap (Scutellaria baicalensis)

A better idea is Chinese skullcap. It has been shown to block the effect of the enzyme 5 alpha-reductase. This is the one that creates dihydrotestosterone (DHT), the "male estrogen," which is strongly associated with the development of prostate enlargement (benign prostatic hyperplasia) and prostate cancer.

Peuraria mirifica - A Page from the Women's' Book

The male prostate is an estrogen-sensitive organ. Yet men accumulate estrogens as they age, as I said above.

A good tip to block those estrogen receptors is to take the new wonder herb from Thailand: *Pueraria mirifica*. We call this HRT, meaning *"herbal remedy from Thailand"*!

Miroestrol, the active ingredient in *Pueraria mirifica*, has a stronger affinity for estrogen receptors than estrogen itself and 3000 times more than soy isoflavones. It is so powerful that the region in Thailand where it is grown has the lowest incidence of breast cancer in the world.

What's the point? To block those receptors by having them bound by miroestrol. It has other great anti-aging properties too:

- Serves as an anti-wrinkle agent for aged and wrinkled skin
- Darkens white hair and increases hair growth
- Helps with memory loss
- Increases energy and vigor, more reflexive bodily movements
- Alleviates sleep disorders

Men should take 80 mg a day (half the female dose). Beware of fake *Pueraria*. Almost everybody is claiming to have it - even China. These are the wrong forms of *Pueraria*. The only safe source I know of, guaranteed to be the real plant, is from www.longevityplus.com. Their product is "Beyond HRT."

However, *Pueraria* does not take the place of good diet, exercise, and cutting down on alcohol and losing plenty of weight.

In addition, men are urged to consider:

Zinc, at least 15 mg daily. It increases testosterone levels.

Chrysin (from the passion flower), which is well known to inhibit an enzyme called aromatase (Kellis JT Jr. et al. 1984). Aromatase converts testosterone to male estrogen. Bodybuilders have used chrysin as a testosterone-boosting supplement because, by inhibiting the aromatase enzyme, less testosterone is converted into estrogen (our former state governor Arnie can't be wrong – can he?).

Carnitine. Both testosterone and carnitine improve sexual desire, sexual satisfaction, and nocturnal penile tumescence, but carnitine is more effective than testosterone in improving erectile function, nocturnal penile tumescence, orgasm, and general sexual well-being. Carnitine was better than testosterone at treating depression.

Cruciferous vegetables. Cruciferous vegetables, such as broccoli and cauliflower, contain isothiocyanates and glucosinolates, which act as antioxidants and potent inducers of phase 2 proteins believed to suppress prostate cancer formation.[3]

One extra tidbit, before we close: In males, estrogen is present in low concentrations in blood, but can be extraordinarily high in semen and as high as 250 picograms/ml in testicular fluids, which is higher than serum estradiol in the female.

Tossing Away the Risk!
Men could reduce their risk of developing prostate cancer through regular masturbation, researchers suggest.[4]

They say cancer-causing chemicals could build up in the prostate if men do not ejaculate regularly.

And they say sexual intercourse may not have the same protective effect because of the possibility of contracting a sexually transmitted infection, which could increase men's cancer risk.

Australian researchers questioned over 1,000 men who had developed prostate cancer and 1,250 who had not about their sexual habits.

They found those who had ejaculated the most between the ages of 20 and 50 were the least likely to develop the cancer. The protective effect was greatest while the men were in their twenties.

Men who ejaculated more than five times a week were a third less likely to develop prostate cancer later in life.

Fluid Emission Could Be the Key
Previous research has suggested that a high number of sexual partners or a high level of sexual activity increased a man's risk of developing prostate cancer by up to 40%.

But the Australian researchers who carried out this study suggest the early work missed the protective effect of ejaculation because it focused on sexual intercourse, with its associated risk of STIs.

Graham Giles of the Cancer Council Victoria in Melbourne, who led the research team, told *New Scientist*: "Had we been able to remove ejaculations associated with sexual intercourse, there should have been an even stronger protective effect of ejaculations."

The researchers suggest that ejaculating may prevent carcinogens accumulating in the prostate gland.

The prostate provides a fluid into semen during ejaculation that activates sperm and prevents them sticking together.

The fluid has high concentrations of substances including potassium, zinc, fructose, and citric acid, which are drawn from the bloodstream.

But animal studies have shown carcinogens such as 3-methylchloranthrene, found in cigarette smoke, are also concentrated in the prostate.

"Flushing out"
Dr. Giles said fewer ejaculations may mean that the carcinogens build up.

"It's a prostatic stagnation hypothesis. The more you flush the ducts out, the less there is to hang around and damage the cells that line them."

A similar connection has been found between breast cancer and breastfeeding, where lactating appeared to "flush out" carcinogens, reduce a woman's risk of the disease, *New Scientist* reports.

Another theory put forward by the researchers is that ejaculation may induce prostate glands to mature fully, making them less susceptible to carcinogens.

Dr. Chris Hiley, head of policy and research at the UK's Prostate Cancer Charity, told BBC News Online: "This is a plausible theory."

She added: "In the same way the human papillomavirus has been linked to cervical

cancer, there is a suggestion that bits of prostate cancer may be related to a sexually transmitted infection earlier in life."

Anthony Smith, deputy director of the Australian Research Centre in Sex, Health and Society at La Trobe University in Melbourne, said the research could affect the kind of lifestyle advice doctors give to patients.

"Masturbation is part of people's sexual repertoire.

"If these findings hold up, then it's perfectly reasonable that men should be encouraged to masturbate," he said.

References
1. Marielle H. Emmelot-Vonk, MD; Harald J. J. Verhaar, MD, PhD; Hamid R. Nakhai Pour, MD, PhD; André Aleman, PhD; Tycho M. T. W. Lock, MD; J. L. H. Ruud Bosch, MD, PhD; Diederick E. Grobbee, MD, PhD; Yvonne T. van der Schouw, PhD. Effect of Testosterone Supplementation on Functional Mobility, Cognition, and Other Parameters in Older Men: A Randomized Controlled Trial. *JAMA*. 2008;299(1):39-52.
2. Kris-Etherton PM et al. 2002; Talalay P et al. 2001.
3. Cavallini G et al. 2004.
4. BBC News Site, 16 July, 2003, 23:11.

ALZHEIMER'S DISEASE... SOMETHING YOU DON'T WANT

The 1990s marked the end of the so-called *"Decade of the Brain."* We are facing a new millennium of brain dysfunction, with Alzheimer's disease leading the field of causes. There are presently an estimated 4.5 million Alzheimer's patients in the US; other developed countries, such as the UK, follow proportionately. Experts are estimating that within 30 years more than half of the population over 85 will suffer with Alzheimer's disease.

Drug treatment is controversial (which means basically useless); tacrine (Cognex), the most widely prescribed drug, has been refused licensing in several countries, since there is no evidence it does any good, despite aggressive marketing persuading doctors to prescribe it. Sadly, a number of drugs are known to make the problem worse, such as L-dopa and acetaminophen (Tylenol).

Yet, despite the gloom, it is not widely known that Alzheimer's is a preventable disease and can even be reversed to a degree, sometimes remarkably so. One has to approach it the right way.

Risk Factors

Certain studies have shown that exposure to electromagnetic radiation significantly increases the risk of Alzheimer's, or makes it rapidly worse. This means working with or near computers, VDUs, and similar equipment. But also, of course, it means that mobile phones are adding to the risk.

Good scientific studies have tied Alzheimer's disease to plasma homocysteine levels. Increased amounts of this important biomarker in the blood spells trouble for the heart and for the brain. However homocysteine levels can be readily brought to normal, using vitamin B6, B12, and folic acid supplements. I usually add TMG (trimethyl glycine) 1,000 mgs daily. Few doctors approach important diseases from a nutritional perspective, yet in this case it can be wonderfully helpful.

An important study at Heidelberg University showed that, in a large proportion of Alzheimer's cases, the mechanism is failure of small blood vessels in the brain (this would lead to brain starvation and degeneration).

An important modern treatment, chelation, is known to be very good at restoring the function of older blood vessels. For this reason, it is an important treatment for heart disease, strokes, and anti-aging. But the great benefit to Alzheimer's can be understood.

Another part of the puzzle is exposure to toxic metal poisoning. Aluminum was thought to be a main offender. Actually, fewer people think that today.

Mercury poisoning seems a far more likely culprit, according to studies carried out at a Texas hospital. But whichever is correct, the good news is that chelation can remove these toxic metals from the tissues. This has been done effectively for over 50 years. Modern switched-on doctors have recognized the value of chelation for Alzheimer's and other degenerative disorders caused by metal poisoning.

Treatment Modalities

It is vital to understand that all good general health issues are also good news for a tired and deteriorating brain. Exercise, sound nutrition and avoidance of stress are all critical factors.

But certain specific treatments have been shown to be highly beneficial. For example, one study showed that **vitamin E was BETTER than a drug or placebo in reducing the symptoms.** The value of B6, B12, and folate have already been alluded to above.

In a very important study published in 1997 by the *Journal of the American Medical Association*, **Gingko biloba** was shown not only to prevent Alzheimer's degeneration, but it actually improved many of the cases, compared to the placebo (all the more remarkable, in that the AMA has always been opposed to natural and nutritional therapies!).

Also helpful are **glutathione, N-acetyl cysteine** and **alpha lipoic acid**. These are powerful brain antioxidants and have remarkable effects on mental performance and cognition, so much so that otherwise healthy individuals notice considerable improvement too!

Which finally brings us to intravenous antioxidant therapy, also known as chelation.

It is a specially compounded formula, administered intravenously (as a drip) weekly on an outpatient basis (takes around two hours). It is quite painless and easy. There are now literally hundreds of thousands of successful cases, attesting to its safety and effectiveness. Its ability to remove toxic damaging metals has been pointed out. It also can reverse age-deterioration. Specifically, it can reverse the cross-linkage of proteins that leads to wrinkles, stiffness, and poor movement function.

Following the groundbreaking work of Dr. David Perlmutter in the USA, it is now appropriate to add a substance known as glutathione, which is administered intravenously. He has observed what he calls the "glutathione miracle" and seen patients with severe Parkinson's disease within one hour be able to stand, walk and move their arms around normally. He has used glutathione extensively in cases with Alzheimer's and other dementias, multiple sclerosis, and strokes. Interestingly, glutathione administered this way stops diarrhea and irritable bowel disease in its tracks.

Chelation is a kind of *"elixir of life."* For Alzheimer's patients (and their suffering families) it could restore the whole meaning of life.

THE BODY MATRIX - CAN YOU CREATE A WHOLE NEW YOU?

What do I keep tellin' ya? Stay alive! The world is changing fast; medical science is advancing by leaps and bounds.

The time will soon come when you don't have to die because your kidneys are shot or you had a heart attack or stroke. We can regrow limbs or organs. You could even go back to normal…or better: back to how you were when you were younger and healthier.

How? By regrowing our bodies; or at least key parts of the body that have been damaged.

It's already happening. You heard me!

The tissue structure of our bodies, called the matrix, was once thought to be mere scaffolding; something to which cells were stuck. But it much more than that: the matrix is an aware, intelligent structure that can program itself to regenerate any organ, from bone to brains. Scientists are just now learning to tap into its amazing powers of growth and tissue construction.

Your job is to keep healthy till this new science is perfected. I can help you with that. Get my truly prophetic book *How to Get Healthy for Your Next 100 Years*.

A Remarkable Bandage
For example, Elizabeth Loboa of the North Carolina State University in Raleigh, is a materials engineer who has developed a special kind of self-destructing super-bandage capable of healing infected wounds quickly, without scarring or standard antibiotics.

You apply the bandage and then the special material degrades until nothing is left but your own, newly regenerated, healthy cells. Call it a super-Band-Aid!

Some researchers have already succeeded in building entire organs from scratch, and the new technique may one day play a role in repairing damaged brains.

Earlier this year, Harald Ott of Massachusetts General Hospital in Boston built the world's first functioning home-grown kidney, a wildly complex organ that stem cell researchers have always assumed needed to be grown from scratch using numerous different cell types.

Ott was astonished to find that, although he fed only two types of cells into a

decellularized kidney matrix – blood-like stem cells into the blood vessels, and endothelial cells into the labyrinthine plumbing that filters the blood – all of the different kinds of cells formed in the sites where they were supposed to.

"It's pretty exciting stuff," says Suchitra Sumitran-Holgersson of Gothenberg University in Sweden. "We're trying to create a whole new human being."

Well, let me tell you where they need to pay homage: to Nature. She's smart; very, very smart. Give her the tools and get out of the way, is my advice!

The Body Matrix
No, not a computer-simulated reality; just the basics of tissue structure. This is the stuff that remains if you strip away the living cells from, say, a blood vessel, an organ or a bit of skin. This scaffolding gives the various parts of our body their detailed shape and solidity.

That was all it was thought to do. Early experiments at organ regeneration used detergent to strip cells way from this matrix and then used it as an inert chassis or a template. It was repopulated with stem cells, which grew back the original organ.

But—and don't I keep telling you this is the ONLY medicine—scientists finally started to get rid of their preconceived ideas and look at Nature herself. It finally became obvious that the structure of the matrix is secondary; it has many functional roles.

While it consists mainly of inanimate structural proteins such as collagen and elastin, it also contains signaling proteins that coax the right cells to be in the right place at the right time. For example, hook-like molecules called fibronectins and integrins provide tailored "molecular Velcro" for specific cells.

Once the right cells have been summoned, the matrix can coax them to turn into bone, muscle tissue, or fat cells. The secret, apparently, lies in what they are subjected to once inside the matrix. For example, high tension in the matrix's structure will persuade any incoming stem cells to become muscle or bone. Place them into a saggier matrix and they become fat cells.

Finally, having convinced cells to develop into the right kind of tissue, the matrix nourishes them so that they continue to mature into larger structures. Its material even contains potent growth factors that help blood vessels to form, providing nourishing oxygen for the growing organs.

The way is wide open for an amazing, unforeseen future. The kidneys worked so well in rats that Ott is now using similar techniques to develop other organs; it is projected that hearts, lungs, esophaguses, larynxes, livers, small intestines, and pancreases will soon be able to be recreated.

Let me repeat: you won't just get back the crappy organ that just failed. You get a whole new one, 100% working and filled with youthful vitality!

Now you see why I am urging you just to do what's needed, stay healthy, and stick around for a whole new you…

What About Regrowing Muscle Tissue?
Muscle is not quite so easy. Damaged muscle can regrow to some extent, but if a severe injury destroys too much of one specific muscle group, scar tissue prevents it from growing back. Such an injury—for example vehicle crash trauma or battle wounds—usually mean amputation and a prosthesis.

But what if you could use the matrix to attract and grow muscle from a person's own cells?

Already a trial in which matrix taken from a pig (qualitatively quite like human tissue) has been used to regrow big chunks of muscle in six people who had lost more than half of a muscle in road accidents or other trauma.

The early results have been astounding. Six months later, the pig matrix is gone, replaced by a completely new, natural matrix from the volunteers' own bodies – with muscle to match.

Ron Strang, a 28-year-old US Marine whose quadriceps muscle had been destroyed by a roadside bomb in Afghanistan, volunteered.

Strang couldn't even get out of a chair without assistance, but after surgical clearance of all residual scar tissue and replacing it with a strip of matrix, the results were sensational.

"I go out hiking," Strang says, "and I'm able to ride a bike." He has also taken up football and basketball. This is a guy who before treatment couldn't stand!

Even Bone
Building muscle is one thing. But what about rebuilding shattered bone? That's what Carmell Therapeutics in Pittsburgh is trying to do. They have chosen matrix material that is effectively a highly concentrated blood clot. The success of recent animal studies prompted them to begin a trial in human volunteers.

The dough-like substance carries high concentrations of growth factors known to promote bone repair. In a year-long trial in South Africa, this "bone putty" was applied to the broken shin bones, or tibiae, of 10 volunteers.

The accelerated healing the group has seen should help them win approval for larger trials, planned in Europe, and work on other bones.

Renewing Blood Vessels

Synthetic matrix can also be used as a template to build body parts far stronger than those that Nature provides. One group that could benefit enormously would be the millions of people who undergo kidney dialysis every year.

Dialysis is rough on the body: you need to be hooked into machines that cleanse the blood three times a week, with a large arm vein punctured. To do a few days of the kidneys' work in a few hours, blood must be forced through the system quickly. This heavy use often makes the veins collapse, so doctors have to continually reopen them.

It's harrowing and painful.

Now we have customized natural vein matrix parts that are stronger than the real thing. To do this, scientists first crafted a fast-decaying biodegradable polymer into a tube exactly the dimensions of a vein, but with a thicker vessel wall.

Then they coated this tube with human smooth-muscle cells. Within days, the cells completely replaced the biodegradable tube with a matrix of natural collagen, identical to a patient's own.

After stripping off the cells, these tubes were then surgically implanted in the patient, and served as the vein for dialysis.

The results have been so positive, we will soon see artificial blood vessels grafted as coronary bypass arteries.

Your Brain, Too?

It's almost the holy grail of regenerating organs. Will we be able to recreate brains, as good as new? I hope so, otherwise there is no future for politicians!

Seriously, though, it's theoretically possible.

Greg Bix of the University of Kentucky in Lexington discovered a key component of the matrix that could promote brain repair all on its own: a signaling molecule released from brain matrix that has been damaged by stroke, called perlecan domain five (DV). It promotes the growth of new blood vessels. When Bix injected DV into mice and rats who had deliberately been given strokes, the results were astounding. "In a fortnight," he says, "you couldn't tell they'd had strokes."

Until the Time Comes...Here's What you Can Do

It's true... we are all growing older. But that doesn't mean we have to age. Until the time comes when more research has been done and the new science of the matrix has been perfected, your job is to stay healthy.

You are certain to live far longer than you once planned, so why not do it well and enjoy your "Third Age" years to the fullest?

In my remarkable book, *Get Healthy For Your Next 100 Years*, I tell you all the latest science, organ by organ, system by system, explaining what you need to know and what you need to do to stay healthy longer. Go here, I have the science, if you have the willingness to learn it…visit: www.alternative-doctor.com/gethealthy

COULD STARDUST FIGHT AGING AND OBESITY?

You know, science can be tricky. Even with the best intentions and complete honesty, facts emerge that make it look like someone has been fudging all along.

Take obesity. There could be said to be a "science of obesity" today.

We know a lot about it; including the metabolic syndrome, the dangers of belly fat, the inflammatory nature of visceral fat, and how all this can lead to degenerative liver disease (fatty liver causes over 50% of cases of cirrhosis; alcohol abuse only 6% of cases).

Fat ages us fast. It also causes progressively earlier death. **Obesity is a killer…**

But wait a minute! It's not all like that; lots of holes have appeared in the old story. In fact, scientists have now started to refer to "metabolically healthy" fat or healthy obesity (really!). It seems that not all obesity is the same.

The concept of "metabolically healthy obesity"—that is, individuals with a body mass index (BMI) above 30 who do not have metabolic-syndrome factors that put them at risk for cardiovascular disease events—is not new, but is only now being more widely recognized by experts.

Metabolically healthy obese individuals have smaller waist circumference (pear vs. apple shape), high insulin resistance, and are "fat and fit," but there are no standardized cutoff points to identify metabolically healthy vs. unhealthy obese individuals.

So without any helpful test (as yet), it's difficult to spot these different individuals, for whom the normal advice might be wrong. Not that anyone is saying it's OK for them to remain overweight; just that they are not subject to the same "rules" as other overweight individuals.

A Far Better Measure Than Body Mass Index

Part of the problem is the definite confusion caused by the so-called BMI measure **(body mass index).** According to this test, Michael Jordan, one of the world's greatest athletes (National Basketball Association), is technically obese!

A better measure by far is waist circumference, especially in normal or moderately obese individuals; if yours is over 40 inches (male) or 35 inches (female), that's bad news. Blood tests shed light on the probable risk factors of obesity far more than simply weighing one's self on the bathroom scales.

For example, insulin levels are revealing. When insulin resistance sets, in the tissues cannot metabolize glucose properly; the result is that glucose is turned to fat and dumped in the tissues. Insulin resistance is shown by sampling blood levels after a sugar-loading challenge test.

Other problem issues include **inflammation, which is the number one aging phenomenon in our bodies**. Markers for widespread inflammation include c-reactive protein (CRP), adipokines, interleukin-6, and TNF-alpha

Eye-Catching Twin Study

What caught my eye this week is a study of identical twins, published online October 6 (2013) in *Diabetologia*, where each pair had one lean twin and one obese twin (so that gets rid of the genes issue!)

The identical twin pairs were aged 22 to 35 years old with a mean difference in weight between twin pairs of approximately 17 kg (37 lbs.); in other words quite a lot.

The researchers examined detailed characteristics of metabolic health, including subcutaneous, intra-abdominal, and liver fat (as measured by magnetic resonance imaging or spectroscopy), plus oral glucose tolerance, lipids, adipokines, and C-reactive protein. They also assessed mitochondrial function and inflammation in subcutaneous adipose tissue.

In half the twin pairs, the obese twins turned out to be as metabolically healthy as their lean counterparts, with low levels of liver fat, good glucose and insulin-sensitivity profiles, and little sign of chronic inflammation in their adipose tissue.

But the remaining eight obese twins had the classic hallmarks of unhealthy obesity, with marked insulin resistance, dyslipidemia, and a fatty liver (more than a 7-fold increase in liver fat compared with their lean twin), as well as up-regulation of chronic inflammation in their fat tissue.

That's very dangerous.

These obese, metabolically unhealthy twins also had significantly greater insulin production in response to an oral glucose tolerance test, greater levels of C-reactive protein (CRP), higher levels of LDL (bad) cholesterol, and lower levels of HDL (good) cholesterol than their lean twin, PLUS a tendency toward hypertension.

What Was the Difference?

Not totally clear, but the results suggest that metabolically healthy obesity is characterized by an adipose tissue that maintains normally functioning mitochondria, does not exhibit inflammation, and is able to handle the excess energy by making more fat cells and not just bigger fat cells.

That's according to lead author Jussi Naukkarinen, MD, PhD, from the Obesity Research Unit, University of Helsinki, Finland.

More fat cells for the same amount of fat means less fat per cell (adipose). That could be significant.

Then the study goes off the rails: according to the authors, no medication currently exists for the specific purpose of preventing adipose tissue inflammation or to promote mitochondrial health for efficient processing of food into energy, but it is possible that such treatments could be developed, the researchers say.

This is wrong. You can beat down inflammation, using a host of herbs like curcumin, along with omega-3 fatty acids. They don't even think of these things because they are not "medication." But the result will be valuable to you.

Eating Stardust Is Good for You

As for the mitochondria and keeping up their numbers and performance, you could turn to PQQ. Let me explain…

Today, scientists recognize mitochondrial dysfunction as a key bio-marker of aging. To take one instance, researchers have recorded evidence of 50% more mitochondrial damage in the brain cells of humans over 70 than in middle-aged individuals.

Mitochondrial dysfunction and death are now definitively linked to the development of virtually all killer diseases of aging, from Alzheimer's and type 2 diabetes to heart failure. And, of course, "metabolically unhealthy obesity," as you have just read.

The good news is that mitochondrial dysfunction can be reversed. The scientific literature is now filled with studies documenting the therapeutic power of CoQ10 to boost mitochondrial health and bio-energetic capacity.

And the new kid on the block is an enzyme called **co-enzyme pyrroloquinoline quinone or PQQ for short.**

Actually, when I say "new kid," I'm way wrong. PQQ is present in interstellar stardust and this has led some experts to hypothesize a pivotal role for PQQ in the evolution of life on Earth. I am reminded of the words of the Woodstock song lyric:

"We are stardust, we are golden, we are billion-year-old carbon, …"

PQQ has been found in all plant species tested to date. Neither humans nor the bacteria that colonize the human digestive tract have demonstrated the ability to synthesize it.

This has led researchers to classify PQQ as an essential micro-nutrient.

But perhaps the best news of all is that PQQ promotes the growth of NEW mitochondria. In one study, published in the *Journal of Nutrition*, researchers fed mice a diet supplemented with PQQ, and the test animals grew a staggering number of new mitochondria in just eight weeks. That's a very powerful anti-aging capacity indeed. PQQ is truly "stardust" come to Earth for us!

You can get PQQ from The Life Extension Foundation. But a better idea might be to get a supply of Dr. Al Sears' Ultra Accel, which combines CoQ-10 and PQQ in one easy capsule.

HOW TO AVOID A FATAL BLOOD CLOT: EYE-OPENING STUDY EXPLAINS WHY LOWERING YOUR BLOOD VISCOSITY IS CRUCIAL

...And What You Can Do to Keep Your Blood Youthful & Live Until You're 100 Years Old!

When will the pendulum swing away from the nonsensical obsessive focus on lipid metabolism and move to viscosity and clotting? Most fatal cardiovascular events are blood clots, not fat sludge!

Now a new study from Edinburgh University in the UK has shown conclusively that blood viscosity (its free-flowing liquid vs. sludging characteristic) is crucial. It is NOT the quality of artery walls that matters; it's the quality of the blood itself.

Raised blood viscosity is at least as important as two old favorites: blood pressure and "bad" cholesterol (LDL) in predicting death by heart attack.

PLUS: THEY SHOWED IT'S MORE IMPORTANT THAN SMOKING AS A RISK FACTOR.

This is so obviously important that only doctors making money off the outdated nonsense of chasing cholesterol levels for a living will fail to act on this research and incorporate it in patient care.

Big Pharma will try to smother the research, because cholesterol-controlling statin drugs are still their number one profit-earner, worldwide.

Study Details...

The Edinburgh Artery Study, as it's called, looked at a random population of 1,592 men and women aged 55 to 74 years, who were followed over a mean period of 5 years. After adjustment for age and gender, the levels of blood viscosity and a related measurement were consistently raised in patients who had experienced a bad cardiovascular event, such as heart attacks or stroke. [1]

In a seminal report just prior to the publication of the Edinburgh Artery Study, Louisiana State University pathologist Gregory Sloop proposed that blood viscosity is the one unifying mechanism that pulls together and makes sense out of all currently accepted cardiovascular risk factors, including LDL cholesterol, high blood pressure, diabetes, obesity, and smoking. [2]

Moreover, numerous other published studies have confirmed the link between blood viscosity and the following cardiovascular risk factors:

- Hypertension (3-6)
- Hyperlipidema: positive correlation with LDL cholesterol, total cholesterol and triglycerides; negative correlation with HDL cholesterol (7-13)
- Diabetes, insulin resistance syndrome, and obesity (12,14-18)
- Tobacco smoking (6,19-21)
- Male gender vs. pre-menopausal women (12,14-18)
- Aging (12,21,24)

In his report, which was titled *A Unifying Theory of Atherogenesis*, Dr. Sloop indicated that blood viscosity was uniquely suited to predict the entire course of cardiovascular disease because blood viscosity accomplishes the following:

1. Accounts for the morphological similarity of atherosclerotic lesions associated with many diverse risk factors.
2. Explains the anatomic distribution of lesions throughout the body.
3. Provides a role for platelet activation by turbulent blood flow caused by hyper-viscosity.
4. Includes an explanation of the protective role of HDL "good" cholesterol (i.e., HDL has been shown experimentally to lower viscosity). [2]

Blood viscosity holds certain similarities to blood pressure.

Like blood pressure, the viscosity of blood changes during each cardiac cycle and is reported using two numerical quantities: systolic and diastolic viscosity.

However, while blood pressure is parameter of the circulatory system as a whole, blood viscosity is a parameter specific to the fluid flowing through the system.

Therefore, viscosity can be said to precede pressure and therefore to be more fundamental than pressure.

What's to Be Done?

You need to make sure that, if you are in medical care, your physicians are using viscosity measurements to monitor your risks.

If they are not, demand they do or change to a different physician. Otherwise you will join the army of 50% of citizens who die of cardiovascular events.

Do NOT accept Coumadin as a means of controlling clotting risk because:

1. It's dangerous in its own right (a whole other story)
2. It's solving the wrong problem (it does nothing for viscosity)

Take plenty of omega-3s, as we always tell you. It's anti-inflammatory, slows blood clotting, and, if you like, "thins the blood."

Be sure to discontinue it before dental or surgical treatment, otherwise the dentist or surgeon will have trouble stopping the bleeding! That's how good it is.

If you have already had an adverse event, get Dr. Garry Gordon's "Beyond Chelation Improved" formula (BCI). Dr. Gordon boasts $10 million of published research behind showing that it eliminates those fatal CV events, because BCI lowers blood viscosity.

While taking BCI, no one has suffered a fatal cardiovascular event or stroke in over a decade.

"No matter how serious the clinical picture is (i.e., high-grade LAD vascular occlusive disease, diabetes, lipid issues, high CRP) my patients are all routinely protected against MI and stroke," Dr. Gordon says (personal communication, Sept. 27, 2013).

Finally, invest in a PEMF device and use it on yourself regularly. The PEMF-100 is the one I would recommend. Immediately after use, microscopic examination of the blood shows that the "sticky" parcels of red cells have broken up and the blood is much more free-flowing.

Ten to fifteen minutes a day could keep your blood youthful for many decades to come!

If you can't afford the considerable expense of one of these devices, find a local practitioner who has got one or is willing to buy one for his or her practice. Book yourself in regularly for sessions.

PEMF devices are the future, according to doctors like Garry Gordon.

References

1. Lowe GD, Lee AJ, Rumley A, et al. Blood viscosity and risk of cardiovascular events: the Edinburgh Artery Study. Br J Haematol 1997; 96:168-173.
2. Sloop GD. A unifying theory of atherogenesis. Med Hypotheses. 1996; 47:321-5.
3. Smith WC, Lowe GD, et al. Rheological determinants of blood pressure in a Scottish adult population. J Hypertens 1992; 10:467-72.
4. Letcher RL, Chien S, et al. Direct relationship between blood pressure and blood viscosity in normal and hypertensive subjects. Role of fibrinogen and concentration. Am J Med 1981; 70:1195-1202.
5. Devereux RB, Case DB, Alderman MH, et al. Possible role of increased blood viscosity in the hemodynamics of systemic hypertension. Am J Cardiol 2000; 85:1265-1268.
6. Levenson J, Simon AC, Cambien FA, Beretti C. Cigarette smoking and hypertension. Factors independently associated with blood hyperviscosity and arterial rigidity. Arteriosclerosis 1987; 7:572-577.
7. Sloop GD, Garber DW. The effects of low-density lipoprotein and high-density lipoprotein on blood viscosity correlate with their association with risk of atherosclerosis in humans. Clin Sci 1997; 92:473-479.
8. Lowe GD. Blood viscosity, lipoproteins, and cardiovascular risk. Circulation 1992; 85:2329-2331.
9. Rosenson RS, Shott S, Tangney CC. Hypertriglyceridemia is associated with an elevated blood viscosity: triglycerides and blood viscosity. Atherosclerosis 2002; 161:433-9.
10. Stamos TD, Rosenson RS. Low high density lipoprotein levels areassociated with an elevated blood viscosity. Atherosclerosis 1999; 146:161-5.
11. Høieggen A, Fossum E, Moan A, Enger E, Kjeldsen SE. Whole-blood viscosity and the insulin-resistance syndrome. J Hypertens 1998; 16:203-10.
12. de Simone G, Devereux RB, Chien S, et al. Relation of blood viscosity to demographic and physiologic variables and to cardiovascular risk factors in apparently normal adults. Circulation 1990; 81:107-17.
13. Rosenson RS, McCormick A, Uretz EF. Distribution of blood viscosity values and biochemical correlates in healthy adults. Clin Chem 1996; 42:1189-95.
14. Tamariz LJ, Young JH, Pankow JS, et al. Blood viscosity and hematocrit as risk factors for type 2 diabetes mellitus: The Atherosclerosis Risk in Communities (ARIC) Study. Am J Epidemiol 2008; 168:1153-60.

15. Jax TW, Peters AJ, Plehn G, Schoebel FC. Hemostatic risk factors in patients with coronary artery disease and type 2 diabetes - a two year follow-up of 243 patients. Cardiovasc Diabetol 2009; 8:48.
16. Ernst E, Weihmayr T, et al. Cardiovascular risk factors and hemorheology. Physical fitness, stress and obesity. Atherosclerosis 1986; 59:263-9.
17. Høieggen A, Fossum E, et al. Whole-blood viscosity and the insulin-resistance syndrome. J Hypertens 1998; 16:203-10.
18. Carroll S, Cooke CB, Butterly RJ. Plasma viscosity, fibrinogen and the metabolic syndrome: effect of obesity and cardiorespiratory fitness. Blood Coagul Fibrinolysis 2000; 11:71-8.
19. Ernst E, Koenig W, Matrai A, et al. Blood rheology in healthy cigarette smokers. Results from the MONICA project, Augsburg. Arteriosclerosis 1988; 8:385-8.
20. Ernst E. Haemorheological consequences of chronic cigarette smoking. J Cardiovasc Risk 1995; 2:435-9.
21. Lowe GD, Drummond MM, Forbes CD, Barbenel JC. The effects of age and cigarette-smoking on blood and plasma viscosity in men. Scott Med J 1980; 25:13-7.
22. Kameneva MV, Watach MJ, Borovetz HS. Gender difference in rheologic properties of blood and risk of cardiovascular diseases.
23. Clin Hemorheol Microcirc 1999; 21:357-363.
    Fowkes FG, Pell JP, Donnan PT, et al. Sex differences in susceptibility to etiologic factors for peripheral atherosclerosis. Importance of plasma fibrinogen and blood viscosity. Arterioscler Thromb 1994; 14:862-8.
24. Coppola L, Caserta F, De Lucia D, et al. Blood viscosity and aging. Arch Gerontol Geriatr 2000; 31:35-42
    Meridian Valley Lab http://meridianvalleylab.com/the-link-between-blood-viscosity-and-cardiovascular-disease

A NOVEL TECHNIQUE FOR CLEANING YOUR TEETH

A very friendly US correspondent of mine, who prefers to remain strictly anonymous, wrote to me after I mentioned the misery following my recent dental work ("Medicine Outside the Box," Jan. 3, 2014). What he said was news to me and could be useful to millions of people! I'll let him tell it in his own words…

I have always had amazingly strong and good teeth with almost no cavities. One dentist referred to them once as teeth of a bull elephant. But a few years ago I started getting a lot of plaque and periodontitis.

I tried everything from SCENAR to all sorts of herbal mouth washes, toothpastes, water pick, mechanical toothbrushes, and laser treatments.

The result was that I ended up losing my molars on both sides. So suffice it to be said: I've been through a bit of the dental pain and disappointment you describe. But this battle didn't end completely even after losing some of my teeth!

I find all of this to be personally embarrassing, but I happened to mention my dental battle to an old friend who is very knowledgeable in natural remedies. Surprisingly, he said that he wished I had told him sooner because he most likely could have saved my teeth, not to mention thousands of dollars in dental bills and all the pain. He told me to simply brush my teeth with nothing else but some organic raw coconut oil. After looking closely at the ingredients of all my toothpastes (even the "natural" ones) I figured I certainly couldn't hurt myself trying something like organic raw coconut oil.

The complete protocol is not to initially swallow the melted coconut oil as the teeth are being brushed, but reserve it in the mouth so that when finished brushing, the saliva and coconut oil mixture can be used to swirl around and between the teeth like a mouthwash. Then the whole mixture can either be spit out or swallowed. (Dieters will spit it out and others will swallow for the coconut oil benefits.)

I did this protocol, along with the dental "brush tapping" method you once wrote about, (the *Tooth Wizard*, download a free eBook from here: http://www.toothwizards.com/shop.html) and the results were dramatic. My entire mouth starting quickly responding wonderfully and now my remaining teeth are back to being as strong as a bull elephant's.

Better Than a Mouthwash
Evidently (and according to my friend) raw coconut oil has all sorts of natural antibiotics and natural healing powers. It seems to leave the healthy flora alone while destroying all the infectious bacteria.

I've been brushing with nothing but raw coconut oil for a few years now and have been totally free of any problems as well as I've found that it seems to greatly inhibit even the creation of plaque.

The only other thing I can tell you is purely subjective. When I first starting brushing my teeth with coconut oil and swallowing my throat would become raspy or sore. But this inflammation would slowly dissipate after approximately 10 minutes. After a few weeks, this reaction in my throat stopped altogether.

Therefore it's my guess as to what was happening (and this may be psychosomatic) is that, as the coconut oil was pulling the toxins and infections out of my mouth, my throat was reacting to a film of these same things after I swallowed. Now that my mouth is healthy, I no longer seem to have any detectable reaction in my throat.

HOW TO FIGHT CANDIDA AND PAINFUL YEAST INFECTIONS
Get Sensational New Additions to the Candida Story Right Here…

Everyone has heard about *Candida*. The problem exists but it's unlikely that *Candida* is the real cause. *But how can you fight Candida?*

People get sick–of course they do–but *Candida* isn't the cause, unless you are dying of terminal AIDS or cancer.

The *Candida* hype is from sources about 30 years out of date. I pointed out the many other candidates as causative organisms in one of my books as long ago as 1992. The truth is, there are dozens of potential culprits.

Even food yeasts are capable of fermenting foods and producing most, if not all, of the symptoms of fatigue, brain fog, etc.

I repeat: *Candida* is very, very rarely to blame. It just doesn't show up–you can't find it in stool samples, where it would be OBVIOUS if the *Candida* story that's being peddled was correct.

Sensitivity tests only tell you that you encountered it. Well, we all do! *Candida* is everywhere, like germs in the soil! It's on your skin and under your fingernails right now!

Fight Candida – Arm Yourself with the Right Information

The sad thing is, even good (otherwise good) holistic practitioners get this wrong, too. They fall into the lazy trap of reading other people's books and websites and parrot it back to patients.

You are about to learn the full story from a master in the field. This is so way beyond typical housewife, how-I-cured-myself publications.

You will be impressed as everything is backed by up-to-the-minute science, plus I reveal what works and what doesn't from my direct personal experience.

What you want is the cutting-edge science. That's what I do. I eat, sleep, drink, and think cutting-edge stuff. It's my equivalent of oxygen and food!

The truth is, what we used to call dysbiosis has become the number one health hazard of our modern world. It's far more terrifying than just the simplistic "*Candida*" model. You'll be shocked.

It's something that threatens our very DNA; it's something that is made so much worse by our modern toxic lifestyles; it's truly THE disease of the 21st century.

I have no hesitation is telling you that you need to know and UNDERSTAND this phenomenon. It's got nothing to do with just being tired and lethargic; **if you have EVER taken an antibiotic, you'll be at risk. If you have EVER eaten bread or drunk alcohol, you'll be affected.**

Read more and get yourself a copy of my book, *Beyond Candida*, to get everything you need to know about this common, overlooked, misdiagnosed health problem.

Visit: www.alternative-doctor.com/candida

Get your copy now and understand the whole journey, starting with how to fight *Candida*, and then beyond…

THE BRAIN AND GUT CONNECTION – LINKED TO ALZHEIMER'S DISEASE

Yet another study, published in the September 2012, issue of *Neurology*, has linked low vitamin D levels with significant health issues — in this case, poor cognition.

People with Alzheimer's disease (AD) had lower concentrations of vitamin D than those without AD and better cognitive test results were linked to higher vitamin D concentrations.

According to the main author, Cynthia Balion, PhD, a clinical biochemist and associate professor, Department of Pathology and Molecular Medicine, McMaster University, Hamilton, Ontario, Canada, the results provide sufficient evidence to warrant further investigation to determine whether a cause-and-effect relationship exists.

She's right, of course. Just because the two are associated doesn't mean low vitamin D causes cognitive problems. It might mean, for example, that people with malabsorption (a common problem, due to bowel inflammation) are short of all nutrients and because of the inflammatory process also get Alzheimer's—essentially a disease of brain inflammatory decay.

You'll learn more about this brain and gut connection in my book, *Fire In The Belly*. I was a pioneer in this area in the 1980s and 1990s. (Visit: www.alternative-doctor.com/firebelly)

But, for the time being, vitamin D is dirt cheap, I think **we should be taking it as a protective**. You need it anyway. There is no longer any reasonable debate about whether vitamin D protects from cancer: 4,000 – 5,000 IU will cost you less than $10 a month. We need to aim for blood levels of at least 40 nmol/L (nanomoles per liter). 75 nmol/L or more is better. That means getting cooperation from your doctor to arrange the tests. Any doctor who allows a patient to continue before 40 nmol/L blood levels of vitamin D is criminally negligent. There's just too much science out there now, proving the benefits of vitamin D.

Cynthia Balion is right again: We now need to do good interventional studies and see whether or not giving vitamin D helps people at higher risk for developing cognitive decline; maybe it even improves those already showing signs of being on the slippery slope to dementia.

"How exactly vitamin D protects the brain is not clear, but research suggests that vitamin D acts as a neurosteroid," said Dr. Balion.

At the molecular level, the brain can synthesize the active form of vitamin D [1,25(OH)D] within several cell types and regions, predominantly in the hypothalamus and large neurons in the *substantia nigra*.

Also, many genes are regulated by vitamin D, which contributes to neuro-protection by modulating the production of such things as nerve growth factor, and regulating neurotransmitters.

It's a miracle! Our guts are a hotbed of inflammation, which affect systemic health in all our other organs and tissues. Find out how to protect yourself from *Fire in the Belly* today.

[SOURCE: *Neurology*. 2012;79:1397-1405]

WHY ANTIBIOTICS MAKE YOU FAT
Do you know this hidden cause of weight gain?

Have we been missing something all these years? Obviously, the main cause of weight gain is overeating. But is there something behind that—something driving the overeating—that nobody has noticed?

I think so—and now people are beginning to recognize its importance.

Other Causes

We know that MSG in food is addictive and causes people to overeat.

We know that eating carbohydrates is highly addictive, with people being driven by blood sugar spikes, followed by a drop in blood sugar. Refined carbs are the worst.

A few of us pioneers back in the 1970s and 1980s discovered that **food addiction is often related to food allergies and that too drives people to binge eating**. In fact, it's the chief mechanism behind eating disorders; if only more people knew it.

We know that insulin resistance (the early stage of diabetes) blocks glucose uptake by cells, which is then diverted to the liver and stowed away at fat.

We know that psychological hang-ups can lead to "comfort eating."

But there is something else? You betcha…

Antibiotics!

I could kick myself for not thinking of this, decades ago. But we know that farmers feed their livestock on antibiotics, to make them grow. Pigs, lambs, and sheep can be up 40% bigger and fatter, because of this antibiotic treatment. But we never thought "well, that must apply to humans too"… *duh!*

Of course it applies to humans.

If we feed ourselves incessant antibiotics, exactly as happens to young kids these days, due to the idiotic parental obsession with getting "treatment" for every cough, cold, snotty nose, and sore throat that comes along, we are raising our kids exactly the way farmers fatten their herds!

Does this make sense? When somebody lays it out in front of you, then it's easy to join the dots: we are dooming our citizens to be grossly overweight by the unnecessary use of dangerous and powerful antibiotics.

Scientific Proof

To investigate whether overusing antibiotics could also play a part in the rise of obesity, researchers fed infant mice low doses of penicillin to mimic doses given to farm animals. After 30 weeks, penicillin-fed mice were between 10 and 15 percent bigger and twice as fat as drug-free mice.

When the team looked at the mice's gut bacteria, they found that the antibiotic-fed mice had a different complement of bugs than the untreated mice. Low doses of antibiotics had seemingly shifted the balance of certain gut microbes, reducing the numbers of *Lactobacillus*, which is a "good" bacterium linked to a lower risk of cancer recurrence.

This is the classic "dysbiosis" I write about. But the problem is actually much bigger than that (see below).

First, the researchers wanted to prove it was the altered bowel flora to blame, not some other pathway affected by antibiotics. So they turned to germ-free mice, which are bred in a sterile environment and have no gut bacteria. These mice were given gut bacteria transplanted from the mice fed antibiotics and, just five weeks later, the once germ-free mice were 35 percent larger than mice with a regular microbiota.

There is more: in the initial experiment, the biggest mice were those that had started antibiotic treatment from birth. Even mice that were given drugs for only four weeks ended up as large as mice on antibiotics for the full 30 weeks.

This suggests that gut flora may be most vulnerable to disruption in the earliest moments of life. Children are exceptionally at risk, exactly as I said above.

But still: it's even worse!

Antibiotics used to treat children may also have a detrimental effect on their immune systems.

Readers of my book, *Fire in the Belly*, (visit: www.alternative-doctor.com/firebelly)

have already been introduced to the concept.

It's one of the biggest breakthroughs in understanding the full importance of the human microbiome (sometimes you will see the scientific word microbiota). It means the composite of all the microbes living in your gut: bacteria, viruses, protozoa, molds, and even parasites. It's important to us and directs how our body responds to challenge.

The bugs down there in the warm and dark of our intestines actually educate the newborn's immune system and teaches it what to do. It's very important that a child is inoculated, at birth, with this gift from Momma's bowel. Without it, the child will grow up with a malfunctioning immune system. He or she will grow up with food allergies and other miseries.

Of course, if Momma already has messed up bowel flora, from the days when SHE took antibiotics, than the child is not given the "real deal" but dysbiotic organisms instead.

In a separate study in mice, this same research team mimicked the short courses of higher-dose antibiotics that young children tend to receive for infections, to see if this typical manner of administering antibiotics was bad. They found that levels of important T-cell signaling chemicals were abnormally low, meaning the immune systems were compromised.

But it's worse even than THAT!

We now know that the microbiome also educates the brain and nervous system. It's incredible but true. Again, without healthy bowel flora, a child's neurological growth is stunted. This may even be the real cause of the rise in autism. Bad bowel flora (including the notorious measles virus found in the gut by Andrew Wakefield) may result in the abnormal physical signs of autism spectrum disorder.

It's all new and wildly different from anything we imagined back in the 1980s, when doctors like me were sounding the alarm but we didn't have the least idea what was happening and why; only that we must stop taking so many antibiotics and try, with probiotics, to get our gut flora back to normal.

It's so very important to all of us to stop using antibiotics, except as a life-saving necessity. You need to learn and understand alternatives. If you haven't already got a copy, you may want to go over and get my encyclopedic compilation of safe, natural antibiotic alternatives, *How To Survive In A World Without Antibiotics* (visit: www.alternative-doctor.com/wwa).

Weight Gain

So, back to where we started, which is that antibiotics dispose to significant weight gain. As use of this class of drugs has soared in recent decades, so has the incidence of obesity.

In other words, **our epidemic of obesity is probably driven by antibiotic overuse**; especially the feeding of food livestock with antibiotics.

Let me emphasize that it's a real effect; no question. Another recent study, from Copenhagen University Hospital in Denmark, followed the development of 28,000 babies. The results showed that those infants given antibiotics within the first six months of life were more likely to be overweight at age 7, even if their mother had a healthy weight.[1]

It's Down to the Quality of Your Sh*t

OK, I'm being deliberately provocative (as usual!) The scientific word for shit is feces (proper English spelling faeces, since it's a Greek word, not an American word).

It's an important health-quality issue. For example, feces that float in the toilet pan and stick to the sides contain undigested fat; often it signals liver disease, since bile is needed to emulsify fats, to enable digestion.

But the actual makeup of our feces, in terms of the organisms present, has emerged in recent years as possibly the number one health issue. As I said in *Fire in the Belly*, it's probably true that most or all diseases have an element of this problem.

Hippocrates, 2,500 years ago, was in no doubt. He remarked that…

"All diseases start in the gut."

Now we understand the concept of our human microbiome (the DNA makeup of the other passengers in SS Human), we can see there are very far-reaching consequences indeed from the unwise or careless use of antibiotics. You may want to worry more about what's coming out of your backside than what you put in your mouth! You know, Winnie the P.…

[SOURCE: This man, Martin Blaser, is where I got most of the scientific info: http://www.med.nyu.edu/biosketch/blasem01/publications]

Reference
1. *International Journal of Obesity*, DOI: 10.1038/ijo.2011.27.

WHY NO ONE WANTS TO TALK ABOUT PARASITES

A man died in California of a massive infection with parasitic worms that spread throughout his body, including his lungs. He was probably infected in Vietnam, one of the countries where this particular worm is found.

The worms, a species called *Strongyloides stercoralis*, had remained dormant until his immune system was suppressed by steroid drugs used to treat an inflammatory disorder.

Strongyloides stercoralis worms are most commonly found in tropical and subtropical areas of the world, although they've also appeared in the Appalachian region of the United States. Typically, they infect people in rural areas such as Brazil, northern Argentina, and Southeast Asia, and may currently infect as many 100 million people worldwide.

Compare that with lung cancer: less than 2 million.

Strongyloides is nasty. I covered it in my comprehensive life-saver manual, *The Parasites Handbook* (visit: www.alternative-doctor.com/parasites). Between 80 and 90% of patients will die of this worm, once the infection has been released in the so-called "hyperinfection" stage, also known as disseminated *Strongyloides*.

This is when the adult worms are producing eggs and the larvae emerging from the eggs are invading the intestinal wall and disseminating to multiple organs in the body. The rate of infection just accelerates and a "worm storm" is whipped up inside the victim's body.[1]

Medication can help treat infestation with the worms, but it doesn't help when the hyperinfection reaches an advanced stage.

This unfortunate man was being *"eaten by worms,"* even before he was dead and put in the ground. Rather ironic.

The trigger in this salutary case was steroids. The patient was given massive doses of steroids to treat a condition called temporal arteritis. This suppressed his immune system and released the parasites from natural control. The man's case emphasizes the importance of testing patients who might be infected with parasites, before giving them drugs to dampen the immune system. The problem is that most physicians are not taught about this disease. Their ignorance could cost you your life.[1]

To get yourself informed about parasites and its effects on your immune system, you MUST get my book *The Parasites Handbook* (visit: www.alternative-doctor.com/parasites). It's the most comprehensive, written overview of the whole subject, in terms suitable for and easily understood by the lay person.

Reference
1. March 21, 2013, *New England Journal of Medicine*.

GET TANNED, NOT SKIN CANCER! THE SAFEST SUNSCREEN
First, You Need to Get the Sunscreen Facts Straight…

Vivien and I are traveling in Europe for the summer and now we have been sweltering in a record-breaking heat wave. As temperatures soar, in a place where air-conditioning is not standard, folks are beginning to suffer badly.

---
1 "worm storm" is not an official term, but describes very well the last days of a person's life.

The low-salt diet patients are starting to pass out on the streets, as usual.

But everyone risks sunburn.

We climbed a Lake District peak and—because it took two hours longer than expected—we took a hammering from the UV rays.

By coincidence (there are no real coincidences) I just got an article from my good friend Denie Hiestand, anxious to straighten out my followers on the real facts of sun blockers, and just this morning I read the most stupid, ignorant, and dangerous article on sun protection by a woman called Karyn Meier and sent out by David Riklan's "SelfGrowth.com."

She should quit; Riklan should be ashamed. I have never seen such a flagrant example of "research by Googling" and coming up with wrong stuff— dangerously wrong stuff.

Let's start with her falsehoods and nonsense and finish up with the truth. Silly Karyn Meier believes the official industry myth of SPF factors (skin protection factor). Her ignorance truly stands out when she tells us to be sure to use a factor of 15 or over.

Those of you who read my writings will know that going higher than factor 15 is a total waste of effort and money. 93% of the Sun's rays are filtered out at factor 15; even going up to factor 100 only gets you an extra few % protection.

But it's far worse than that. If she knew anything at all, she would know that **sun creams CAUSE SKIN CANCER**. The Sun does NOT, repeat DOES NOT cause skin cancer.

In fact, as I wrote in *Virtual Medicine*, over a decade ago, people who avoid the Sun are the people who get skin cancer; it's a proven and published fact, in a peer-reviewed journal, but totally ignored by the know-alls, who just circulate the universal medical myths (or "experts" like Meier, who just Google for their "facts").[1]

Get out into the open air, let the sunlight pour down on you and you'll not suffer. Hide from it and your skin becomes like a tinderbox, that will burst into fire if you do finally get to see the Sun.

By contrast, Denie Hiestand tells the real truth about all those "slip, slap, and slop" sunscreen products, in a way you all should know…

Two Kinds of Sunscreen
Sunscreens come in two basic formulations. One contains chemical compounds as the **active ingredients** and the other contains **natural organic compounds**. The two work very differently.

How the Chemical Ones Work
All chemical sun blocks work by "absorbing' some of the sun's radiation. The chemicals lock the rays up into their structure, thus the skin is not directly impacted by the sun's radiation, as much. Great idea, one would think.

However, by locking up or concentrating this radiation into the chemical molecules, we are turning these molecules into miniature nuclear power plants, which then radiate back at us and cause immense damage. One could call it "point blank" radiation of the skin cells.

Think about it: under normal sun exposure without a sunscreen, the sun's rays get absorbed by millions of skin cells as well as penetrating the body tissue under the skin. Therefore, the radiation from the sun becomes dispersed over millions of molecules of skin and body tissue (which is the way we are designed to receive the sun's rays).

No single cell gets overloaded with concentrated radiation.

On the other hand, when you put on a chemical "radiation-absorbing" sun block, you are concentrating the radiation into a very small amount of surface skin cells by way of the chemicals in the cream sitting on and in the cells.

Using any type of "radiation-absorbing" chemical as a sunscreen actually increases the radiation impact on surface skin cells to a highly dangerous level that can, and often will, lead to skin cancer.

You do not have to be a rocket scientist to understand why skin cancer has gone up 92% since the sunscreen industry incorporated chemical "radiation-absorbing" compounds into sunscreens.

I often quote the fact that New Zealand and Australian farmers, who work 365 days a year in what can arguably be described as the most intense sunlight anywhere, and by-and-large never use sunscreens, have the lowest incidence of skin cancer in the Western world.

Yet, their city cousins, who slip, slap, and slop sunblock creams on (at a higher level than any population in the world), have the highest level of skin cancer on earth.

Go figure!

Now to the Organic Compounds & How They Work...

There are two common forms of so-called natural or organic sun blocks, *titanium dioxide* and *zinc oxide*. However, titanium dioxide is not really "natural." It is a "di-oxide" and thus a processed and manipulated group of molecules and there are reams of research showing real concern for their effects on long-term health.

This leaves zinc oxide, one of the safest and longest-used natural compounds known. Its use in skin protection and repair goes back to the Australian aboriginals and the tribes of Africa.

Zinc oxide works as a sunscreen by the simple process of radiation "reflection." The zinc molecules do not "absorb" radiation, but reflect it back out, harmlessly (just like a mirror). That is why zinc oxide looks white, as full spectrum sunlight looks pure white to our brain.

Thus, when a sun cream incorporates natural zinc oxide in its formulation, most of the sun's rays will never impact the skin cells and there is no concentrated or residue radiation in the zinc molecules to "fry" or radiate the skin, as in chemical "absorbers." Zinc oxide is also the only compound that covers the spectrum of rays from 260nM to 400nM, which includes most of the UVC range, and the entire UVB, UVA 2, and UVA 1 spectrum.

No other natural or chemically approved sunscreens, match this.

Can It Kill You?

However, some people have a vanity issue and do not like the white look on their skin. To overcome this vanity resistance, a chemical company developed a non-whitening zinc oxide-based product.

They did this by finely grinding the zinc and then subjecting the molecules to a chemical process that "cloaked" the "reflecting" ability of the natural zinc with a chemical called triethoxycaprylylsilane. This is a silicon-based compound and that should put you on the alert.

Triethoxycaprylylsilane reduces the radiation "reflecting" component of the zinc and makes it into more of an "absorbing" compound. It is now not true zinc oxide because the molecules have been modified by coating and infusing it with a nasty new chemical.

There has been no long-term testing of triethoxycaprylylsilane and we do not know how the body will react in the long run. The fact that the FDA says it is safe does not impress me: the FDA said Vioxx was safe and that killed upwards of half a million people before they (reluctantly) acted.

Just be aware that any company that says they are using "non-whitening zinc oxide" are using a chemically laced, processed, and modified form of zinc that is now not zinc oxide.

In the EU, products that have the coated and modified zinc in them have to list triethoxycaprylylsilane on the INCI ingredient list of the product.

Sadly, this is not the case in the USA, Australia, or New Zealand. The public has no idea they are putting this untested new chemical on their absorb-able skin.

In my view, there is only one form of safe, natural sunscreen and that is unaltered zinc oxide. This is the only sunscreen component that should ever be used for sunscreen.

A natural sun cream ("environmental protection" cream) with 8% zinc oxide will give an SPF of over 15. So always look for the % of natural zinc oxide on the label.

Reference
1. *The Lancet*, Vol. 363, Issue 9410, Pp. 728–730, February 28, 2004.

THE NATURAL HEALING SCIENCE OF TISSUE CLEANING
What Is Homotoxicology?

Tissue Deep Cleansing

Despite a clumsy name, *homotoxicology* is a wonderful natural healing science. It is a therapeutic branch that enables deep cleansing of the body tissues, removing old toxins, disease processes and degenerative debris, leaving the fluids clean, fresh, and able to function as intended.

Based on homeopathy, but not quite the same thing, homotoxicology is the brain child of German doctor Hans-Heinrich Reckeweg (1905-1985). Knowing homeopathy and drawing on a vast knowledge of herbal lore and medicines, he compounded a store of remedies that trod a line between folk medicine and basic plant pharmacology. In the course of time it has proved itself so well that tens of thousands of German doctors use it in daily practice, although it is less well-known in the rest of the world.

It has been also called the **German system of homeopathy**, though this is slightly comical, since the original system of homeopathy was also invented by a German, Samuel Hahnemann.

The Matrix in Health and Disease
Whereas so much molecular medicine is aimed at the cell, as if it were the sole seat of disease, Dr. Alfred Pischinger, then professor of histology and embryology in Vienna, saw with great insight that the extracellular fluids were the key to health.

These fluids, which Pischinger called the "**matrix**," or ground regulation system, because it supports everything else, brings nutrition, oxygen, hormone messengers, and other vital substances to the tissues and removes excretion products, toxins, and the residue of old diseases.

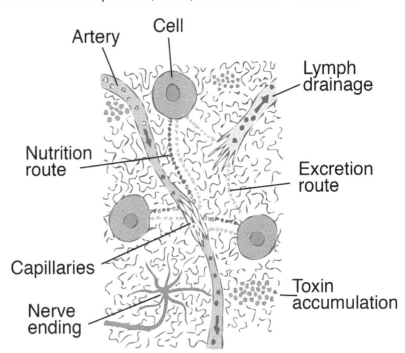

Cells may be important, but not a separate entity, because they cannot exist without being nurtured in this matrix. Reckeweg pursued Pischinger's matrix model and devised ways to use natural substances to support, clean, and revitalize the extracellular matrix. Most of the classic homeopathic remedies are still there, though used slightly differently.

I have reproduced a diagram of the matrix here. It's the best I could find. I hope it sheds some light.

It shows the matrix being fed by blood from the heart and drained away by venous blood and lymphatic drainage (doctors tend to forget this aspect of tissue hygiene).

The connective tissue cells are floating in the extracellular fluid. The whole is supplied by the nervous system, which helps regulate it. But many chemical messengers also control this matrix: hormones, of course. Also cytokines (literally means cell motivators).

Homeopathic Mixtures
The key variation is the use of mixtures, which classic homeopaths frown upon. But Reckeweg ignored the dogma and carried out decades of practical research, demonstrating conclusively that the formulations worked and worked well. He made compounds that would support the liver and kidneys, that would work against flu, diabetes, and women's problems, that would

stimulate metabolism, tone up the immune system, retard tumors, repair inflammation, act as pain-killers, and so on.

In other words, these are function-based medicines. The mixtures give rise to yet another name you may encounter: "complex homeopathy." Not all remedies are mixtures of substances however; some are single remedies in a mixture of potencies (called a "chord," after the musical term for several notes sounding at once).

There are key advantages to using potency chords:

1. Deeper action
2. Fewer initial aggravations than classical dosing
3. Doses can be repeated
4. Broader spectrum of effect
5. No problems selecting the appropriate potency
6. No problems in assessing the duration or spectrum of action
7. Mixing high and low potencies produces an effect that lies somewhere in between: rapid onset (low potency) and long-lasting action (high potency)
8. Faster action
9. Potency stages retain their own effects

Formula

To give an instance of this mixture modality and explain it more clearly, let us consider in detail one of Reckeweg's original compounds, called *Tonsilla compositum*. It contains 30 remedies in all, some herbal, some mineral, potentized vitamin C, and powerful healing substances called nosodes, which are based on original disease processes but diluted many times (quite safe). In addition there is the "message" or "formula" for healthy key tissues, to help the body get its act together in harmony, as it should be (we call these remedies "sarcodes," a term which should not be confused with the disease sarcoidosis).

The full list is as follows:

Healthy Organ Tissue (from pig)
Lymph glands
Tonsils
Bone marrow
Umbilical cord
Embryo
Spleen
Liver
Hypothalamus
Adrenal gland hormones

Hormones
Thyroxine
Natural cortisone

Nosodes

Psorinum-nosode ("Black Death")
Fever toxin

Intermediate Catalyst
Acidum sarcolacticum (sarcolactic acid)

Herbal Sources
Pulsatilla (wind flower)
Conium maculatum (spotted hemlock)
Gallium aparine (goosegrass)
Echinacea augustifolia (coneflower)
Aesculus hippocastanum (Horse chestnut)
Dulcamara

Coccus cacti
Gentian
Geranium

Minerals
Calcium phosphate
Kalium stibyltartaricum (antimony potassium tartrate)
Mercurius solubilis (mixture containing essentially mercuroamidonitrate)
Barium carbonicum (barium carbonate)
Sulfur

Vitamin
Acidum ascorbicum (vitamin C)

Homeopathic Trials

A popular homeopathic external application manufactured by HEEL, Traumeel, has been studied for its efficacy in the treatment of sprained ankles. This combination of 14 remedies in 2x to 6x potencies was given to subjects with sprained ankles.

After 10 days, 24 of the 33 patients who were given the homeopathic medicine were pain-free, while 13 of 36 patients given a placebo experienced a similar degree of relief. This same medicine was also used in the treatment of traumatic hemarthrosis (joint swollen with blood) and was shown to significantly reduce healing time as compared to a placebo. Objective measurements of joint swelling and movement and evaluation of the synovial fluid at injury were assessed.

A study of 61 patients with varicose veins was performed double-blind and placebo-controlled. Three doses of a popular German combination of eight homeopathic medicines were given daily for 24 days. Measures were venous filling time, leg volume, and subjective symptoms. The study found that venous filling time improved in those given the homeopathic medicines by 44%, while it deteriorated in the placebo group by 18%. Other measures also had significant differences.

Six Steps to Cancer and Death

Reckeweg devised an ingenious model of disease he called progressive vicariation (progressive, in this sense, means getting worse). The first three are excretion, reaction, and deposition. The poisons cause the body to first start to reject the toxin - excretion.

We look on a runny nose or diarrhea as healthy ways to get rid of the toxins, and these processes should not be blocked, but aided to conclusion. If excretion is not effective, the body will start to react to the toxin and symptoms will result. If the process continues, then there is accumulation of the toxin or the deposition phase. From here on, things start to become serious.

In the next phase, impregnation, the toxin becomes more permanently embedded in the matrix. Next comes the degeneration phase, where cells, tissues, and organs become damaged and start to die and decay. Finally, we enter the de-differentiation stage, where malignant tumors are the norm! Death can be expected to follow.

We can summarize all this in a simple table like this:

LOCALITY OF TISSUE CHANGES	DESCRIPTIVE TERM
Humoral phases In the fluids of the body	Excretion phase
	Reaction phase
Matrix phases In the connective tissues	Deposition phase
	Impregnation phase
Cellular phases In the cells and organs	Degeneration phase
	De-differentation

NOW you understand the term **homotoxicology**. It is the investigation and removal of auto-toxins, that is, self-generated toxins that accumulate within the body and cause damage. NOT homeopathy, as such, you will readily see. But a keenly related discipline.

Unlike orthodox medicine (sometimes called allopathic, in contrast), we take the view that it is possible to reverse some of this degeneration process. Wherever you start, you can always improve it, sometimes quite a lot.

WARNING: common sense says that the further down this series of phases you go, the harder it is to reverse the process. I've seen homotoxicology remedies work miracles. But you cannot expect to cure everything if there has been a lifetime of abuse and overload.

How Can Homotoxicology Help Against Cancer?
Homotoxicology has a lot to offer in the battle against cancer. I have explained how progressive deterioration of the body's own cleansing system leads to gradual compromise of the defense mechanisms.

Eventually, as the process nears an end and the "biological age" of the body tissues (the biological vitality of the tissues, as opposed to the calendar age), neoplasms or cancer changes are seen as almost inevitable on this model. It makes sense, then, that reversing this process will gain valuable points in the fight against a tumor. The more you help the body recapture its lost biological age, the better it can compete with the invasive cells. It's like turning back the clock!

A basic attack would be to use a detox formula and liver support (there are several), Lymphomyosot or a similar mesenchyme cleanser, and a general anti-viral (more and more cancers are being found to have a viral basis), specific detoxes for acquired vaccine abuse of the immune system (a complex job, requiring skilled medical advice), then tissue stimulants, such as glyoxal and Psorino-heel, and finally, as the situation warrants it, some viscum preparation. I use HEEL's own Viscum compositum, and alternate it with an *Echinacea* complex (again, this is a compounded formula, with 25 other ingredients than the *Echinacea*).

How Can Reckeweg's Cures Help Against Aging?
Two ways. Firstly, life-long use of these remedies is a better way to enable healing. The majority of treatments conventional medicine uses are simply ways of **suppressing the disease**, not aiding nature in bringing about a cure.

Aware doctors have already observed that this simply drives the pathological process underground, only to emerge in later life as a chronic and often degenerative disease. Homotoxicology not only helps cure the disease, it removes the whole process so that, as it were, there is no mess left behind to haunt the invalid in years to come.

Secondly, there are a number of compounds that will support organs and keep them vibrant and efficient until late in life. Thus there is Hepar compositum to help the liver and Solidago compositum or Populus compositum to stimulate kidney drainage. Cerebrum comp. is great for the aging brain and Ovarium comp. and *Testis* comp. may help in maintaining the vitality of sex hormones until much later in life. *Aesculus* (horse chestnut) and *Cretaegus* (hawthorn) have been known since times immemorial as cures for arterial and heart problems; now we have Aesculus comp. and Cretaegus-heel.

Kreb's Cycle Catalysts

But that is not all. Reckeweg was very modern and compounded formulas based upon knowledge of the citric acid or "Kreb's cycle," the intra-cellular process which generates all our energies. Each of the 10 steps of the citric acid cycle needs a special "catalyst" or enzyme, which results in a new intermediate substance (it is called a cycle because eventually it goes back to where it started and runs continuously). Reckeweg found that his method worked just as well on each step of this life-giving cycle and stimulating "intermediate catalysts" are now a key part of homotoxicology. It is one of the great boosts against the slowing-down process of aging.

The energy cycle I am talking about is only as efficient as its weakest link. It makes sense, therefore, to give remedies that assist each stage of the process. Some catalysts are very specific and have important, far-reaching consequences. For example: *Acidum DL malicum* is a fantastic detox compound. It also helps oxygenation and so is good for the heart and circulation, but also for respiratory and skin problems. It should be given only with *acidum fumaricum* D6 (fumaric acid at potency 6X).

Here are some conditions that can benefit from intermediate catalyst therapy:
- Paresis, neuralgia, toxic neuritis, vegetative dystonia, migraine
- Eczema ("neurodermitis"), itching (including pruritus vulvae), psoriasis, vitiligo, pemphigus, scleroderma
- Bronchial asthma
- Gastric and duodenal ulcer, hepatosis, cirrhosis of the liver and injurious hepatic disorders, pancreopathy
- Kidney disease, e.g., nephrosis and chronic nephritis
- Myocardial impairment, angina pectoris, treatment subsequent to myocardial infarction, arteriosclerosis, cerebral sclerosis
- Hormone dysfunction and dysregulation of endocrine glands, e.g., diabetes mellitus, over- and under-active thyroid
- Pre-cancerous and de-differentiation phases (previously: neoplasm phases) within any tissue whatsoever
- During and after X-ray and radioactive exposure (several enzymes, e.g., maleate dehydrogenase, are sensitive to radiation)
- Blood manufacturing disorders: thrombocytopenia, leucopenia

Homotixicology Remedies to Try

Depending on local laws in your country, you may be able to prescribe for yourself. Very many of Reckeweg's remedies are available over the counter and by mail order.

Formulas to try are as follows:
- Immune Function: Echinacea comp., Engystol, Lymphomyosot
- Detox: *Berberis homaccord*, *Nux vom. homaccord*, Lymphomyosot
- Organs: Hepar comp (liver), Solidago comp (kidneys), Populus comp (kidneys)
- General Defenses: Tonsilla comp, Discus comp
- Increasing Cellular Energy: Coenzyme comp, Ubichinon comp.

Homotoxicology Dosing

All these remedies are best given by injection but all can be taken by mouth, with considerable benefit. You simply place a few drops in water and swallow. They can be mixed together. Some formulations require that you dissolve the remedy in a liter or so of water and drink that throughout the day, then skip two days and repeat (one day on, two days off, if that's easier).

NOTE: I have used throughout the product names of major German manufacturers HEEL (*herba est ex luce*, which is Latin for "plants are from light"). There are other quality producers of complex homeopathy products and we must mention in particular also Dr. Reckeweg (company name), Noma, and US firms BHI and Futureplex. Each produces a manual/catalogue, which explains the rationale of their formulations in detail.

IF I HAD MY LIFE OVER AGAIN…
Written by an 85-year-old man, dying of cancer.

Taken from Leo Buscaglia's video
"Only You Make the Difference"

If I had my life over again I'd not be afraid of more mistakes next time -
In fact I'd relax a lot more
I'd limber up
I'd be sillier than I've been on this trip
In fact, I know very few things I'd take so seriously
I'd take more chances
I'd take more trips
I'd climb more mountains
I'd swim more rivers
I'd sit and watch more sunsets
I'd go more places I'd never seen before.

I'd eat more ice cream and fewer beans
I'd have more actual troubles and fewer imaginary ones
You see, I was one of those people who lives prophylactically and saintly
and sensibly
hour after hour, day after day.
Oh I've had my moments and if I had to live all over again
I'd try to have more of those moments- in fact I'd try
To have nothing else but wonderful moments

Side by side by side -

Instead of living so many years ahead of my time.
I was one of those people who never went anywhere
Without a thermometer, hot water bottle, gargle, raincoat and a parachute.

If I had to do it all over again
I'd travel lighter next time
I'd play with more children
Pick more daisies
I'd love more if I had my life over again
But you see - I don't.

SECTION 2

TAKING CARE OF YOUR MIND, SOUL, & SPIRIT CAN HELP YOU LIVE LONGER

Whether you are experiencing life is as a parent, remembering times as a child, or if you're just a big child at heart, I'm sure you can't fail to be moved by the following poem by Maria-Anne Pike:

A Life in Your Hand

If a child lives with criticism
He learns to condemn

If a child lives with hostility
He learns how to fight

If a child lives with ridicule
He learns to be shy

If a child lives with shame
He learns to feel guilty

If a child lives with tolerance
He learns to be patient

If a child lives with encouragement
He learns to be confident

If a child lives with praise
He learns to appreciate

If a child lives with fairness
He learns justice

If a child lives with security
He learns to have faith

If a child lives with approval
He learns to like himself

If a child lives with honesty
He learns to be truthful

If a child lives with lies and deceit
He too learns how to lie and deceive

If a child lives with acceptance and friendship
He learns to find love in the world.

As you get older, it is all too easy to get in a rut - with fixed viewpoints, stuck emotions, ways of being that others can see clearly but you just think are "right." A life full of safe solutions.

But if you start to shut out new experiences, or if you take less interest in new things, so your capacity for enjoying life diminishes. You stay in your comfort zone, and as you get older, your comfort zone gets smaller and smaller. This is harmful because you not only stop doing things that scare you, but you also stop doing things that give you pleasure.

Feeling good is not just a luxury; it is a vital necessity for good health and long life.

There is scientific research that supports this. In 1973, Dr. Ronald Grossarth-Maticek undertook an experiment on more than 3000 elderly Germans. He measured how often they felt pleasure. In 1994 he followed up and found that those with the highest scores were 30 times *more likely to be alive* and well than those with low scores.

How satisfied are you?

Which of the following statements best sums up your life?
(a) It has its ups and downs but is mostly fulfilling
(b) There must be more to it than this
(c) I spend most of my time wishing it would change

How often does your job, family or social life force you to do things you don't really believe in?
(a) Very rarely
(b) Sometimes
(c) All the time

How do you feel about your body?
(a) I'm in good shape and satisfied with my appearance
(b) It's not bad but I would like to feel better
(c) I hate the way I am and want to change

Which best describes your social life?
(a) I have plenty of friends and try to get out as much as possible
(b) I would love to have a wider social circle and go out more often
(c) I hardly see any of my friends anymore and never seem to have time to socialize

Is your life mentally stimulating?
(a) Yes
(b) Sometimes, but I would like to be stretched more intellectually
(c) I feel as if I'm vegetating. Everything is so unchallenging

How did you score?
Mostly (a) - You manage your life pretty well. You know life can be better still because you know from past experience that what you get out of life depends on what you put into it - there are no limits.

Mostly (b) - As you're fairly satisfied with your life, you may be inclined to put off change. But unless you take some risks, you'll never realize your true ambitions. Consider your answers and think about new ventures and things you can do to make a difference.

Mostly (c) - You're not happy with your life - it needs a complete shakeup. It's time to sit down, take a deep breath and plan some big changes.

Get the Life You Want!

Changing your life for the better isn't easy. You know what you want but getting it seems a lifetime away. Family commitments, financial problems, and fear of the unknown can all hold you back - but going for your goals can give your life the boost it needs. Happiness often depends on how close you are to what you would like to be. Here, we take the first steps towards finding the new you.

Make a list of things you used to enjoy in your last year at school - aim for 10 or 15 activities. Put a tick next to those you still enjoy. From the others, pick one activity and do it in the next week - *yes, do it!*

Force yourself out of the comfort zone. Taking steps to push out the boundaries of your experience will ensure that you continue to enjoy life. Think of an activity that you normally wouldn't consider, such as taking a cold shower. Each day turn the water from hot to cold while you're under the shower, and gradually lengthen the time you stay there each day until it's a minute or more. After a week, turn on the cold water for just 10 seconds - it should seem easy: Your comfort zone has expanded.

Of course, this takes self-control. For this week, every time your lazy or scared self wants to say "No," say "Yes." It should be quite an educational experience.

Decide What You Want

Write down five things that are really important to you: they might include a nice house, loving supportive partner, the chance to travel, a good job, etc. Now look at your current life and see how it matches up. These questions can help you pinpoint problem areas:

- What are you doing that you want to do?
- What are you doing that you don't want to do?
- What are you not doing that you want to do?

In the light of this information, clarify your goals. Be specific - before you can plan how to achieve a goal it needs to be stated in a way that is realistic, measurable, and time-targeted.

Your action plan should be broken down into manageable chunks - the steps you know you can make that, one by one, will take you to where you want to go.

Unpredicted obstacles may arise, so it is important to stay flexible and to think laterally. Life is a game - think of it like that and don't take anything too seriously. Enjoy the challenges life offers!

Can you remember the last time you had a moment of pure joy?

It is possible to change your life so that you have that delightful feeling as often as you want.

What Makes You Happy?

Write down a list of things that make you excited, however big, small, likely or unlikely. Then work to make them occur more often. And appreciate the good things you take for granted - your child's hug or a good book. Look for moments of joy and savor them. Recognize how many happen every day. Feeling good can be a way of life, not just an occasional accident.

Take Care of Your Health

Eating well and getting plenty of exercise will raise your spirits. Lack of nutrients will get you down, so don't skip meals or make do with junk food. Physical exercise is known to stimulate endorphins that lift depression and anxiety - so walk, swim, run, or do whatever you like doing best.

Smile!

Smiling triggers happy feelings in the brain and reduces stress. Even if you don't feel happy or confident, just behave as though you do and soon you will. Find the joy in your life and you'll be more attractive and nicer to be around; people will be nicer to you too - and you'll smile some more! Joy is infectious but so is misery; therefore don't have anything whatever to do with people who dampen your spirits, invalidate your achievements, or tell you what to think.

Make the Most of Your Resources

Beware of "must-abation," the belief that you must have a new relationship, a better job, and a bigger house before you can be happy. Extremes of thought only set you up for failure. Remember, what you want is what you've not yet got but what you need is all around you! Don't chuck the baby out with the bathwater, work to improve things.

Get Positive

Write down every negative thought you have over the course of a week, whether it's "My family don't appreciate me" or "I look dreadful." Negativity is a habit and we often don't realize we're doing ourselves down. Under each negative thought you've written, see if you can spot an alternative way of looking at it that isn't so negative. See if you've exaggerated the situation, overly generalized, if you are being unnecessarily intolerant or thinking in "should" and "ought-to" terms.

Recognize All Possibilities But Expect Success

There's a world of difference between expecting failure or rejection - so as not to be disappointed when it occurs - and recognizing it as a possibility. It's sensible to look at a situation from all angles and to have a backup plan to fall back on if need be. People who do this will often see failure as another step on the road to eventual success; but by expecting and envisioning success, there's less likely to be a failure. You naturally move towards whatever you envision. Those who dwell on the worst-case scenario, on the other hand, and give themselves worry and stress, tend to be devastated when it actually happens, even though they've been predicting it.

Assert Your Rights

Think of things which you have a right to, e.g., "I have a right to an evening out with my friends from time to time." Think of rights that every human being should have, such as, "I have the right not to be bullied." Now, protect your rights with your life, and watch your integrity and self-esteem grow.

Nurture Your Relationships
Take time and trouble over your friends and your partner. Talk and laugh with them and - especially - listen and understand their points of view. Don't make being right more important than a friendship. People with a few close friends are more likely to be happy than those with many mere acquaintances.

Give Yourself Some Time
For most of us, life is fast-paced. Be sure to put aside a little time every day for yourself - relax with a book, in the bath, or sitting in the garden with the sun on your face. Think of some things that make you happy - worrying solves nothing. And at nighttime, go to bed early enough that you get enough sleep to feel your best the next day.

Put Things in Perspective
When something's gone wrong, it's tempting to believe that nothing will ever go right again. Put it in perspective - things go wrong sometimes, even when life's really good. Life is for learning and, without mistakes, you learn very little. Notice when you exaggerate or generalize about an issue - "It's unbearable ..." or "Everyone thinks ..." - and rephrase your thoughts more realistically.

Take Control
Instead of feeling overwhelmed by a task, break it down into small segments that you know you can do and start on the first one. If you have lots of incomplete jobs, list them in order of priority and tackle the most important job first. This way you have a sense of achievement at each step - and you'll soon find yourself getting a whole lot more accomplished. Production equals morale.

Communicate
If you have a problem, the thing to do is to communicate: find out the information you need to get the full picture, so that the solution becomes apparent. If you're upset, you need to communicate and say how you feel. If you've done something wrong, again you need to communicate this. Spot where you're backing off from what you then need to do or say and, as the saying goes, "Feel the fear and do it anyway." You'll be glad you did!

Be Creative
Making something come to life that you have envisioned - whether a painting, a wonderful meal, a dress, an invention, a business plan - is infinitely satisfying. And you'll feel pleasure every time you think of it. If you want to be happy, get active - at work, within the family and the community. You will feel happier when you're participating in an activity, whether it's just playing with a child or helping organize a worthwhile event.

Live for the Moment
Joy is often about living in the moment, being absorbed in what you're doing, not brooding on the past or guessing your future. Decide what YOU really want and then go for it. This may mean a job, a friendship or a hobby. It can take courage but it's worth the risk. Then give yourself wholeheartedly to the present moment.

You Deserve It
Self-esteem comes from demonstrated competence. Everyone has skills but not everyone uses them. So use your skills - find out what you're good at and do it. Tell yourself that you deserve all the praise that comes your way and wallow in it!

These are all things you can do for yourself to fill your life with enjoyment, pride, affection and enthusiasm. There will probably still be issues causing anger, sadness, anxiety, guilt, or frustration that remain. The mind is complex and heavily conditioned into patterns of behavior and fixed thinking that require a course of practical training to resolve. And there are many life skills you may want to improve and new ways of thinking that you might not have considered.

QUICK TIPS FOR BUILDING SELF-CONFIDENCE

Self-confidence is the central issue of personal growth. Here are the best ways to enhance the quality of your life, and it's important to us that we find the most effective means for you to tackle this issue of self-confidence.

Everybody could do with a confidence boost sometimes, so to start with, here are a few tips...

1) Feel Good When You Want

For times when you need a quick boost to your self-confidence or self-esteem, find three things that make you feel good. These could be memories of good times, a piece of music, a holiday souvenir, or a person's face - use photos if it helps. Practice thinking about them and bringing them to mind.

Because of the way emotions "attach" themselves to memories, you will quickly train yourself to feel good when you want - a great help in developing self-confidence that lasts.

2) Beat Self-Consciousness

Learn how to keep your attention off yourself – self-consciousness is the No.1 enemy of self-confidence. You can do this easily by following these steps...

1. If you notice you have become self-conscious (you can usually tell because you start to feel anxious), choose something "everyday" that you can see and study it in detail. For example: examine a door, look at the different textures and shades of color, wonder about who made it and how, and so on. The important thing is that you're learning how to keep your attention off yourself.

2. If you feel self-conscious in a social situation, it's usually because you don't have enough to do! Focus on what your purpose in the situation is. Whether you're there to:
   - Find out if you like the other people in the situation
   - make others feel comfortable
   - find out some information
   - make business contacts
   - and so on...

It's easy to feel self-conscious if you have nothing to do and it's much more difficult if your attention is occupied by a task. Think how comfortable you have been with others when you're all working toward a common goal. The common goal of socializing could be making friends, it could be the exchange of mutually beneficial information, it could be whatever you want it to be!

3) Don't Take Undue Criticism - Even From Yourself !

Challenge your own assumptions. For example, take note that:

1. Confident-looking people have bad moments too.
2. Just because you feel under-confident doesn't mean other people can tell.
3. If you're saying things to yourself like *"You're no good at anything"* then rest assured, you're wrong. Everyone can compose a sentence, get successfully to the store, eat without choking. Don't let yourself make sweeping statements about yourself - in the long run it is this sort of thing that can really damage your self-image.

Building self-esteem is not just about thinking good of yourself, it's about not thinking bad for no reason!

4. Just because you have felt bad about yourself in the past doesn't mean you're always going to feel that way. I have seen hundreds of people surprise themselves once they have learned how to build self confidence in a way that it stays built!

Persevere and don't expect everything at once. Really learn how to develop your self-confidence by following these tips. The small wins soon build up and you start to have major positive changes in your life - believe me, that's how it works. Beating low self-esteem is a wonderful thing, and it's much easier than you'd imagine.

MENDING THE FRAGMENTED SELF

I turn now to the shaman model of healing called *soul retrieval*, not merely as a curiosity, but in considerable awe and respect for a tradition as old as consciousness and twice as old as other healing arts! It has worked so well for so long among so many peoples, it is in every sense a **Super Healing Technique**. The fact that most of the proponents are supposedly less sophisticated than ourselves does them less than justice and probably turns our blind eye of prejudice away from what may ultimately prove to be the best of all wellness approaches.

Journey with me and see if you agree…

Soul Retrieval

Quite simply, there is *no real health without true being*. We are not a body; therefore to treat only the body is to miss much of the impact and purpose of the healing arts.

In the words of Sandra Ingerman, US career-shaman, "For shamans the world over, illness has always been seen as a spiritual predicament."[1] Her lovely book is subtitled *Mending the Fragmented Self*, which says it all. Mechanistic reductionist science has little currency here.

One of the most succinct models for dis-ease in this domain is the "loss of soul" or soul parts. You might prefer the term "life particles" to soul parts. The concept is of parts of the self being torn off and getting lost. This would typically take place at times of extreme suffering.

Today we often find soul loss is a result of such traumas as incest, abuse, loss of a loved one, surgery, accident, illness, miscarriage, abortion, bad drug trips, and military combat. Even witnessing traumatic events, such as a crime scene or bloody death, can cause loss through shock and horror. Coma, of course, is the most extreme form of soul loss.

People will often describe feeling as if they are incomplete after the calamity; "Something died inside me," "I don't feel myself anymore," "I left my heart behind," "I don't feel all here," "I'm aching and empty inside," and so on. The hippies used to have an expression "feeling untogether," which is a rather poetic way of putting it, though in their case it was often self-inflicted by recreational drug abuse.

What seems to happen is that the patient loses some of their resources when the part or parts flee. Certain skills, qualities, or other desirable character traits are no longer there and so he or she cannot act out these aspects of the self. The same is true in reverse, of course, and the skills and knowledge present at the moment of schism return remarkably when the retrieval procedure is completed. But the break is very real and the homecoming particles sometimes have to be brought up to date regarding what has happened to the patient in the intervening years in order to fully integrate.

Sandra gives a checklist of symptoms, which might point to soul loss. I reproduce them here:

1. Do you ever have a difficult time staying "present" in your body? Do you sometimes feel as if you're outside your body observing it as you would a movie?
2. Do you ever feel numb, apathetic, or deadened?
3. Do you suffer from chronic depression?
4. Do you have problems with your immune system and have trouble resisting illness?
5. Were you chronically ill as a child?
6. Do you have gaps in your memory of your life after age 5? Do you sense that you may have blacked out significant traumas in your life?
7. Do you struggle with addictions to, for example, alcohol, drugs, food, sex, or gambling?
8. Do you find yourself looking to external things to fill up an internal void or emptiness?
9. Have you had difficulty moving on with your life after a divorce or the death of a loved one?
10. Do you suffer from multiple personality syndrome?

If you answer **yes** to any of these questions, **you may be dealing with soul loss.**

"Important parts of your essential core self may not be available to you. If so, the vital energy and gifts of these parts are temporarily inaccessible."[2]

History of Shamanism

The basic technique is remarkably similar and cogent in societies throughout the world that practice soul retrieval. Typically, the shaman was the one who did the travelling to other realities to look for the missing part or parts and invited them home.

The technique I now propose to describe is easily done by the subject, with or without accompaniment. I believe it strengthens and educates the person more if they are held less passive and invited to actually EXPERIENCE the procedure for themselves. There is the additional advantage that the person acting as shaman does not need the same depths of transcendental skills. The therapist does not need to visit other worlds or speak to spirits (though it's fine if you can do that successfully).

No ceremonies are needed. We are better off without them. There is always the danger that the methodology becomes identified with the ceremony. This makes it easy for cynics to scoff. If there is drumming, they will argue that drumming cannot make the psyche whole; if there are scents and candles, critics will suppose that there was a trance state. Of course, it is the reintegration that makes the person whole, not the accompanying music or rituals.

In addition, there is no reason to blindly observe ritual and history, beyond its proper context. It seems right to take older practices and modernize them in accordance with later learning. To do otherwise is to accord too much significance to the act and not enough to the knowledge process. Yet there are people who think to change procedures or improve them is to be "wrong" and that one has become somehow disrespectful.

Gestalt

Since this brief tract will be read by people from many disciplines, a general overview would be appropriate.

The psyche, spirit, or soul is creative, at least insofar as we experience what we want to experience, (often) independently of outer reality. That there are many aspects to the way we react to our surroundings is simple but adequate evidence of a multiple-viewpoint personality. The modern gestalt view that we are a sum of parts and integrated as a greater whole is more or less sufficiently self-evident as to be regarded as axiomatic.

People are naturally whole and integrated. We have all the qualities and resources we need. This needs interpreting with care, however, since we do sometimes find the missing part far into the past (previous incarnation). Such a person was not born whole in this life.

The idea of losing a part of oneself seems quite natural, once the spiritual model is entered. People readily grasp the metaphor of losing a part of "self" leaving it behind in some other place or some other time. Occasionally we find the part has drifted off into other realities (magical zones and fantastic environments).

If you don't like the notion of a soul (many people object to the word because of its identification with a restrictive religious context), you can still get the idea of a personality in many parts. Gurdieff spoke of many "I"s. To lose one is to lose a part of one's self; to be less than whole. Some people experience many "I"s as an everyday reality. The fact that they tend to be considered mad and treated as such may have more to do with prejudice than exact psychology. However, it is worth observing that such individuals do tend to have difficulty coping with themselves and ordinary reality, so it is not a state one would like to share with them, even if it is true that they are seeing deeper into the reality of our nature.

Definitions for Soul Retrieval

"Lost," in this context, means can't contact or integrate with the part. The practitioner will readily learn that the person ALWAYS knows where it is. A "part" means an awareness or energy entity - a grouping of personal qualities, attitudes, abilities, and emotional feelings that is not complete in itself but can have some of the characteristics of a whole being.

When this part is lost, the person also feels they don't have those qualities or abilities. For example, a child heavily abused may be incapable of love in later life - because her ability to experience it fled under the duress and is still missing.

Neuro-linguistic programming (NLP) is an approach to communication, personal development, and psychotherapy. Its creators claim a connection between the neurological, language, and behavioral patterns learned through your experiences and that these can be changed to achieve specific goals in life.

NLP has a technique called re-imprinting, in which the subject is asked to revisit old and painful areas and re-establish them WITH THE MISSING RESOURCES. It seems to me that this is very little different from a soul-retrieval; merely different terminology and a different model.

Either what we do is merely a metaphor and actually works mechanically as described in NLP. Or, quite validly, NLP provokes the missing soul part back to life and leads to a natural (almost inadvertent) soul reintegration.

Make up your mind after you have done a few!

Soul Giving and Soul Theft

The usual cause of this phenomenon, which might logically be called dis-integration, is some powerful emotional trauma. Very little matches up to the psychic violence of losing a loved one, whether through death or infidelity and separation. Sometimes the things a person says give the game away. We hear expressions like "That man took away my soul," "She stole my heart," "I'll always be with you in some meaningful way," and so on.

The very essence of a loving relationship is that ego boundaries go down and we share "as one." So it is quite natural for bits to end up in the wrong place after a marriage or relationship breaks up. Sometimes a person goes off with a piece of a loved one, stealing it, clinging to it for their own needs, usually to avoid the sense of desolation that follows. This leaves the part unavailable to the owner and is a major infringement or transgression. In other cases, the person leaves behind a part of their own soul, a sort of gift (usually unwanted). What manifests here is that the person who is dumped with the gift continues to manifest traits they don't really want; these have come from the departed one. Removing the stuck part and sending it back to its owner is both a kindness (for them) and a release for the patient in question.

It may be obvious from what material you are offered while working that such a phenomenon has taken place. Great compassion and insight is needed in these tricky situations. You often feel like you are dealing with more than one patient! Discuss matters with the client and get her agreement and understanding.

When to Do Soul Retrieval

The most fruitful time to do self reintegration is after you have been cleaning up a stressful event or area of a person's life. The actual technique you are using doesn't much matter, provided it drains off or, as we say, "reduces" the adverse emotional and spiritual energy (sometimes also called "discharging"). From this sort of regression approach, done properly, you usually get a resurgence and the individual brightens up considerably. It is as if black energy has been cleaned off and they have been freed up from an area where their attention has been stuck for so long.

However, it is sometimes obvious that, despite the benefits, the individual is still to a degree stuck there. He or she feels "better" or even "great" but they are not congruently clear of it and you can see that doubt or dispersal still lingers.

This happens when a part of the self was shed and the loss has not been spotted. A full recovery would need retrieval of the missing part and reintegrating it.

The detailed and highly effective procedure is given below.

STEP 1. PRELIMINARY

An incident is encountered and reduced by some kind of therapy or de-stressing procedure (abreaction).

A soul retrieval step would be considered if:
the person wasn't balanced, content and whole afterwards; or…

it was "logical" that the soul broke up or parts were lost (NDEs, severe injury, shock, dreadful emotional harm such as abuse cases, threat, etc).

STEP 2.

Ask: "During this incident, did a part of you leave?" or
"At that time (long period) did a part of you fade or leave?"

If the person says "No" and she has no reality on this concept, you have nothing to do.

If she says "Yes," continue.

IF THE NEXT ACTION IS NEEDED, PUT ON YOUR BIG-HEARTED SHAMAN'S HAT, CREATE A HUGE AMOUNT OF LOVING SPACE THAT ENFOLDS YOUR SUBJECT. TALK GENTLY, WISELY, AND CALMLY. PROCEED AS FOLLOWS:

STEP 3. LOCATING THE MISSING PART

If she is convinced that a part of the soul left, explain that "We will do a journey to locate it."

The part could be in ordinary or non-ordinary space and maybe in the past. Bearing in mind that you are the shaman - you can participate in the search if you wish. You may even see where the missing part is, before the subject finds it. In shamanic practice, the shaman makes the journey alone and retrieves FOR the person. We find that aware individuals do best if they make their own journey.

"Where does it seem to be?"

It could have the age, emotions, and attitudes that were appropriate at the time it left. Get into gentle communication and rapport.

Say to the part "We are here to help you."

STEP 4. SEPARATING THE MIXTURE (SOUL MIX)

Almost invariably, there are other soul parts, from other beings, mixed up with the subject's own. These would usually be people involved in the original event (see also SOUL GIFTS and SOUL STEALING later).

Tell your subject: "Look at it (the soul part) - are there other parts or energies present?"

Instruct her to unravel "who" is involved. Separate them out, being kindly and gentle. Once unraveled, it will be easier to see who is there.

STEP 5. HANDLING THE PARTS.
NB: Always do the person's own part last, when all the others are gone, otherwise it would be rude.

Explain that we want to send each part back home.

"Who do we take up first?" There will be appropriateness in this, as in all other stages.

Have him or her locate the being with part(s) present, as they are in real time-space (if dead, use other-reality). Have him or her thank the part for its good intentions. Then:

Have the subject mock up "hands" and put the part cupped into one hand and the real-life being in the other. He or she now simply brings the hands together gently. The part will be perceived to have rejoined and leave.

Check for more parts and repeat.

STEP 6. THE SUBJECT'S OWN PART.
Ask "What happened that caused you to separate?"

Ask "Would you like to return?" but don't invite it yet.

Possibly ask "What resources can you bring that will be beneficial?" but don't imply barter.

SHIFT OF ATTITUDE: All this has been done with a loving, calm, and gentle manner, with a BIG safe space. Now switch back to therapist mode.

STEP 7. IS IT WANTED?
Focus on the subject (not the part): "Would you like it to return?"

Ask "Do you have space for it?"

Possibly ask "Will you honor this part if it comes back?" Discuss the possible implications of this.

STEP 8. ASK IT HOME.
Back to shaman mode:

Run out the part's distress if necessary, otherwise you might bring it along.

Then ask it home. Get the subject to cup the part with "hands" and draw it in, willingly, welcomingly, and non-judgmentally. Nine times out of ten it will just come in.

Tell the subject "I would like all your cells to wake up and receive this energy back." Warn her it often fizzes and scintillates. THERE WILL USUALLY BE SOME HEAVY EMOTIONS RUNNING AT THIS POINT. I have seen patients sob and sob and sob; but eventually the storm calms and the sun begins to come out once more. Simply wait for a sensible moment to break off and go onto the final stages.

STEP 9. GROUNDING
Now take your subject out to open ground and in contact with the earth.

- Do the Gaia step. Have the subject make contact with the earth's heart, feel the physical connection, and ask the Earth Goddess to renew her energies and sustain them.

STEP 10. POWER ANIMAL
Now go on to produce the power animal learning. It is very simple; you don't have to visit another world to find the power animal. Have the person in their new state of awareness run a few swift paces across the earth, leap high into the air, and then take up an instinctive gait upon landing. Usually they burst into some kind of stylized movement.

Ask her what animal it feels like.

Tell her to honor and respect this new power animal and use it OFTEN. It's a use-it-or-lose-it gift. The secret to using your power animal is to take some time (often) to LOOK OUT FROM THE ANIMAL'S OWN EYES AT THE WORLD AND SEE WHAT NEW HIDDEN SIGNALS APPEAR.

STEP 11. FINALIZATION
The whole process of reintegration and adjustment can take days, weeks, even months. Many things will change for the individual. Most of it is very holistic and personal, but there may be real psychological initiatives too.

It is vital that you instill one or two warnings. The new soul part which came home is often very disoriented. It may have been alone and isolated for decades and be very uncertain of its new environment.

DO NOT ALLOW YOUR SUBJECT TO DRIVE OR WORK MACHINERY FOR A FEW DAYS. Accidents can happen.

There may also be strange emotional reactions, some of them unpleasant. Ask her to stay calm and talk gently and reassuringly to the new part, as if educating a child (which is basically the case).

Problems with Soul Retrieval
If it gets stuck or won't come home:

1. Check for other parts that may be stuck to it. Clean them up and then try again.
2. The part may need more understanding of the present-time situation (explain to it).
3. Try negotiation: "What would it take for you to come home?"

If still no response, try running its incident again.

Ask again: does the subject really WANT it back? Would he/she honor it and use it? Talk through any rejection, fears or doubts.

An Example
To get more of a grasp on how this can go, let me outline a soul retrieval session. The patient was a 35-year-old female aromatherapist with severe ME. There was no couch, no music, no psycho-galvanometer; just the patient sitting in an upright chair, relaxed, with her eyes closed. I decided to begin exploring the psychological aspect of her eczema, which continued unresolved. Exploration of life issues revealed the fact that she had been left somewhat bereft since her grandmother had died painfully of cancer a few years previously. Father was evidently quite

controlling and domineering and perhaps grandmother had been to a degree able to intervene and protect her, if not physically, then with mental resources at a distance.

We reduced the force of the death and bereavement. There were tears. From what was said, it was obvious that the patient was still very connected; her images were of "sailing away in a boat" with grandmother. A soul loss was discussed and this seemed real to the patient, who was very aware of higher consciousness issues (but knew nothing of the soul retrieval model).

On the day in question I reoriented her to the issue of grandmother and asked directly: At that time did a part of you leave? She affirmed yes. I asked her gently "Reach out and find it … in this space, other space or any universe or dimension, wherever." After quite some time she reported having made contact. I asked her where is the part? She said, "Up among the stars, playing with grandmother." I told her to say hello and tell it, "We are here to try and help." Again, this took some time, but eventually she nodded that this had been done. I asked what was happening and she said that grandmother was laughing and playing with the soul part

I said to thank grandma for her good intentions but to ask her respectfully if she would be willing to give back this soul part. The request was denied and grandmother continued to laugh and play. I was careful not to think any judgmental thoughts about grandmother's attitude, in case these were imparted telepathically, and closed down the session.

So I instructed the patient to ask grandmother if she would be willing to speak with me directly - I explained there was no need for magic or mysticism: the patient would be acting as a relay messenger for my words. Yes, grandmother was willing, I was told.

So I asked the patient to explain to her "I am trying to help you (the patient) and that you might need the resources of this other part in order to fully regain your well-being." Grandma apparently understood but was reluctant. I said, "Please tell her from me that she might want to move on to another incarnation and work on some more karma." But grandma hesitated and didn't think this was possible. I asked "Is there anything standing in the way of you taking a new incarnation and coming down here again with us?"

The answer was that there was a black sticky cloud hanging around, making it difficult. As a shaman, I knew right away what it was and had the patient ask her: "Is this the pain and unhappiness surrounding the final disease?" The answer was yes. The patient now told me Grandma had stopped laughing and fooling around; that she had started to cry and felt confused. Grandma simply didn't know what to do.

Via the patient, I explained that I wanted both of the ladies to carry out a task for me, which was to pour glowing bright energies on the blackness and blow it away: "Gold is best but white or blue will do fine." I thought it was a good idea to get the patient helping in this task too, since she loved her grandmother so much and would clearly want to help.

Considerable time passed, in which I watched various facial and energetic phenomena. I encouraged them both with various comments and was kept informed as it was melted away. After a long pause, I checked and was told that it had gone but it kept coming back. So I said to explain to grandmother that this black mass was her creation but that it was not her self. She should separate from it and stop putting it there. She had done that bit of karma and wouldn't need it again in the next incarnation, I told her. Yes, she now understood this.

I now turned attention to the missing part and had the patient speak directly to it and ask: "Would you like to come back?" In reply, it said it was unsure. So I left it for a moment and asked the patient: "Would you like the part to come back?" She said yes but I told her not to invite it home yet. I then had her turn back to Gran and ask her: "Would she be willing for the part to come home, that you need it?" Progress; Gran was now fully in agreement!

Back to the patient; I said to her to explain to the part that everything was now OK but that it would now be holding Gran back if it clung on, that she needed to wrap it up here and move on to her next stage of karma. It agreed, reluctantly, to come home.

Setting the stage ready, I had the patient tell Grandma to mock up some beautiful loving hands, ready to hand back the soul part and to mock up some loving hands of her own, ready to receive the part. Ready? Everyone was now poised. "Now take it from her, with love, and say thank you, and then start to pull it towards you."

After some struggle with this move, it was obvious there was still some resistance. I asked the question : "Ask the part what would have to happen for it to be happy to come home?" It answered, "I want to be able to see grandma when I wish to." A little bit of horse trading was called for here. So I had the patient tell it that Grandma needed to move on, that she had her own purpose to lead, and that, if she was truly free, she could come down here to earth again and be with those who were dear. I explained that there were many loving couples who meet up this way in successive lifetimes and that might be a good answer. I told the part that I had a patient who was the incarnation of her own grandfather.

This seemed to do the trick and the patient at last started to reel it in gently. As the part arrived, I saw her face suffuse with a beautiful glow and a smile. I had her welcome it and show it love. This was a very special moment. All that remained was to sign off with Grandma. I told the patient to go out to her again and say that the time was close for the last farewell. "Not this moment, but please decide what course you want to follow and I'll leave it to you to break the connection and I will know. And I hope to see you again soon."

Everything seemed OK and, although she was clearly emotional, the patient was smiling with love and sentiment. I ended off and, after giving her the warnings referred to above, took her out for some Gaia energy and a grounding. It seemed like just a matter of moments, but the whole thing took about 90 minutes. The following week she reported sparkling fizzy energies, which lasted for several days before calming down.

References
1. Ingerman S, *Soul Retrieval*, Harper San Francisco, 1991, p. 17.
2. *Ibid.*, p. 23).

ACCEPTANCE AS A TOOL TO PERSONAL GROWTH

There are two fundamental rules of rational living. These equate to a happy life, not only in terms of the "feel good" factor. They also work well as foundations for personal growth, competence, and efficiency, in work, play and relationships.

Following these rules will lead you towards a "stress-free" emotional environment, meaning no unwanted hostilities.

The keynote is acceptance. Not the sissy feeble-mindedness of those who cannot oppose their misfortune and so decide it is "good" for them, but acceptance as the powerful spiritual strength of those who are able to withstand the buffeting of many adverse forces that surround them, yet remain firm, facing true north, centered and strong.

Rule 1. Whatever happens, be able to accept the experience willingly and get the best out of it you can.

If you could accept anything at all which befell you, you would never be unhappy. Think about this.

Rule 2. Cause only those experiences that other people can easily accept.

It is fine to say, "If they don't like it, it's their problem" when you do something they cannot tolerate. But it will certainly be YOUR problem too if these are people with whom you have to live and work! They will become a source of negative feelings and energy that kick back against you.

If you want to experience the challenge of living with friends, colleagues, and family members you have disturbed emotionally, then by all means stir them up; do plenty that is beyond their ability to accept. You will have a hell of a tough time! However, it is far smarter to create the kind of environment around yourself that is a pleasure to live in. In which case, you cannot violate Rule 2.

Acceptance Definition

I was shocked to find how poor the dictionary definitions were for the word "acceptance." Most used the word "accept" or even "acceptance" in their definition! *Webster's New International*, for example, says the act of accepting; state of being accepted or acceptable; also consent to receive. That's poor indeed. The *Funk and Wagnall Dictionary* uses the exact same definition, word for word (dictionaries often copy each other)!

Dictionary.com does better:

1. the act of taking or receiving something offered.
2. favorable reception; approval; favor.
3. the act of assenting or believing…

But then you have to look up "assenting" and perhaps "favorable." It's such a crucial thing to have our key words clarified that I'll help you out here (I think I was a lexicographer in a past life somewhere!)

- Acceptance means the act of or state of mind of…
- Allowing something to happen
- Allowing it to be
- Not resisting or rejecting
- Consenting or approving, without changing it
- Receiving with favor
- Saying YES to
- Not arguing with or speaking against
- A willingness for something to be the way it is…

The key concepts here are willingness and consenting. It means something more than just "putting up with" something. That's tolerance. Acceptance is a warmth and positiveness about whatever it is you are accepting. It's an act; you DO acceptance.

The breadth of a person's acceptance is a very good measure of their overall sanity. An individual with a very low tolerance level is not for this world, which is harsh, random, forceful, and painful.

Beyond a person's threshold of acceptance, he or she experiences increasing discomfort and unhappiness. One way to reduce your stress levels, then, is to extend your threshold of tolerance. This next step will show you how.

The Acceptance Rubric

Try this simple but healing procedure… on yourself, on others around you, with anyone you can be a Samaritan to!

1. The first step is to identify and NAME the situation or area to improve.

Start by making of list of areas in your life where you would like to reduce the stress you feel. That means anywhere in which you feel doubt, frustration, overwhelm or fatigue.

Now choose one area of your life and acknowledge its limitations. How would it be if you could accept that part of your life, just as it is, now, without even changing it?

2. Using the Solutions Focus technique of "scaling," figure out where your acceptance is on a scale of 1 – 10 in respect to that difficulty.

So: "On a scale of 1- 10, what is your acceptance of that situation/problem/ person, whatever…?" If you are doing it with other people, don't worry about oddball answers like, 11 out of 10 or minus 50 out of 10. Take them as what they are: just figures of speech, rather than numbers.

If numbers don't mean anything to you, just use words, like "a lot," "a little," "massive," and so on.

3. Now ask the million-dollar question: *"Are you willing to allow your acceptance of that (whatever) to increase?"* You are not going to try to force a better outcome, but simply be willing to let it happen.

You want a "Yes," of course. If it's OK, then say, "Let your acceptance increase" or if you are doing it alone "I allow my acceptance of this situation to increase."

4. Then check: "What is your level of acceptance of (whatever)… now?"

5. Get a new number and again ask: "Am I willing to let my acceptance of that increase?"

Repeat 3 and 4, over and over. Notice how you may feel calmer, lighter, and more at peace as the acceptance numbers rise.

Important: It must be made very clear you are not trying to fix the problem. The outcome is not the disappearance of the problem or difficulty; the outcome is accepting it, fully and freely. But don't be surprised if it becomes a teeny bit less of a problem!

Finding It Hard?

If you bog down (or the person you are working with bogs down), try breaking it up: "What part of that problem or area can you accept?"

Ask if it's OK to allow acceptance of part of the problem area to increase. Let it rise. Then go to another area or part of the situation that can be accepted. Raise acceptance on that. Sooner or later, the whole will begin to shift, not just the parts.

If you can't get any change, then you are resisting (or the person you are working with is resisting). In that case, call up the resistance: name it! Then ask:

"On a scale of 1 – 10, what is your acceptance level to this resistance?"

Work on that acceptance, let it rise, and pretty soon the resistance will melt. Then go back to acceptance of the original issue and that should rise, too.

Again, you are not solving the problem, you are working on acceptance!

Remember: that part of your mind that is resisting is trying to protect you in some way. There is no need to ask what or how; but at least honor it. Don't spit and snarl; thank the part for trying to help you! Accept your resistance and then it will begin to melt.

There are tons more rubrics like this one: simple techniques or strategies that turn life around. Note: I don't dabble in explanations. Let others write the stuffy books on that. I do fixes! That's what you really want.

Time to get yourself an instant copy of the new book *BOOM!* I've released it in digital format, so no excuses, OK? Visit: http://alternative-doctor.com/healyourlife

FINDING THE GOOD IN EVERYTHING, NO MATTER HOW PAINFUL

It's not easy getting sight of the Sun in dark and stormy skies. But you can actually turn anything into a triumph, if you make an effort to frame it with a different perspective.

When my first wife Pauline ran off suddenly, I was bereft and thought the happy part of my life was over. It took me years to get over the shock. For a long time, I thought bitter thoughts about the man who had taken her from me, using lies and deceits, as I structured it in my mind.

Now, if I ever met him, I'd shake his hand and say, "Thank you!" I'd express my full gratitude because, if that painful split hadn't happened, I would never have met my beloved second wife, Vivien. It was worth any degree of misery to get her as the prize!

It crashed my career for many years. But in the end, I enjoy what I do more, with less stress, and earn more money than I ever did in the old days (let me here insert my gratitude to my first wife, who supported me and helped build my international reputation in the 1980s. It would be surly and dishonest not to acknowledge it).

I didn't do it quite right though…I waited. Instead I should have got out a pen and paper almost right away and listed: "the benefits of my wife being gone from my life"! There were plenty to list. I just couldn't see them at the time.[1]

This is fun: a few months after she left, a visitor had me stand at the front door and shout to the world, at the top of my voice, "Next!"

Now I would generalize this as a technique anyone can use: no matter what disaster scenario you are facing, figure out what's GOOD about it. Write a list because it has been many times proven that writing in your own hand has a far more powerful psychological impact than just thinking about something.[2]

You can find the good in everything, if you try. It may take a little digging. But, as with controlling the flow of water, there are moments when you unblock a channel and a whole flood of stuff comes into the light.

Listen, even terminal cancer. Many people I have met had cause to bless the fact they got cancer. It brought them up sharp, made them re-appraise their lives and, in many cases, the changes were healing and curative. It's a scary way to get to a good place but the result was, ultimately, positive.

To do this, you have to believe that there is always good somewhere, in everything. Jews being killed by Nazis…bad. But then the West got lots of capable scientists that found a new life and new freedom in the USA—people like Werner von Braun, whose rocketry skills put a man on the moon; or Einstein, who was then free to work unmolested and give us keynote philosophies, as well as exciting science.

War is always bad. But there are good aspects. In WW2 we got radar, developed under fear and threat. But today it has saved millions of lives and keeps ships and aircraft safe.

Even for Germany, it holds true. Germany lost the war, supposedly, but today they are the richest and most powerful nation in Europe. One can indeed ask the question: did they really lose the war? They developed rocket craft and there is an argument they, not the Americans, put the first man on the moon!

All Things Considered

In your own life, if you got fired…bad. But now you might have time to pursue things that mean more to you than the workaday job and the stressful commute.

You could take up painting or write that novel, at last! Less money? Yes, but that's not necessarily bad, all things considered.

---

1   I don't mean that to sound nasty. I mean it was up to me to look at things differently and see what positive things had come to pass, like being free to travel to places she didn't like; no more upsets and arguments to disturb my writing; no monthly PMT headaches to live with; the chance to have wild flings with lovely younger women (plenty of those), and so on…

2   See the writings of James W. Pennebaker.

After my first wife left, my whole financial prosperity collapsed. But then I didn't have to work so hard to pay a big mortgage and 12 staff. I slipped off to Spain and goofed around in the sun! I wrote my book *Virtual Medicine* in just 12 weeks. Get the idea?

The real point is that it's your choice how you view things.

In the words of Shakespeare:

"There is nothing either good or bad, but thinking makes it so" Hamlet, Act 2, Scene 2).

Events are only negative from your limited perspective. All you have to do is change your view and everything improves, as if by magic.

All this is mixed up with other important perspective changers, like gratitude and forgiveness. You can change the whole world around you by letting go of disappointment, bitterness, anger, and resentment.

They say revenge is good; a dish that is better served cold (premeditated). Oh no, it's not. It's a disgusting meal that will poison all your life if you let it. And the "triumph" of revenge does not taste good…ever.

Or not for more than a fleeting moment, before you come to the realization that you hurt THEM but it didn't, in the end, make you feel any better whatsoever.

That means he or she beat you in the end. Revenge is the loser's path.

Better to reframe the supposed hurt in more positive terms. It makes you feel good and that's an even better way to spite your enemies! That means YOU win in the end!

Today I can easily picture the dismay on my first wife's lover's face, when I hug him and say, "Thank you!" because a number of things were done at the time which made it clear that the pair intended to make it more damaging and painful than it need have been. It will spoil their fun to realize I benefited immensely from the outcomes.

Bernie Siegel quotes from a wonderful essay in his book *Love, Medicine and Miracles*, which always makes me weep. It's called *"Lessons from the Art of Surgery"* by New York surgeon and prize-winning author Richard Seltzer, in which he describes observing the loving presence of a god:

The young woman speaks. "Will my mouth always be like this?" she asks.

"Yes," I say, "it will. It is because the nerve was cut."

She nods, and is silent. But the young man smiles.

"I like it," he says. "It is kind of cute."

All at once I know who he is. I understand and lower my gaze. One is not bold in an encounter with a god. Unmindful, he bends to kiss her crooked mouth, and I am so close I can see how he twists his own lips to accommodate to hers, to show her that their kiss still works. I remembered that the gods appeared in ancient Greece as mortals, and I hold my breath and let the wonder in.

What kind of man could have found it in his heart to say that his wife's twisted face was kind of cute? No bitterness or anger from him, that his beloved is hurt. Truly, he must have been a god…

TRUE HAPPINESS IS FOR LIFE, NOT ONLY JUST FOR THE HOLIDAYS!

What do you take me for, an idiot?

— Charles de Gaulle, when a journalist asked him if he was happy.
Happiness.

Happiness feels good—but it's also health-building. You'll live longer if you enjoy life!

But I'm talking about real happiness. During the December holidays, we hear messages like "merry" Christmas. For most people that means getting drunk with cronies and finally barfing up in the toilet. That kind of "happiness" is not what I'm talking about.

I mean real, VAST, all-embracing, and lasting happiness. The kind that comes at you in a tidal wave of joy. Walk with me, while I talk…

Profound Happiness & True Happiness
The truth is, it's not always easy to tell, in a complex world, which course of action will do the most good, over the widest range, to the maximum delight of the most people!

That's why I say, *"Happiness is the new wisdom"*!

It's a smart philosophy, as well as a good-natured person's approach. For sure, it's not an approach where dogma works. Always do what it says in such-and-such a book, chapter 17, verse 23, is NOT the way to get good outcomes in life.

That's especially true when said books were written thousands of years ago, by people who never knew the meaning of science; never saw a computer, motor car, or a cell phone; had little or no music and poetry; and whose focus in life was killing anyone they didn't like… who were, in fact, a bloodthirsty bunch of primitives.

I have some better markers for achievement and happy outcomes than that!

**Take My 12 Channels of Being.
They Are Also 12 Acts of Being.**
It's like zoning life into different energy and activity channels, where you can compare input and output in each, and also one against another, to be sure you are getting close at least to a properly balanced life.

Without it, you can end up with a life that seems very purposeful and worthwhile…for a time… but then you suddenly realize you sold yourself short and you are missing out on major leverages to happiness.

Take the story of Millard Fuller. He was a millionaire, had the ambition to make $10 million, and possessed the skills and resources to do it. He had a luxurious home, a cabin on a lake, 2,000 acres of land, speedboats and luxury cars. He was a huge success…wasn't he?

Well, he also had chest pains, from stress, and his marriage was falling apart, because his wife and kids never saw him. It was a one-channel "success"; the other 11 channels were all but ignored. Millard was certainly not happy. Neither was he healthy. He had a heart attack and could have died.

His story ended well, because he got back to balance in HIS 12 Channels Of Being. Millard gave up his jet-setter lifestyle and in 1976 he set up Habitat For Humanity. He gave his new life to a bigger picture, which now included everyone else! Happily, it also included his wife Linda and the rest of their published story you can read at leisure.

All I am arguing is that it's smarter to figure it out ahead of time. No use getting the message as you are waking up in the after-life, is it? No use running out of time due to age, the years wasted and lost, now wishing you had spent each valuable minute differently.

Be smart: get happy! But profoundly happy, not shallow trickery and treats that bring shallow and short-term reward.

Let's see what that really means.

Sharing with Others

First of all, dispose of the ingrained American attitude that money is the monitor of all success. It can be on the table; maybe even in the first five or six important things in your life. But only as the instrument; never as the end in itself.

I'm not suggesting the cliché of giving all your money to the poor; I am suggesting that it has nothing whatever to do with happiness.

Actually, that isn't quite true: scientific studies make it clear that if you don't have enough to feed and clothe yourself and find shelter, then sufficient money to acquire these basics is a happiness factor.

But—here's the kicker—as soon as the basics are taken care of (and that's for most of us in the Western world), more money does NOT bring more happiness.

Wealth and happiness are not inextricably linked, as get-rich gurus like to teach. It's clear to anybody who isn't greedy by nature that rich people are no happier than the rest of us; neither are they less happy. It's just irrelevant.

What seems to count far more is getting the sensations out of life that thrill and stir you.

Getting involved with things that matter to other people is a great way to discover new avenues of happiness.

Be a Real Winner

Being profoundly happy is one way of saying you are one of life's winners.

I mean a real winner; not some Darwinian lunatic who takes satisfaction in grabbing from others, cutting off other drivers in traffic, always trying to be "first" in line, beating out others for that promotion or grabbing that innocent guy's gal!

In the words of the Bob Dylan song: *"And the first one now will later be last, for the times they are a-changin'…"* It was a song to herald a new world, which hasn't happened yet, but I believe is daily getting closer.

I'm talking about a real class of winner: one who takes the whole world up with him (or her). In a way it's defined by my *12 Channels of Being*: different zones of life in which to get involved, make a mark and reap the rewards.

Funny thing is, if you give up something you want, to give someone else what they want, you get such a reward, it was like you didn't give up anything!

Just keep being kind to yourself and the journey is a no brainer. As psychologist

David Lykken says:
A steady diet of simple pleasures will keep you above your set point. Find the small things that you know give you a little high—a good meal, working in the garden, time with friends—and sprinkle your life with them. In the long run, that will leave you happier than some grand achievement that gives you a big lift for a while.

RIGHT-LEFT BRAIN MYTH

We all love the metaphor of right- and left-brain thinking, but I've been pointing out for years that it's just not true. Everyone uses both sides, all the time. Women who speak (no, fill in your own joke here…) are using their left brain, not their right brain. Men who visualize how things could look are using their right brain, not their supposedly masculine left brain.

Nevertheless, there is a widely held belief that people use one side of their brain more than the other and that this influences their personality traits. For example, left-brained people are said to be linear, logical, and detail-oriented, while right-brained people are creative, caring and thoughtful.

We need both sides equally and what really matters for optimum performance is integrated right- and left-brain function, plus lowered brainwave states. Alpha is especially relaxing and, while theta is more relaxing still, you could not drive or use computers and machinery while in that state.

Integration of brain function is easily influenced by modern audio equipment, such as binaural beats or isochronic tones.

The right- and left-brain thing is simply a myth. It was started, remember, by Roger Sperry looking at the function of severely damaged brains, with the corpus callosum (the bridge between the two brain halves) severed. Sperry got his Nobel Prize, but this anomaly has nothing to do with how healthy, intact brains actually function.

Now a new study from the University of Utah simply confirms what I have been saying. Brain scans show no evidence that people are predominately right- or left-brained.

For the study, neuroscientists analyzed brain scans from more than 1,000 people, aged 7 to 29, and examined thousands of brain regions for indications that people are more likely to use either the right or left side of the brain, but found no signs that this was the case.

The metaphor and language of so-called right-brain thinking and left-brain thinking is harmless enough and, in any case, it's not going to go away. But for the good of your soul, know the truth!

[The study was published in the Aug. 14, 2013, online edition of the journal *PLoS One*.]

SECTION 3

ROMANCE KEEPS YOU HEALTHY: LOVE & SEX

Two persons who have chosen each other out of all the species with a design to be each other's mutual comfort and entertain - men have, in that action, found themselves to be good- humored, affable, discreet, forgiving, patient, and joyful, with respect to each other's frailties and perfections, to the end of their lives.

- **Joseph Addison (1672-1719)**

FINDING LOVE IN EVERYTHING

One of the greatest sayings I ever encountered, and one that changed my life the most at the time, was that *"True freedom is liking what you do, not doing what you like."*

As a number one unruly individual who hated authority and conformity, it was a completely new way of looking at the balance between independence and involvement in life.

Peter Caddy, one of the founders of Findhorn, was fond of quoting his Rosicrucian teacher Dr. Sullivan:

Learn to love the place you are in, the people you are with, and the work you have to do.

The point is, of course, to **FIND SOMETHING you can love about the place you are in, the people you are with, and the work you are doing.** Just forget the negatives and smile. This seems to me to encompass much the same philosophy.

But we can go further than that and say that everything in life becomes wonderful, worthwhile, pleasurable, and meaningful if we put love into it. If you find that you cannot flow love into what you are doing, then it isn't worth being involved with. If your task isn't something you love doing, then it isn't spiritually valuable to you.

The computer people have the term GI-GO. It stands for 'garbage in - garbage out'. In other words, what you get out is only a reflection of what you put in. Life is exactly the same as a computer in this respect. If you can pour love into whatever you have your attention on, it comes back to you. By that I don't just mean the old idea of someone will love you or the boss will give you a raise, though that's possible and a valid part of the formula. But what is overlooked - and it spoils the beauty of this bit of wisdom - is that: YOU GET IT BACK INSIDE YOURSELF. Something lifts and glows inside that gives you a tremendous feeling of lightness, joy, and involvement that simply never comes if you're in a grumbling just-a-job mood.

What then of the mundane tasks, like washing up and shopping for groceries? Well, they have to be done, so why not put love into these, too? You have a perfect opportunity to develop spiritually, so these moments can become a sort of exercise in personal growth. Instead of wasting precious moments of your life complaining and trying to avoid needful assignments, why not cultivate the skill of putting love into these too?

Of course it does help to know that your life is focused. If you are drifting from day to day, with no true purpose, then you cannot see the web-like inter-relationships between each simple task of the moment and your big life picture. If you haven't got a bigger picture, nothing makes sense, anyway.

So experiencing boredom, laziness, and lack of involvement is a very good pointer to the fact that you need to shape up your life and make something of it; **work out some meaningful goals and start to work towards them.**

The reverse of this is equally true: when you know what you want to do and are working for it, every act becomes a statement of commitment, achievement, satisfaction and SUCCESS! Every small task becomes delightful as well as necessary, because it is taking you to where you want to be.

Cooking and Eating
One of the great times to evince love is while you are preparing food. There is a saying that the food tastes better if the chef puts some love into it.

Well, you can test this out for yourself and you will find it is true! More than that, mealtimes are those moments of the day when there is time to take a little pause and feel relaxed, gentle, and human. You can share it with friends where possible. If you all involve yourselves in the meal preparation, that's even better: someone to cook, someone to prepare food, someone to lay the table, put out candles, crockery etc., with LOVE. It all adds a great deal to the pleasure of eating.

If all this is new to you, try one or two simple alterations in your style while cooking.

Put on music and dance while you peel vegetables; or swirl round once, like a dancer, as you move from place to place in the kitchen; or just make one or two graceful gestures with your hands as you fling in the condiments!

Exercise in Love
If you are tired, inactive, lacking involvement, or feeling resentful about what you are doing, stop and look for love. It is vital for the peace of your soul and the good of your heart and mind that you find it. Sourness and hating what you do is the very opposite of life's true principle of happiness. It will lead to trouble in the long run, and it can be BIG trouble - such as heart disease, cancer, and an early death. I'm speaking now as a doctor.

If you can't find love in what you do and who you are doing it with, then it is time for a change. In the meantime, find something that you love; something to make you get up and do it before work; something to rush home for at night, so that you can get started with it. A really good hobby might fulfill this requirement.

Creating Loving Relationships

And of course, if a relationship isn't meeting all your needs for love, it's time you acted. Love between two people is something to be tended and nurtured, like a flower. It is a complete and deadly folly to think that love that is vivid and exciting will last forever. It will hardly last a month, if you don't go on creating it. Love running on autopilot isn't love at all. **A LOVING RELATIONSHIP NEEDS TO BE CREATED ON A CONSTANT BASIS.**

This doesn't mean you need to keep re-inventing it all the time. It does mean you need to output the love, make a sign, an act, a gesture, a word, SOMETHING that generates that magic. If you don't, then we have that unfortunate state that we label "taking things for granted."

Many relationships end this way. Sometimes one can sympathize:

- Pressure of work
- Lack of time
- Anxieties about money

Or even some other difficulty may mean that the expressions of love are forgotten or almost obscured by the bigger problem that demands attention.

The fact remains that if love is not created constantly, it will begin to die.

Again, to reverse the view, if one flows love at a problem, it will tend to vanish. Each individual must support the other and be part of the solution, not part of the problem. There is nothing more powerful about a loving relationship than the way that the two together can conquer seemingly insurmountable difficulties. It is a version of Buckminster Fuller's SYNERGY; two people acting in one accord are much MUCH more powerful than just the sum of the two separate energies.

There is scientific truth to the saying *"Love conquers all."*

Love is like life; it could be the same as the life energy itself. As beings, our spirit nature is love. You will never see a spiritual person who doesn't emanate considerable love and tolerance. So to love what we are doing and who we are with is simply to give life and expression to our deeper nature. By the same terms, to not feel love or have an expression of it is to shrivel and die as persons. We are depriving our inner being.

I can sum all this up in fewer words than either of the key quotes above by saying: BEING REALLY TRULY ALIVE IS LOVING EVERYTHING THAT YOU EXPERIENCE.

The doctor in me is prescribing you love; lots and lots of it. Have an abundance of this blessed feeling in your lives, so that you know the true happiness that love can bring.

WAVES THAT THRILL (SEX IS NOT INTERCOURSE)

The moment of penetration and subsequent orgasm, for all its exquisite intensity, is but a *small* aspect of sex. True sex is not merely an act but a mind process, which pervades all our conscious thinking. At times it is a faint tremor, at other moments it swells to an urgent and demanding feeling. It becomes an imperative. There are many degrees to sex.

It rolls to and fro like a tide. High water may be the times of nakedness and caress, with tumescence and ultimate release. But sex is there even in the ebb. It is an echo, a sigh, a fading chord that breathes its blessing on all our hours spent together.

When my love is not there, I feel the rhythm of the tide. When I know she is coming towards me, I feel the current beginning to stream. There is excitement, a tremble, vibration in the waters. I feel her before she is there. These are moments of intense anticipation that are as meaningful as the full message. To want only the roaring high tide is to miss the beauty, the lust, the magic, which is present there at low water also.

The peace, the trust, the comfort, contain the voice of distant longing and earlier fulfillment or that which is to come.

Love speaks to us in these rise-and-fall rhythms, as a kind of music. But it is never truly absent. A brief silence, indeed, may a part of the melody, in the same way that a pause in the music can add poignancy and meaning to a tune.

Love Facilitates
Love helps one work better. It generates energy, especially the creative sort. This is surely connected with the procreative drive. One's product and results are bettered. The environment is made more whole and secure. The healing power of love is undisputed.

There is thus a responsibility for those in love. Love is so powerful; you hurt others when there is a storm. Remember to fix it quickly afterwards. Even better, try to avoid strife in the first place. Give out your goodness and make a fruitful show of it.

Making Waves
The loved one is your all and your everything. You need to show them that. The touch, the gesture, the word that fills you up starts an energy reaction. It emanates outwards, like ripples in a pond, and can be passed on to others. It is nurturing for them, too.

It's great to see people light up around love. A special couple with that particular feeling for each other have a kind of radiant light, a warmth, an energy that can inform others around them. Have you observed the reactions of the faces turned towards such a couple? There can be no

doubt that something is passed on. Don't hide it. Make waves!

WHAT DOES LOVE MEAN?
Someone sent me this in an e-mail one time and I have no idea who compiled it.

Slow down for three minutes to read this. It is so worth it.

What Does Love Mean?
A group of professional people posed this question to a group of 4 to 8 year-olds: *"What does love mean?"*

The answers they got were broader and deeper than anyone could have imagined. See what you think:

"When my grandmother got arthritis, she couldn't bend over and paint her toenails anymore. So my grandfather does it for her all the time, even when his hands got arthritis too. That's love." Rebecca - age 8

"When someone loves you, the way they say your name is different. You just know that your name is safe in their mouth." Billy - age 4 (I love this one)

"Love is when a girl puts on perfume and a boy puts on shaving cologne and they go out and smell each other." Karl - age 5

"Love is when you go out to eat and give somebody most of your French fries without making them give you any of theirs." Chrissy - age 6

"Love is what makes you smile when you're tired." Terri - age 4

"Love is when my mommy makes coffee for my daddy and she takes a sip before giving it to him, to make sure the taste is OK." Danny - age 7

"Love is when you kiss all the time. Then when you get tired of kissing, you still want to be together and you talk more. My Mommy and Daddy are like that. They look gross when they kiss." Emily - age 8

"Love is what's in the room with you at Christmas if you stop opening presents and listen." Bobby - age 7 (Wow!)

"If you want to learn to love better, you should start with a friend who you hate." Nikka - age 6 (we need a few billion more Nikka's on this planet)

"Love is when you tell a guy you like his shirt, then he wears it every day." Noelle - age 7

"Love is like a little old woman and a little old man who are still friends even after they know each other so well." Tommy - age 6

"Love is when Mommy gives Daddy the best piece of chicken." Elaine - age 5

"Love is when Mommy sees Daddy smelly and sweaty and still says he is handsomer than Robert Redford." Chris - age 7

"Love is when your puppy licks your face even after you left him alone all day." Mary Ann - age 4

"I know my older sister loves me because she gives me all her old clothes and has to go out and buy new ones." Lauren - age 4

"When you love somebody, your eyelashes go up and down and little stars come out of you." (what an image) Karen - age 7

"Love is when Mommy sees Daddy on the toilet and she doesn't think it's gross." Mark - age 6

"You really shouldn't say 'I love you' unless you mean it. But if you mean it, you should say it a lot. People forget." Jessica - age 8

And the final one -- Author and lecturer Leo Buscaglia once talked about a contest he was asked to judge. The purpose of the contest was to find the most caring child.

The winner was a 4-year-old child whose next-door neighbor was an elderly gentleman who had recently lost his wife. Upon seeing the man cry, the little boy went into the old gentleman's yard, climbed onto his lap, and just sat there.

When his Mother asked what he had said to the neighbor, the little boy said, "Nothing, I just helped him cry"

When these kids grow up, maybe the world won't be such a bad place after all!!

DOES VIGOROUS SEX CAUSE MEMORY LOSS?

OK, I don't normally share secrets of my intimate private life with the public. But—you know me—wherever there is a lesson to be gleaned and it does somebody some good, somewhere, then I'm right there.

A few weeks ago I had an alarming episode that doctors call *"transient global amnesia" (TGA)*. It's sudden but **temporary memory loss following some strenuous or stressful event.** In my case it came on after passionate sex with my beloved wife.

All of a sudden, I couldn't remember what we were doing or why. I knew who I was but wasn't sure about the lady with me! For several hours I was quite confused about recent events and couldn't get a grasp on things. I remembered shopping at the local supermarket but not what we bought.

It may result from the deactivation of the brain's temporal lobes and/or thalamus (the part of the brain that serves as a center for the relay of sensory information).

Usually occurring in otherwise healthy persons, TGA triggers memory loss from external stresses such as strenuous exertion, high levels of anxiety, sexual intercourse, immersion in hot or cold water, and other similar conditions.

It was quite scary for me but absolutely frightened my wife out of her wits. She assumed I had had a stroke or some serious event and from the first imagined that she'd lost me, for good. I kept saying "Goodbye!" and "I love you!", just in case these were the last few moments of my life.

Hours later my memory came back and although I am still a little vacant about those few hours (I can remember maybe 60%), my considerable intellectual powers are not diminished in the least.

In fact, the curious thing is there is almost never any residual damage. What's more, it's rare to experience this TGA more than once; certainly three times maximum in a lifetime. Only 3% of people who have a TGA will ever get it again.

There are no ethnic associations or inherited conditions associated with TGA. Men experience the condition more often than women. In addition, the occurrence of this type of amnesia rarely happens before middle age, with about 12 out of 100,000 people ever experiencing the condition before age 50. The most likely ages in which to experience TGA are the 50s and 60s. I'm 65 next birthday (and feel around 30 years old).

So if anything like this has happened to you, be comforted. If it happens to you in the future—*don't panic!* You won't know what hit you; but your spouse, friends, or loved ones can be reassured that it's not serious.

Only thing is, it could be a stroke or embolus. So being seen in ER or by an emergency physician is still a good idea.

Anyone who quickly goes from normal awareness of unfolding reality to confusion about what just happened requires immediate medical attention. If the person experiencing memory loss is too disoriented to call an ambulance, call one yourself.

Although transient global amnesia isn't harmful, there's no easy way to distinguish the condition from the life-threatening illnesses that can also cause sudden memory loss. In fact, sudden amnesia is much more likely to be caused by a stroke or a seizure than by transient global amnesia. A medical evaluation is the only way to determine the cause of sudden memory loss.

Doctors base a diagnosis of *transient global amnesia* on the following signs and symptoms:

1. Sudden onset of memory loss, verified by a witness
2. Retention of personal identity despite memory loss
3. Normal cognition (ability to recognize and name familiar objects and follow simple directions, for example)
4. Absence of signs indicating damage to a particular area of the brain (limb paralysis, involuntary movement, or impaired word recognition, for example)
5. Duration of no more than 24 hours
6. Gradual return of memory
7. No evidence of seizures during the period of amnesia
8. No history of active epilepsy or recent head injury

[list from the Mayo Clinic]

I hope this reassures many people that fit and well human beings, with competent minds, can have what appears to be a disaster unfold and yet it is 100% survivable and without residual damage.

Still, it gave me a glimpse of what Alzheimer's must be like. Don't want to go there. **Take your coQ10 and omega-3s.**

20+ WAYS TO SHOW LOVE

These ways to show love make up a code of behavior and, as such, cannot be enforced upon anyone. The word "burden" is chosen advisedly, though it need not have a negative connotation. It means merely it should not be undertaken lightly. Hence, it is a burden of responsibility to those who wish to invoke its powers.

However, such a code of agreement and the expression of ways to show love between two lovers can also be a source of reason and joy in their lives together. Indeed, if a relationship doesn't inspire these values it is hardly worthy to be called such.

20 Ways to Show Love
1. Above all, live in the present time, not existing as a blur with past events, past people and places, past dreams and past habits. Love is NOW!
2. Develop the climate of communicating freely and encourage the other to do so at all times.
3. Listen helpfully when the other is burdened with care, avoiding antagonism or criticism, even if it hurts you. Add comments only if invited (and not much of even then).
4. Ensure that both partners share the responsibility of solvency and security. Do not leave it "up to the other."
5. Apportion the work within the home and connected with living together equally. There should be no excessive load falling on one or the other individual.
6. Apportion the work within the home and connected with living together equally. There should be no excessive load falling on one or the other individual.
7. Never disparage your partner behind his or her back, especially to gain sympathy or advantage. Honor, praise, and defend your lover against all criticism and calumny by others.
8. Be worthy of the other's trust. Tell him or her the truth and harbor no secrets that you wouldn't wish known. Faced with doing something you wouldn't want your partner to know, stop and consider: you are about to betray his or her trust. Seen in those terms, you probably wouldn't want to do it anyway.
9. Be model adults with offspring. As a man, allow them to perceive male courtesy, wisdom, and strength. As a woman, show them your guile, grace and capacity to love and nurture.
10. Discuss all problems in private and never attack, hurt, or shame the other in public (this means not in front of the children or any other family members, as well as strangers).
11. Forgive quickly and return the tone to love and calm as soon as possible after a quarrel. Do not harbor grudges or resentment towards your lover EVER. It is a folly, which reflects on yourself to consider your loved one in some way flawed.
12. Never use sex – or the withholding of sex – for spite, gain, or punishment of the other party. Sex is a joy given by Higher Power to inform your lives and not a tool for crude human leverage.
13. Share the creation of a safe space as a way to show love in which each person, and any offspring, can flourish, express themselves freely, and feel cherished.
14. Never put material values or family property before people values. A relationship based on material worth is demeaning and lacks substance.
15. Be both loving and lovable. Show interest in the other's world and remember to be less than demanding about your own interests.
16. Understand and support the growth of the other's spiritual and mental domain, as well as his or her physical, property, and legal rights.
17. Look as beautiful or handsome as you are able, since you are in effect your partner's main "scenery,"
18. Waste no time and. as often as possible, in varied and non-mechanical ways, demonstrate your love and commitment.
19. When looking for ways to show love, seek to give your lover values that they could not have otherwise attained without you.
20. Be competent, tender, loving, and sincere in that acme of human relations – the orgasm. Whoever does or doesn't "score," both parties respond to affirmations of love, pride, rejoicing, and pleasure at this time. NEVER, NEVER utter unkind or destructive words at these moments.

Be sure you are willing to defend and protect the other, being willing if necessary to put yourself in danger. God forbid it ever happens, but if you failed at this when called upon, you would be unworthy of romantic sexual love at its deepest and most convincing. This final point is important. Biology still applies somewhat to our society. Though we live sheltered lives, occasionally the issue of life and death does surface to challenge people and is one of the ultimate ways to show love.

THE CUDDLE HORMONE (CAN I GET SHOTS?!)

Oxytocin was once thought to be an exclusively women's' hormone and involved only in setting up uterine contractions during labor and squeezing the uterus empty after birth.

Now we know both sexes have it and it performs a great role in love and bonding: so much so that it's sometimes called the *"love hormone"* or the *"cuddle hormone."* Lots of it gets released at orgasm, in both sexes. Hmmm. Like to get regular injections for that, wouldn't you!

The basic point, in Nature, is that the mother will bond with her newborn and love the child. Her nurturing desires are what will take care of the little baby for months, even years, to come.

With this new understanding of its essentially psychological role in humans, scientists have started to study the impact of oxytocin on a variety of social situations and interactions.

New research presented at the 2010 annual meeting of the Society for Neuroscience in San Diego has also traced oxytocin's effect in boosting trust and empathy (to the point of increasing the wish to donate to charitable causes) and in reducing anxiety and stress.

Also, the higher your oxytocin blood levels, the higher your happiness and well-being, at least for women.

And, perhaps not surprisingly, those women with higher oxytocin had more sex with fewer partners, reflecting more long-lasting relationships. They were likely to be liked by other people.

But the researchers were reluctant to allow that these findings might translate to men. However, the study leader did admit to an earlier study, which focused on men and found that men treated with the love hormone were more generous after watching public service ads.

Those on placebo donated to 21% of the ads, those on oxytocin 33%. Moreover, the men given the hormone donated 56% more money to the causes than men in the placebo group.

Oxytocin seems to control the balance between self and others in the brain.

Of course, cynical advertisers are onto the power of oxytocin. Why are puppies in toilet paper commercials? Because pitchmen know people feel good about puppies -- hopefully so good their brains will release oxytocin. That can make them more likely to buy the product.

But that's exploitation, not science.

Autism

Some people even feel it could help with autism. There is some human research that has found improved social function in people with autism after treatment with the hormone. In the future, targeting the oxytocin system in people with autism may be useful, especially when combined with behavioral therapy.

Predictably, there are the naysayers. Despite some of the promising new findings, Sue Carter, PhD, professor of psychiatry at the University of Illinois at Chicago, was quick to warn: "People are trying to treat autistic kids [with oxytocin] in the absence of [definitive] research."[1]

It could have long-term negative effects. Well, she's right of course. But you feel she's coming from a party pooper perspective (try saying that three times fast!), rather than worthy scientific caution.

Reference
1. Sue Carter, PhD, professor of psychiatry, University of Illinois, Chicago. Neuroscience 2010, San Diego, Nov. 13-17, 2010.

10 REASONS MEN DON'T WANT SEX AND WOMEN HAVE TO FIGHT TO GET IT

This theme was circulated in 2006 by WebMD but without the women's interest. Yet it seems to me that a man not wanting sex is the woman's problem as much as the man's (or more so). Maybe he's OK with no passion but that's frustrating to the partner.

My reading demographic is mainly middle age and boomers, so this should be a topic of interest to many readers. I have chosen the ones I consider to be the most important 10; not the same as WebMD's selection.

The first question to ask is: is there really a problem at all? It's widely held that men are all hungry studs and will want sex at every available opportunity. That really isn't true for most men. Once the wild passion of new romance wears off, a more realistic agenda for regular sex may be relatively infrequently.

Also, the woman may be negative about sex. If she gives out the wrong signals, saying she is not interested, a sensitive man may respond by quenching his own desires. It's still a problem. But I always say, you have to get the real cause to be able to make any successful change.

I recall a patient complaining that her husband wasn't up for much sex; I told her to bring him along and I'd fix him. So I did! He jumped her bones and she came back to me, very distressed. "It was disgusting," she complained, "I'd rather go shopping than have sex at my age."

Poor guy, I thought!

ALL THAT SAID, HERE'S A LIST OF THE 10 MOST COMMON REASONS WHY MEN MAY NOT WANT SEX

Medications. Some drugs are notorious for killing libido. Blood pressure medication and antidepressants are the two main culprits. But, again, I have seen many other substances do it. It's often an individual thing. So if libido is low, discuss coming off medication. Try to solve the problem that required medication, instead of just masking it with drugs.

Along with meds comes alcohol and recreational drugs abuse. These are just as bad. You remember Shakespeare's oft-quoted joke (from Hamlet) that alcohol provokes the desire but takes away the performance. Well, after a while it gets worse than that: alcohol takes away the desire too. Street drugs are often as bad. If you are in an active loving relationship, you should not be abusing drugs and drink, for your partner's sake. Stop doing it.

Fatigue. Next comes lack of adequate rest and sleep. When we are younger, men will often stir from sleep, or put it off, even when tired, for the delights of a sexual encounter. But, as people and relationships age, sex can lose its compelling nature and a good night's rest can be quite tempting. It is possible to be just too tired to be aroused.

Hormonal levels. Our libido comes from testosterone, and as we age, particularly after 50, levels begin to fall to where they affect sex drive. Don't let your ignorant doctor test for total testosterone; it's FREE testosterone that affects our libido. But two feminizing hormones are also relevant and should be checked: prolactin and dihydrotestosterone (DHT). Dihydrotestosterone is simply measured indirectly, as SHBG (sex hormone binding globulin).

Undetected organic illness. This is an astonishingly prevalent causer of sexual dysfunction; it just doesn't get diagnosed enough. If you are partnered with a man who seems to have "gone off" sex, always insist that a doctor take a proper look for physical illness, beyond the causes listed here. Heart disease, diabetes and early cancer are just some causes of physiological stress, which in turn leads to sexual de-tunement.

Obesity. Really, this is a disease state in its own right. You simply cannot be healthy and obese; it's a contradiction. And whatever they say about cheerful fatties, my experience with most is that they are unhappy with themselves and their image. Erotic feelings do not thrive in the presence of this sort of self-directed negativity.

Out of sensory sync with the mate. Failing to meet each other's sensory needs is probably the biggest destroyer of sexual delight. By that I mean that the man loves words, the woman likes only touch; or she likes words ("Talk dirty to me") and he likes visuals (black panties and so forth).

Middle-age disempowerment. The "mid-life crisis" really does exist. It can start suddenly, because of some trivial setback or relatively minor incident, as well as big issues, like failure, redundancy, death of a family member, bankruptcy, etc. The man begins to feel uncertain about his role and achievements. Sometimes a loss of faith is the trigger.

Quarrelling. The longer a relationship survives, the more disagreements build up. It takes great wisdom and tenderness to steer these flare-ups away from permanent damage to the relationship. Some spouses will punish their partner by withholding sex but, for others, it's not a matter of punishment, they just cannot muster sexual feelings when there are unresolved conflicts.

Embarrassment. Poor performance is a source of great humiliation for a man. Moreover, it becomes self-reinforcing: one failure leads to performance anxiety and makes subsequent failures more likely. Typically, a man will avoid sexual activity altogether, rather than face the embarrassment of what he sees as failure.

Sometimes, as I said at the start, there is the question of whether there really is a low sex drive or a dysfunction. One way to test this is masturbation. If the man can muster arousal feelings and a good erection, even without reference to his life partner, then he knows that the "equipment" is working OK. There is just not enough stimulus in normal relations.

That's at least pointing to the right problem, which can then be solved. Item #7 might be the one to focus on.

I'd just like to say a word about masturbation and "other" sources of arousal. These days porn is so readily available on the Internet, many men access it because they find it spicier than the real thing.

Ladies: the problem is NOT the man indulging in porn; the porn is his SOLUTION! The problem is he is not getting what he wants otherwise.

The Internet makes porn so readily available—just a click of the mouse—that many men who might not have sought out other sources of visual sexual stimulation (magazines, videos, movies) have found their way to locate sexual imagery online.

This alarms some sex workers but not me. Porn can be quite arousing and lead to MORE of the real thing. If it replaces physical sex relations, the porn isn't the problem, as I have already said. So porn is NOT one of my top 10.

ARE ORGASMS SEXUAL?

It might sound like an odd question: of course orgasm is sexual, you say. But it may not be as clear-cut as you think.

An interesting study I spotted in a special issue of the journal *Sexual and Relationship Therapy* showed that women could have orgasms, just from exercising. Not very sexy but sounds like good fun!

This type of orgasm I'm talking about is sometimes referred to as a "coregasm" because of its association with exercises that involve core abdominal muscles.

According to study author, Debby Herbenick, co-director of the Center for Sexual Health Promotion at Indiana University's School of Health, Physical Education, and Recreation, the most common activity associated with exercise-induced orgasm were abdominal exercises, climbing poles or ropes, biking/spinning, and weight lifting.

The findings are based on the results of online surveys completed by 124 women between the ages of 18 and 63, who reported experiencing exercise-induced orgasms and 246 women who experienced exercise-induced sexual pleasure. Most of the women were married or in a relationship and about 69% were heterosexual.

The excitement was not just a one-off either; about 40% of the women who had experienced exercise-induced orgasms and exercise-induced sexual pleasure had done so on more than 10 occasions. Most of the women were not fantasizing.

So what works? I knew you'd be asking that!

Abdominal exercises accounted for 51% of exercise-induced orgasms, followed by weight lifting (27%), yoga (20%), bicycling (16%), running (13%), and walking/hiking (10%).

Around 20% of the women said they could not prevent the orgasm. Well, they might have said that just because they were embarrassed. In any case, why would you want to block it? Prudery?

Never mind masturbation: go to the gym and have fun, I say… You can get fit at the same time!

SECTION 4

DEATH CREEPS IN AT THE GUMS - WISE DENTISTRY

WHAT DENTISTS DON'T TELL YOU!

ADVANCED GUM DISEASE MAY RAISE CANCER RISK

TREATING GUM DISEASE MAY SAVE YOUR LIFE

BRUSH YOUR TEETH, LIVE LONGER

Here's a curious fact: *from the start of the 20th century, the number one predictor of death by heart disease was dental abscesses; and, by the end of the 20th century, the biggest predictor of death by heart disease was... no, not exactly abscesses. But a major dental problem, gum (periodontal) infections.*

Now a specific bacteria has been implicated, called *Streptococcus gordonii*. It can enter the blood stream and increase the risk of dangerous blood clotting. It mimics the effect of fibrinogen, which is a major blood-clotting factor.

Fibrinogen activates platelets (cells that are found in blood and involved in clotting), which stick together and form clumps that start the clotting process. The resulting blood clots encase the bacteria, protecting them from the immune system and from antibiotics used to treat infection.

Platelet clumping can result in growths on the heart valves (endocarditis) or blood vessel inflammation that can block blood supply to the heart or brain. If clots take place in a major supply artery, like the coronary artery, you could be in big trouble (sudden death).

These findings were presented at a Society for General Microbiology meeting in Dublin, my old stomping ground, this week.

It emphasizes the importance of keeping gums healthy and getting regular dental care.

Avoid sugar like poison, since that turns your mouth into a food yard for bacteria.

You can consider regular cleanups, using an antiseptic. Don't use Listerine, which is toxic junk sweetened with sorbitol or (worse) sucralose.

But, you can try hydrogen peroxide or, even better, chlorine dioxide protocol (sold as MMS) or a sodium chlorite (same thing) mouthwash, such as TheraBreath, Oxyfresh, CloSYS, or ProFresh.

It's my mission to share with you what dentists don't tell you and secretly hope you never find out!

WHAT DENTISTS DON'T TELL YOU!

There are many more health hazards to dentistry than just mercury toxicity, as this article reveals (excerpted from "Virtual Medicine," as published by *What Doctors Don't Tell You*).

Right at the start of the 20th century, the biggest single risk factor of death due to heart disease was tooth and jaw infections.

Numerous pathology specimens in the medical school museum, showing subacute bacterial endocarditis, cavernous sinus thrombosis, and brain abscesses, testify to just how precarious life could be in the age before antibiotics and what we may face if the present abuse continues. A single unhealthy tooth could lead to an early grave.

Now, at the very end of the 20th century, what do you suppose is among the biggest predictors of death due to heart disease?

Teeth. Well, more exactly, gum disease. This one risk factor has recently been shown to be just as important as smoking, obesity, blood pressure, or an unfortunate family history in determining whether we will die before we should.[1] *Why is what goes on in your mouth so dangerous?*

Teeth sockets are a royal highway for disease pathogens leading straight into your bones and bloodstream. A tooth abscess is really just another kind of osteomyelitis, that is, bacterial bone infection. From there, bacteria migrate to other parts of the body and can cause septic foci.

As biological dentist George Meinig puts it:

These bacteria are kind of like people, if they get to like Seattle or Reno or someplace, they decide that's where they are going to have their home. Well, the bacteria travelling round the body, they may get to the liver, the kidneys or the heart or eyes or some other tissue and they set up an infection in that area. This is why the degenerative diseases occur from the teeth.[2]

[The position is not helped by techniques such as crowning of teeth. It may make them appear cosmetically attractive on the outside. But often these metal or plastic caps do nothing more than cover and hide a seat of purulent infection, waiting to explode at some time in the future when defenses are compromised.]

Back Pressure

The late Patrick Stortebecker, professor of neurology at the Karolinska Institute in Stockholm, Swedish, carried out a series of experiments in the 1960s that I consider highly illuminating and the results are rather scary. He injected tooth bone margins under pressure with radioopaque dyes and then took x-rays of the skull. What he showed was that most head veins do not have valve control and therefore blood could travel backwards into the cranium; his radioopaque dye appeared all over the head, far away from the tooth that had been injected.[3] If the tooth in question should happen to be infected, the results could be very adverse indeed.

Bacterial toxic matter could be propelled into the cranium and there set up an unwanted focus of infection right inside the skull. Stortebecker himself mentioned the obvious risk of cavernous sinus thrombosis and suppuration. This was once a killer condition. The cavernous sinus is a large vein reservoir at the base of the brain and, if it should clot and become filled with purulent matter, widespread meningitis and brain abscesses are the almost inevitable result. Many fatal tragedies from nose picking and pimple scratching took place in former times; those of us old enough may remember that parents tended to frown on this behavior and we were slapped. Now you know there was a scientific reason for the almost universal injunction against pimple scratching.

But that's not all.

Stortebecker had another disease model which is very persuasive. He considered that what he found is the principle factor in pathogenesis of multiple sclerosis. Through extensive research he was able to show that most plaques of nerve demyelination (the unmistakable sign of MS) were located around blood vessels.4 No one else had noticed this important fact before.

Stortebecker speculated that the back pressure on veins had shunted toxic matter into the brain tissues, where it set up foci of inflammation and myelin loss. What was particularly convincing was that MS cases with optic neuritis (leading to blindness) generally had bad teeth and inflammation plaques in the brain; whereas those who had leg weakness or paralysis, with demyelination plaques in the spinal cord, had pelvic or other lower-body disease foci.

[Unfortunately, Stortebecker is gone. Apart from a handful of us, his work is ignored and it is very difficult to interest anyone in the medical establishment. Dentists don't want to even think about it. Doctors say it's a dental problem and nothing to do with them. Another sad example of how specialization makes medicine foolish and ineffective.]

Toxic Dentistry
It is not really stretching the human mind too far to suggest that most **dentistry is, by nature, quite toxic**.

Modern methods rely heavily on materials such as metals, plastics, and polymers, ceramics and prosthetic structures of many kinds. Most of this foreign material is stressful to the body.

It can be a considerable drain on the immune system and therefore a major contributory cause of fatigue and chronic ill health. In this new context, we can only urge people even more emphatically to try to prevent dental problems from starting up. Good diet and adequate teeth hygiene may, even in this day of antibiotics, still be a key life-saver.

Cooked Teeth
Recent research by Ralph Turk and Fritz Kronner in Germany has shown that even the act of drilling a tooth causes severe energy disturbance.6 Turk describes the modern dental turbine rotor as a sort of time bomb and says that its damaging intensity has been completely missed by the vast majority of dentists.

There are many likely reason, not least being the fact that, despite water cooling, the temperature of the dentine rises by as much as 10 degrees after just a few seconds of drilling. In biological terms that is cooking the tooth. This denaturation obviously destroys the viability of the tooth and its ability to resist bacterial invasion.

From over 6,000 cases studied, it was uniformly seen that, as soon as a tooth was visited by a high-speed drill, focal osteitis trouble began in connection with that tooth within two years. It is possible to reduce the damage by taking sensible anti-tox procedures before, during, and after a dental program. Such elementary measures would include vitamin C, charcoal (to absorb toxins), homeopathic support, and immune drainage remedies, such as HEEL's Lymphomyosot or Pascoe's Pascotox (all this is described in detail in my book *Virtual Medicine*, Thorsons, London 1999). (Visit: http://alternative-doctor.com/vm)

Galvanic Fields and Energetic Disturbance

Slightly more bizarre is the phenomenon of electrical fields around certain teeth and the effects of these produce. I remember well the first time I saw Hal Huggins's slides of teeth cut open to show the scorch marks, where electrical current had been running for many years.

Teeth can work like little batteries. This is quite logical: there are two or more metals and a saltwater fluid medium (saliva). This is how Allessandro Volta's original batteries were made; the battery of your motorcar is essentially the same thing.

The trouble starts from the fact that electrical currents actually leech the mercury out of the teeth, because of an effect called electrolysis. This is why patients sometimes complain of a constant metallic taste in the mouth, made worse by hot fluids and salty food (more electrolysis). If that isn't scary enough, then the reader should know that electrolysis is capable of releasing deadly mercury vapor. This goes straight to the brain tissue, where it is highly invasive and toxic.

But the problem is even more complicated. The currents generated by amalgams can be quite considerable and these are being formed very close to brain tissue, which operates at far lower potentials (a few millivolts). I have seen momentary spikes of up to one volt when testing teeth for the electrical effect; this is enough to light a small torch battery. Remember that the brain is really only a few millimeters from the jaw bone, where the roots of the teeth lie, just the other side of the thin cranial bone and the meninges. Thus there is potential for mental dysfunction and this is often found in clinical practice, by asking the appropriate questions.

Casebook...Female, 44 years

The patient had suffered from Meniere's disease: vertigo and vomiting, with intermittent staggering (sailor's gait). She could not think clearly any more, had trouble with her memory, could not see clearly lines appeared not straight. This was accompanied by pain in the nape of the neck. She was unable to continue working due to the severity of these symptoms. Her attending physicians could find no clinical explanation and the patient was told it was all in her head (in a way this was true). Finally, a brain tumor was suspected and tests were required to exclude this grim possibility.

The patient's luck eventually turned and an ENT surgeon referred her to Dr. Helmut Raue, an electro-acupuncture specialist who understands biological dentistry, as this new specialty is called. He measured the teeth galvanically and found 215 microamperes current between the gold filling and a nearby amalgam. One week after having the amalgam removed, all pain had disappeared and her balance had returned to normal. The patient admitted then that she had had suicidal thoughts because of the excruciating pain and baffling dizziness.[6]

The reason that not enough of these cases are being diagnosed and the true picture is not emerging is that patients do not usually consult their dentists with symptoms such as headache, facial neuralgia, dizziness, sleep disorders, and digestive disturbance (just to give a few examples).

Energetic Fields

Electro-acupuncture practitioners are finding teeth foci as a common cause of energetic disturbance. The problem is immensely more complicated than it at first might seem. Several key acupuncture meridians cross the line of teeth as they pass over the face. An abscess or *"transmitting focus"* can actually create pathological results anywhere along the line of that meridian. These are reconnected again with secondary organs and sites. Thus problems with a front incisor tooth may impact on the kidneys, since this meridian passes through the incisors. But the kidneys, in turn, are related to the knee joints. If I see a patient with incisor problems or a bridge in this location I can surprise them by asking about the arthritis of the knees. Try it yourself!

Sometimes the consequences of these interconnections are very surprising and virtually beggar explanation but should make us very wary indeed about the effects of dentistry.

Casebook... Female, 33 years

The dentist had prepared a new crown tooth prosthesis, the type with a post of nickel, which fits in a hole drilled down the center of the tooth, to give support. As the dentist offered the post to its new location on the right upper jaw, the woman let out a squeal: she went blind in that eye! The dentist removed the tooth and she could see again. He offered it back and she went blind again. This was repeated several times until both were quite sure of what they were observing.

She refused the crown and had the tooth removed.

What important about this striking example of what we might call "VIRTUAL DENTISTRY" is that there was an INSTANT reaction; there was no way it could depend on any chemical manifestation, even metal toxicity. Allergies to nickel do occur, though this metal is far less poisonous than mercury. But it would take a little time to develop. The sudden loss of vision indicated clearly that there was neurological dysfunction along the optical pathways due to a field disturbance, probably at the quantum or information level.

This story makes vividly clear what risks we take when we allow metal into our mouths. The resulting disturbance of the body's energy field can have unpredictable and very serious consequences. I try to imagine what would have happened if the woman had not lost her vision immediately but had gone blind over the subsequent few weeks. Almost certainly the correct cause would never have been diagnosed. She may have ended up with harmful and unnecessary interventions, which would fail because they were not aimed at correcting the real problem.

What's in a Name?

NICO is an abbreviation of "neuralgia-inducing cavitational osteonecrosis."

Osteonecrosis means the bone has died or lost its viability as a result of restricted nutrient supply; it is softened and eaten away, like rot in an apple.

Neuralgia-inducing means that it has been postulated as a potent cause of neuralgia of the face, particularly that vicious kind known as trigeminal neuralgia. The trigeminal nerve (emerging at the ear) is largely sensory and supplies the face, jaws, and teeth. A phenomenon known as referred pain means that trouble anywhere within the nerve net can be felt at other places supplied by the same nerves.

Thus NICO is a factor to consider in migraine or any kind of atypical headache. It is worth pointing out that the jaws are the only major bony tissue with important sensory nerve endings.

The cavitational part of the label simply means some kind of cyst or space in the jaw bone, not necessary infected or inflammatory. Quite common is a fatty osteitis, where an old focus of inflammation has finally settled down and turned into a fatty cyst. There may be blood or chocolate matter in the cavity. But the important point that knowledgeable dentists are making is that this is not really an inflammatory process, but tissue destruction caused by insidious loss of blood supply. In that respect, it is more like other textbook bone diseases, where destruction comes from impaired blood and nutritional supply, which in 1915 US dentist G. V Black described as progressive "death of bone, cell by cell."[7]

NICO is not rare. In one population study it was found in 1 in every 4,900 adults. This makes NICO by far the most common osteonecrotic bone disease; once again, specialization means that doctors are not talking to dentists, as they should. NICO has been seen in ages 18-94 but typically it affects people in the 35-65 age range. An individual may have more than one focus of this disease process. It is hard to avoid the conclusion that it is the result of burnt-out chronic infective foci.

It is unfortunate that NICO is usually not visible on x-ray. Many cases are missed even by experienced diagnosticians, since 35-50% of bone loss is necessary before changes become radiographically evident. That is where electro-acupuncture diagnostic screening comes in. I know dentists who are bold enough, and trust good electro-dermal screening practitioners sufficiently, to drill into bone at the site indicated as a reading focus. It is very satisfying to both parties when the cortex is breached and a cavity filled with biological sludge makes its presence known.

Once diagnosed, treatment is currently by curettage of the site, sweeping away all the dead and softened bone, and maybe the first millimeter or so of healthy bone, in the hope that new good bone will form. Coral granules may be used to pack the hole and encourage recalcification of bone tissue. In about a third of cases this radical treatment fails and may even make the problem worse but, according to one writer, only about 10% of patients feel that the process wasn't worthwhile.7 Curettage is rather heroic and I have no doubt that, in the future, something a little less aggressive will be the rule. While NICO is chiefly the domain of holistic dentists, such "commando cures" are rather untypical of holism in general.

What You Can Do
You might be worried about what is written here. This could be with good cause, but don't overreact. The first thing to do is make contact with a biological dentist, as they call themselves. These are advanced dentists who appreciate Price's work and freely use homeopathic remedies, nutrition, and other natural accompaniments to dental hygiene. They also willingly interact with EAV practitioners, preferring the body's own signals for guidance.

Read more and become informed about the issues. WDDTY has always had the view that individuals should take responsibility for their own health care and this applies equally to dentistry. To leave decisions solely to your dentist, if he is of conventional thought mode, is to be subject to yesterday's science and it may do you harm in the long run.

Eat a proper diet, which avoids sugars that cause dental decay and feed micro-organisms.

Use co-enzyme Q 10 supplements (ubiquinone). This has been shown to have unequivocal benefit for periodontal (gum) disease. More teeth are lost due to gum disease than caries.

Large doses of vitamin C seem to be very helpful for periodontal disease and toxicity of all kinds. Take large amounts before, during and after any dental procedures.

References

1. 1Beck J D, Offenbacher S, Williams R, Gibbs P, and Garcia R, Periodontitis: A Risk Factor for Coronary Heart Disease?, *Annals of Periodontology*, Chicago, Vol. 3, No 1, July 1998, pp. 127-141.
2. 2Radio interview of the Laura Lee Show, transcript published in the Townsend Letter for Doctor and Patient, August/ September 1996.
3. 3Stortebecker P., Dental Caries as a Cause of *Nervous Disorders*, Bio-Probe Inc, Orlando, USA, 1986. P. 34.
4. 4Stortebecker P., Dental Caries as a Cause of *Nervous Disorders*, Bio-Probe Inc, Orlando, USA, 1986. P. 116.
5. 5R Turk Iatrogenic Damage Due to High Speed Drilling, paper presented at the Scientific Session at the dedication of the Princeton Bio Center, New Jersey, 13th June, 1981.
6. 6H Raue, Resistance to Therapy; Think of Tooth Fillings. *Medical Practice*: vol. 32, No 72, pp 2303 2309, Sept 6 1980.
7. 7J E Bouquot in Review of NICO, G V *Black's Forgotten Disease*, The Maxillofacial Center, Morgantown, West Virginia, 3rd Edition, 1995.

ADVANCED GUM DISEASE MAY RAISE CANCER RISK

If you've read my book *Virtual Medicine* you'll know that I gave some space to the dangers of periodontal disease. **Today it's probably the #1 marker for heart disease.**

But do you remember, I also talked about dental dangers, with particular reference to the work of Dr. Patrick Stortebecker, of the Karolinska Institute in Stockholm, Sweden?

Stortebecker, a brilliant researcher, was convinced that gum and dental disease can also form the focus for a cancer of the jaw or mouth. I accept this.

In the '80s and '90s I saw dental foci over and over again as the deadly energetic signal on a body with cancer of the mouth region.

Always happy to be 20 years ahead of the curve—Hey, it's where I live!

Now a new study backs up everything I wrote over those years. Chronic periodontitis may significantly raise the risk of head and neck cancer. Periodontitis is advanced gum disease that leads to progressive loss of bone and soft tissue that surround the teeth.

In fact, each millimeter of bone loss due to chronic periodontitis was associated with a more than four times higher risk of head and neck cancer, after taking into account other known risk factors such as smoking, which is remarkable.

This may help explain why head and neck cancer rates continue to climb, although smoking rates have been declining for the last 40 years.

The study also adds to a growing body of research that shows chronic inflammation can affect the risk of cancer, heart disease, diabetes, and other health problems.

The study, published in *Cancer Epidemiology, Biomarkers and Prevention*, compared rates of periodontitis in 226 people with head and neck cancer and a comparison group of 207 people without cancer.

Use your toothbrush often, get dental checkups and teeth cleaning, take CoenzymeQ10, a powerful cure for periodontal disease, and follow everything I said in my book *Diet Wise* to keep your inflammation levels very low.

TREATING GUM DISEASE MAY SAVE YOUR LIFE

People with rheumatoid arthritis (RA) are **eight times more likely to have gum disease than people without this autoimmune disease**. Inflammation may be the common denominator between the two. Making matters worse: people with RA can have trouble brushing and flossing because of damage to finger joints. The good news is that treating existing gum inflammation and infection can also reduce joint pain and inflammation.

Tooth Loss and Kidney Disease

Adults without teeth may be more likely to have chronic kidney disease than those who still have teeth. Exactly how kidney disease and periodontal disease are linked is not 100% clear yet. But researchers suggest that chronic inflammation may be the common thread. So taking care of your teeth and gums may reduce your risk of developing chronic kidney problems.

This follows closely on work by Weston A. Price, which I reported in my book *Virtual Medicine*. Price found that transplanting teeth from diseased rabbits into healthy animals would cause the recipient animal to develop the same disease as the donor beast. If the donor had arthritis, the recipient got it; if the donor had kidney disease, the recipient got that instead; it was surprisingly consistent.

Very strange. Clearly some kind of energetic signal was being transferred from animal to the other - and probably infectious organisms too. Can bacteria have a predilection for certain organs? We need to learn more.

BRUSH YOUR TEETH, LIVE LONGER

Teeth can kill. It began as dental infections lodging bacteria in the heart and causing fatal widespread septicemia in the days before antibiotics. But 100 years later, by the end of the 20th century, it had come around again that, despite antibiotics, significant gum disease (periodontal disease) was a major risk factor for death by heart attack.

Now a brand-new study (May 27, 2010) has re-enforced what I said. **Teeth and gum infections are deadly**.

Researchers in the UK analyzed data from over 11,000 people who were taking part in a study called the Scottish Health Survey. Patients were asked whether they visited a dentist at least once every six months, every one to two years, rarely, or never. They were also asked how often they brushed their teeth -- twice daily, once a day, or less than every day.

The researchers found that 62% of participants said they went to a dentist every six months, 71% said they brushed their teeth twice a day.

After adjusting the data for cardiovascular risk factors such as obesity, smoking, social class, and family heart disease history, the researchers found that people who admitted to brushing their teeth less frequently had a 70% extra risk of heart disease.

What's more, people who reported poor oral hygiene also tested positive for important inflammatory markers such as fibrinogen and C-reactive protein, which themselves are predictors of early death. In other words, if you slouch on cleaning your teeth, you are very significantly more likely to die young. It may seem incredible but the pathways are clear and well demonstrated and the backup science is pretty well irrefutable.

Do you need me to tell you what to do? I think not.

[The study can be found in the journal *BMJ*, published online May 27, 2010].

SECTION 5

CANCER RESEARCH BREAKTHROUGHS

Conflict of interest blocks out real scientific integrity in cancer research.

A study that was published June 15, 2009, in the journal *Cancer* has highlighted what is essentially corruption in the science of cancer research. It's called "conflict of interest": but you and I would call it corruption, bribery, or malicious threats. Not nice words for a not-nice phenomenon, which I've known about for years.

Well, at least the industry is beginning to talk about it.

What it amounts to is that cancer researchers are likely to "find" (or invent) favorable outcomes for research which is paid for by the major drug cartels. Many doctors engaged in research are on stipends from the very company which produces the product they are supposedly "testing."

Some take secret bribes, of course, but then so do Congressmen!

Some investigators at major hospitals and medical schools have their salary paid, indirectly, via drug company funding to their hospital or laboratory post. Who has the guts to rock the boat when it pays the mortgage? Ridiculous idea, you say; responsible drug companies would never threaten the jobs of honest researchers.

Well, if you are naïve enough to think that, wise up. Not only do drug companies threaten to get uncooperative (i.e., honest and objective) scientists removed from their post—they actually do it.

This new up-to-date study puts some figures to the extent to which drug cartels bias what they laughingly call "research." As I am fond of saying, it's not research, but marketing strategies disguised as research.

The analysis, headed by the University of Michigan, looked at more than 1,500 supposedly scientific cancer studies published in eight authoritative journals, including *Cancer*, the *New England Journal of Medicine* and *The Lancet*.

Here's what they found:
Randomized clinical trials that assessed patient survival were more likely to link a survival advantage to the medical treatment being studied when a conflict of interest was present.

- Apparent conflicts of interest (such as industry funding, consulting fees to authors, and co-authorship by industry employees) found simply by reviewing the authorship credits were noted in 29% of studies, while 17% actually declared industry funding.

- Industry-funded studies focused on treatment in 62% of cases, whereas only 36% of studies done without industry funding focused on treatment.

- While almost half (47%) of studies done without industry funding looked at epidemiology, prevention, risk factors, screening, or diagnostic methods, only one-fifth of industry-funded studies looked at these areas.

Any guesses why the drug industry would slew research away from disease prevention? *I'll bet you know.*

A TESTING BREAKTHROUGH FOR HIDDEN CANCERS

Almost every time I write about cancer, I add the injunction to hang on tight….

Things are moving so very fast that, apart from the corruption in the industry, the problem may soon be solved!

One of the most important things we have been in need of is a way to test for cancers l-o-n-g before there is a tumor. Current medical science cannot detect anything smaller than a pea and even bigger ones often get missed.

Scans are a waste of time and very dangerous. A CT scan delivers as much as 500 times the radiation of a standard X-ray, potentially causing an estimated 1.5 to 2% of all cancers in the United States. PET scans are even worse, because the whole body is exposed to radiation.

A study of database records of more than 31,400 patients who had a CT scan in 2007 at Brigham and Women's Hospital or Harvard's Dana-Farber Cancer Center found that 15% of the patients had received estimated cumulative radiation doses that were higher than the radiation exposure from 1,000 chest X-rays.

In other words, **these "screening" methods are likely to create more cancer than they detect**.

What's needed is a chemical screening that can tell, early on, that a patient is harboring a cancer; I mean *very early on*, when treatment is easy and can be accomplished by little more than changes in diet and lifestyle.

Waiting for your orthodox oncology markers to show up is like waiting till you are really in the danger zone. By the time they are elevated, you are in trouble.

What could be better, then?

Well, suddenly a whole rash of cancer marker tests have shown up. Dr. Garry Gordon waxes lyrical about the profile of tests carried out by Dr. Kobayashi in Japan. But now there is more choice than ever.

There's the *Oncoblot test*, the CYP1B1, and Dr. Schandl's *"Cancer Profile."* Each of these is far superior to the AMAS test of the past, which, despite claims, is not highly reliable. It was the best we had for years but that's no longer true.

Let's Look Further into the ONCOblot® Test

The Oncoblot blood test identifies a specific type of protein in the blood, ENOX2[1], which exists only on the surface of a malignant cancer cell. The ENOX2 proteins are shed into the circulation system and can be detected in the blood. These proteins serve as highly sensitive markers for early detection in both primary and recurrent cancer. It's organ-specific, meaning it can often tell with certainty where the cancer is located.

The physician draws the blood and sends it to the lab. Results take approximately 15 business days. The cost is $850.00 at this time (www.oncoblotlabs.com).

But does it work?

Based on analyses of over 800 Oncoblots covering 26 different kinds of cancers with clinically confirmed diagnoses, 99.3% were positive for cancer based on ENOX2 presence.

Of these, the organ site of the cancer was determined correctly in 96% of the samples; there were no false positives and fewer than 1% false negatives.

That's really quite extraordinary.

In-Depth Explanation on PYP1B1 Testing

To gasp the potential of this test it's necessary to do a bit of in-depth explanation.

Let's back up and talk about *salvestrols*.

These are potent plant chemicals and are probably the real reason that raw, healthy plants protect us against cancer, not antioxidants. Resveratrol is the best-known of them.

In a series of papers in *The Journal of Orthomolecular Medicine*, Professor Gerald Potter, head of the Cancer Drug Discovery Group, De Montfort University, Leicester, UK, and Professor M.D. Burke and co-workers introduced the concept of salvestrols and gave them the name. Together they developed the PYP1B1 enzyme test.

Suffice it to say that **salvestrols destroy cancer cells pretty well**. They are highly anti-inflammatory and a sort of botanical police force for the body. One of the reasons cancer and degenerative diseases are increasing so much in the West is likely that food processing and manufacture drastically reduces salvestrol levels (they taste rather bitter and are deliberately removed).

The key to investigating the properties of salvestrols is an enzyme called *PYP1B1*, which does not occur in healthy cells; it's only found in cancer cells, such as breast, colon, lung, esophagus, skin, lymph nodes, brain, and testis. Salvestrols are metabolized by PYP1B1 into a metabolite, which destroys cancer cells. This is an arrangement that suits us very well.

---

1   Don't even ask, you'll be sorry you did: ecto-nicotinamide dinucleotide oxidase disulfide thiol exchanger

We can test for the presence of PYP1B1 and, if it's found, we can infer that a cancer is present. We can then load the system with salvestrols and the PYP1B1 will produce the cytotoxic metabolite and wipe out the cancer. At that point the PYP1B1 will vanish, because only cancer cells have it!

There are NO false positives, the developers claim. If there is PYP1B1, you have cancer. Period.

I expect one day Big Pharma will try to develop a drug to fit into this schematic. But for the moment they remain icily cold towards salvestrol research.

Incidentally, salvestrols are destroyed by fungicides on plants, AND *Laetrile (amygdalin)*. You all know **I do not accept any research that says Laetrile is a valid anti-cancer agent** (except that cyanide kills all cells; that's hardly helpful).

Anyway, here's proof, if needed, that it doesn't work and is destructive, compromising nature's own natural cancer protection.

The results claimed for Laetrile are without exception the results of OTHER actions taken at the same time. No study has ever been carried out investigating only Laetrile in humans.

So far as I know the PYP1B1 test is *not* offered publicly at this time.

Dr. Schandl's CA Profile Testing

Dr. Emil Schandl is certainly a survivor, having lived as a Jew in Nazi Germany, fought in the Hungarian uprising of 1956, and then made it to freedom. He founded American Metabolic Laboratories in Hollywood, Florida.

His profile testing centers around an analysis of six key enzymes, each of which alone might not be so accurate but, taken together, give a very good score rate.

For example, 68% of cancer cases show elevated levels of human chorionic gonadotrophin hormone (hCG). When the measurement was for the enzyme PHI (phosphohexose isomerase, a tumor marker that regulates anaerobic cellular metabolism), levels were elevated in 36% of the patients; with the enzyme GGTP (gamma glutamyl transpeptidase, a sensitive liver enzyme), levels were higher in 39% of patients; and a test for CEA (carcinoembryonic antigen, a general tumor marker, originally designed to monitor colorectal cancers) showed elevated levels in 51% of patients.

But looking at three cancer markers together (hCG, PHI, CEA), 221 positives in 240 breast cancer patients (92% accurate) were detected. Of lung-cancer patients, 127 of 129 (97% accurate) were correctly diagnosed. And with colon-cancer patients, 55 positives out of 59 patients (93% accurate) were correctly identified.

These are great scores.

But Schandl also added two more tests, which are revealing: *thyroid-stimulating hormone* and *DHEA*.

He has tested thousands of patients with this profile with accuracy greater than 90%. When a patient is actually being treated for cancer, Schandl's tests can be used to monitor the success (or ineffectiveness) of ongoing cancer therapy.

ONE OF THE GREATEST MEDICINES OF ALL TIME IS COMING!

Penicillin was big; it has saved billions of lives. It stops infections. There have been some problems; we know… overuse, misuse, and so on. But that's not a problem with penicillin, it's with doctors. The fact remains that penicillin is a towering drug remedy with a miracle history that is awesome to contemplate.

But this is bigger… and you don't need to have an infection to benefit from it. Everyone gets a result!

The truth is, I can't yet tell you all the details, but I have been shown a confidential document that will turn medicine on its head when it's published. In fact I warned one the developers of this cure to take real care; Big Pharma will surely want him dead and has the power and motivation to hire an assassin. It's happened before…

So when I tell you it's at the starting gate, act fast. Get your supply NOW.

Let me tell you how powerful this is:

A lady with pancreatic cancer (the worst), a 3-inch tumor, was told it's over; she would die. But she tried this remedy and within weeks, the tumor was down to half the size. WITHIN SIX MONTHS IT WAS GONE.

Another woman with inoperable breast cancer took this remedy and her tumor too just vanished. The oncologists at The Memorial Sloan-Kettering Cancer Center were flabbergasted as they called her in to tell her the cancer was totally gone.

So What Is It?

There are two key ingredients in this revolutionary discovery; each has effects that seem to focus on both the innate and adaptive immune system, including antigen presentation, cytokine production, and immunoglobulin secretion.

Each has already been proven to work. But when you put them together, you get one of those explosive synergistic things… each one multiplies the other, over and over. It's like 1 + 1 = 2 transformed into 1 + 1 = 88 or 137, or whatever!

I'm looking at the confidential document as I write; I see that one of the ingredients is a fungus derivative; the other is a probiotic (haven't I been telling you for years about the power of shutting down the fire in your belly?)

Probiotics are BIG; and this one is even bigger than lcr35, the famous probiotic from Aurillac in France (*Lactobacillus rhamnosus* 35).

The fungus is a mushroom derivative, already known to science: AHCC. Active hexose correlated compound (AHCC) is an alpha-glucan-rich nutritional supplement produced from the mycelia of shiitake (*Lentinula edodes*) of the *Basidiomycete* family of mushrooms.[1]

AHCC was originally designed to lower high blood pressure. However, researchers at Tokyo University found that AHCC increased natural killer (NK) cell activity in cancer patients, and also enhanced the effects of killer T-cells, and cytokines (interferon, IL-12, TNF-alpha).

When AHCC and BB12 are paired together, that's when this amazing combination emerges. Nobody has seen the like of it before. That's what this confidential document is about.

Soon it will be made public and the whole world will want this combo.

Anti-Cancer Effect

There have been reports of tumor reduction and even cures of cancer using Reishi mushrooms and Chinese herbs. It has been observed that these traditional remedies may work by up-regulation of the immune system.[2]

A study published in the *Journal of Hepatology* compared the outcomes of 113 post-operative liver cancer patients taking AHCC with 156 patients in the control group. The results showed the rate of recurrence of malignant tumors was significantly lower (34% versus 66%). That's down by half!

Patient survival was significantly higher in the AHCC group (80% vs. 52%). That's up by 153%!

It's almost impossible for the naysayers to argue, because actual survival figures were recorded and the patients had all been carefully observed internally at the time of surgery with photographs of tumors and lesions.[3]

Of course the don't-want-it-to-work faction still try to trash the findings.

In Japan, AHCC is the second most popular complementary and alternative medicine used by cancer patients. *Agaricus blazei* supplements are the most popular (but it's quite liver-toxic).

AHCC is widely used in Japan and China. It is used to protect the immune system of cancer patients undergoing chemotherapy and radiation in over 700 clinics and hospitals in Japan alone. Even the Memorial Sloan-Kettering Cancer Center website admits, "In cisplatin-treated mice, AHCC increased its anti-tumor effects while reducing side effects."

AHCC is available to the general public in Japan, Asia, the USA, and the EU without a prescription and many people use it for general health maintenance and treatment of acute infections. Its legal status is that of a "functional food."

The Anti-Aging Potential

I'm also excited about the anti-aging potential of this remedy. It's been a saying of mine for decades that you live just about as long as your immune system lets you; and not a day longer.

The proof of that remark? Look at what happens to AIDS cases. They shrivel, age and die, once full blown AIDS sets in, and it's very rapid indeed; often just weeks.

We sure need our immune system.

It also has antioxidant anti-aging effects. According to the Memorial Sloan-Kettering, one animal study suggested that AHCC has antioxidant effects and may protect against disorders induced by oxidative stress.[4]

Also, in healthy adults aged 50 years or more, AHCC enhanced certain T-cell immune responses. In patients with hepatocellular carcinoma (HCC) and cirrhosis, AHCC has shown beneficial effects on liver function, possibly by regulating nitric oxide (NO) production.

All of this is great for anti-aging benefits![5]

A Remarkable Probiotic

BB12 (*Bifidobacterium lactis* 12) is a remarkable strain of probiotic. Bif makes sense, rather than *lactobacillus*, because about 90% of our natural flora is Bif.

Certain cancers (e.g., colon cancer) can be favored by the introduction of BB12.[6]

In one study, consumption of BB12 for three weeks resulted in doubling of the number of circulating phagocytes, showing phagocytic activity.[7]

Where Do I Get It?

For the time being, Cosway's in England have this product. It's known as Enhanced AHCC®. To get past regulations and appear as a functional food, they call it mushrooms plus yoghurt. Having read this far, you know better than that!

Each sachet of Enhanced AHCC® contains 600mg high-potency AHCC® from shiitake mushrooms (equivalent to 1,000mg regular strength AHCC®) with BB-12®, a powerful, clinically-proven friendly bacteria from Chr. Hansen, Denmark.

References

1. [Spierings, EL; Fujii, H; Sun, B; Walshe, T (2007). "A Phase I study of the safety of the nutritional supplement, active hexose correlated compound, AHCC, in healthy volunteers". J Nutr Sci Vitaminol 53 (6): 536–539]

2. [Wasser S, Weis A, Therapeutic effects of substances occurring in higher Basidiomycetes mushrooms: a modern perspective, Crit Rev Immunol 19: 65-96, 1999]

3. [Matsui Y, Uhara J, Satoi S, Kaibori M, Yamada H, Kitade H, Imamura A, Takai S, Kawaguchi Y, Kwon A, Kamiyama Y, Improved prognosis of postoperative hepatocellular carcinoma patients when treated with functional foods: a prospective cohort study, J Hepatology 37(1): 78-86, 2002]

4. [Ye SF, Ichimura K, Wakame K, Ohe M. Suppressive effects of Active Hexose Correlated Compound on the increased activity of hepatic and renal ornithine decarboxylase induced by oxidative stress. Life Sci. Dec 19 2003;74(5):593-602]

5. [http://www.mskcc.org/cancer-care/herb/ahcc]

6. [Am J Clin Nutr February 2007 vol. 85 no. 2 488-496]

7. [Schiffrin et al., 1997]

COULD THIS BE A LIVING DRUG?

Let me share something I learned from the *New Scientist* journal: fungus furniture!

Again, I'm serious. New Scientist is holding a Christmas competition and the prize is a fungus chair.

It's made from the Reishi mushroom (*Ganoderma lucidum*). The massive block you see is the part that grows underground (the mycelium). These can be very massive indeed; the largest living organism on Earth is a fungus mycelium, growing in Oregon. It now covers 2,200 acres and is 3.5 miles across!

The creator of this fungus furniture is Phillip Ross from San Francisco. He uses a black plastic bag pressed tight against the soma, which cuts off gas exchange, prompting the fungus to form a leather-like layer to encase itself.

The furniture fungus is then killed, so it won't invade the home. It's treated at 670 degrees and coated in lacquer, so spores can no longer form.

No worries about durability; these will outlast normal wares, says Ross.

Ganoderma (Reishi or Lingzi mushroom) is a formidable health ally. It's anti-aging and it attacks cancer, modulates the immune system, wards off heart disease, calms the nerves, and relieves both allergies and inflammation.

It seems that mushroom therapy can **help against cancer in four specific ways**:

1. Stimulates the immune system
2. Helps immune cells bind to tumor cells
3. Actually reduces the number of cancer cells (cytotoxic effect)
4. Slows down growth

Different compounds found in Reishi are responsible for each of these effects.

The Japanese government officially recognizes mushroom cancer therapy as a treatment, whereas in the USA, it's just a folk cure hoax! Go figure.

Cancer Meets Its Nemesis with Mushrooms

Let's talk about some cutting-edge medicine…

Reprogramming human blood cells has put an end to cancers we thought were incurable.

In March 2013, Michael Sadelain at the Memorial Sloan-Kettering Cancer Center in New York announced successfully treating five cases of acute lymphoblastic leukemia (ALL) with genetically-engineered immune cells from the patients' own blood [see, genetic engineering has many uses other than growing dodgy food crops!].

One of the patients recovered in just eight days. Sadelain would probably argue that's the power of the treatment, though I would want to argue that it's due to the magic of Nature.

You know I have always said that, ultimately, all successful treatments are going to have to follow Nature.

Since then a further 11 people have been put into remission. Several other cancers are being looked at.

What is new is the idea of training the body's own immune cells to fight cancer. We all know that cancer is basically a disease of the immune system; it stops protecting the individual and cancer gains a foothold. Cancer is a sign your immune system is dangerously low, most often due to nutritional starvation.

The latest techniques teach T-cells to target cancer cells, while leaving healthy cells untouched. The trouble is that ALL affects B-lymphocytes, also part of the immune system.

That's why it's so deadly. So Sadelain programs the T-cells to wipe out all the B-lymphocytes, whether healthy or not. Then a marrow transplant restores the healthy cells.

The T-cells are already there, armed and waiting, to wipe out any rogue B-cells that appear.

Voila!

This Is Essentially a "Living Drug"
Well, they would use terms like that, wouldn't they? But I'm OK with this term; it's true!

Several drug and biotech companies are developing these therapies. Penn has patented its method and licensed it to Switzerland-based Novartis AG. The company is building a research center on the Penn campus in Philadelphia and plans a clinical trial next year that could lead to federal approval of the treatment as soon as 2016.

Talking with the researchers, "there is a sense of making history…a sense of doing something very unique," said Hervé Hoppenot, president of Novartis Oncology, the division leading the work.

Lee Greenberger, chief scientific officer of the Leukemia and Lymphoma Society, says, "From our vantage point, this looks like a major advance," he said. "We are seeing powerful responses…and time will tell how enduring these remissions turn out to be."

It's a bit high-tech, admittedly. But this is better than the ghastly chemical approach.

But you know…and here's the kicker: fever cures ALL quite often.

We see increased survival time in children with ALL after a high fever.

Unfortunately, most ignorant doctors panic when the fever comes on. They immediately book more chemo, because the immune system "isn't working." That effectively blocks Nature's wisdom.

Fever Can Cure ALL
My idea would be to create a fever, if possible, and sweat it out (not meant to be a pun), watching the child's temperature soar and yet do nothing. It's a hard discipline!

But doctors are missing the powerful insight this effect brings. They go on using the "It's busted" model, instead of shouting "Hooray!" when the fever comes on.

CAN THIS PLANT SUBSTANCE KILL CANCER CELLS?

What is apoptosis? Let me share with you how plants can create a powerful reaction that can cause cancer cells to self-destruct.

If there was a substance that had powerful properties that caused cancer cells to undergo apoptosis (programmed suicide), you would think it pretty remarkable.

You would also expect the medical profession to jump on this "miracle cure" and start promoting it.

Unfortunately, most of the medical profession isn't interested in cures; it's only interested in money. A cured patient is a disaster—the poor doctor loses his income stream. In fact, the profession thinks that a patient who dies slowly and with expensive treatment is the ideal situation, but a cure is a problem.

So, we are on our own here.

So what is this wonder treatment I'm referring to?

What Is Apoptosis and How Does It Work?

It's *lemon grass*; or more exactly, *citral extract*, which comes from lemon grass.

And to be precise about this discovery, what I am saying is that Israeli researchers at Ben Gurion University (BGU) have found that one gram of lemon grass contains enough citral to prompt cancer cells to commit suicide in the test tube. It does this without harming normal cells.

The findings were published in the scientific journal *Planta Medica*, which highlights research on alternative and herbal remedies. Shortly afterwards, the discovery was featured in the popular Israeli press.

Citral is the key component that gives the lemony aroma and taste in several herbal plants such as lemon grass (*Cymbopogon citratus*), melissa (*Melissa officinalis*) and verbena (*Verbena officinalis*.)

The BGU investigators checked the influence of the citral on cancerous cells by adding them to both cancerous cells and normal cells that were grown in a Petri dish. The quantity added to the concentrate was equivalent to the amount contained in a cup of regular tea using one gram of lemon herbs in hot water. While the citral killed the cancerous cells, the normal cells remained unharmed.

As they learned of the BGU findings in the press, many physicians in Israel began to believe that, while the research certainly needed to be explored further, in the meantime it would be advisable for their patients, who were looking for any possible tool to fight their condition, to try to harness the cancer-destroying properties of citral.

The best way to consume the citral and create a pop is to put the loose lemon grass in hot water, and drink about eight glasses each day.

However, don't go crazy and assume it's a done deal. Science is rarely that easy!

One study I found suggested citral might cause cancer, lymphoma, in female mice who were fed citral in their food.

Citral was nominated by the National Cancer Institute for study because of its widespread use in foods, beverages, cosmetics, and other consumer products and its structure as a representative beta-substituted vinyl aldehyde.

Citral is used primarily as lemon flavoring in foods, beverages, and candies. It is also used as a lemon fragrance in detergents, perfumes, and other toiletries.

Male and female rats exposed to significant doses of citral exhibited listlessness, hunched posture, absent or slow paw reflex, and dull eyes. But there was no increased incidence of any cancers.

However, the incidences of malignant lymphoma in female mice exposed to citral at 2,000 ppm was significantly greater than that in the vehicle control group. Tissues most commonly affected by malignant lymphoma were the spleen, mesenteric lymph node, thymus, and, to a lesser extent, the ovary.

The researchers described this incidence of lymphoma in mice as "equivocal" evidence of cancer-causing properties. If the testing was done properly, it should not, in my view, be dismissed as equivocal. It would be grounds for further research.

For you (reader), it depends if you want to go with the rats or the mice!

DOES MUSIC DESTROY CANCER?

Fabien Maman, a French composer and bio-energetic, explored and documented the influence of sound waves on the cells of the body. He was fascinated with energetic healing techniques and wondered if we are really touched or even changed by music. If so, how deeply does sound travel into our bodies? He began a year-and-a-half study, joined by Helene Grimal, an ex-nun who had left the convent to become a drummer.

She supported herself by her profession as a biologist at the French national Center for Scientific Research in Paris. Together they studied the effect of low-volume sound (30-40 decibels) on human cells.

They mounted a camera on a microscope where they had placed slides of human uterine cancer cells. They proceeded to play various acoustical instruments (guitar, gong, and xylophone as well as voice) for periods of 20-minute duration, while they observed the affect on the cells.

Cancer Cells Being Destroyed by Sound

These pictures above were taken while a xylophone was used over a period of 14 minutes playing the Ionian scale (nine musical notes C-D-E-F-G-A-B- and C and D from the next octave above.) "The structure quickly disorganized. Fourteen minutes was enough time to explode the cell when I used these nine different frequencies," says Maman.

The most dramatic influence on the cells came from the human voice when Maman sang the same scale into the cells. In this experiment the cancer cells experienced a total explosion within nine minutes.

"The human voice carries something in its vibration that makes it more powerful than any musical instrument: consciousness. It appeared that the cancer cells were not able to support a progressive accumulation of vibratory frequencies and were destroyed," reports Maman.

His findings in the laboratory setting urged Maman to continue his study, but this time he chose to work with two breast cancer patients. Each woman committed to tone for three-and-a-half hours per day over a period of a month. In one case, the tumor vanished completely.

The second woman underwent surgery to remove the tumor. Her surgeon reported that the tumor had reduced in size considerably and had literally dried up. She recovered fully from the surgery and made a complete recovery. Maman's explanation for this incredible phenomenon was substantiated by the photographs he had taken during his case studies.

He says…

… the cancer cells show evidence of cell nuclei incapable of maintaining their structure as the sound wave frequencies attack the cytoplasmic and nuclear membranes.

The vibration of sound literally transforms the cell structure. As the voice intensifies and time passes with no break in sound, the vibratory rate becomes too powerful, and the cells cannot adapt or stabilize themselves. Therefore, the cells die because they are not able to accommodate its structure and synchronize with the collection of sound.

They cannot live in an atmosphere of dissonance and they cannot become resonant with the body. Therefore, the tumor cells destabilize, disorganize, disintegrate, explode and are ultimately destroyed in the presence of pure sound.

DNA hears music and participates in the phenomena of awareness. Ever since music has been used as therapy, people have suspected that acoustic vibrations have a direct or indirect influence on the human organism, but no scientific proof has ever been advanced. But can music kill cancer cells?!

Indeed, there was not even a satisfactory theoretical approach. But with the work of Szent-Gyorgyi and Herbert Frolich (both Nobel Prize winners) and especially the recent work of Fritz Albert on the biology of light and electromagnetic inter-cellular bio-communication, we know today that the nucleated cells, by the way of physical and vibratory configuration of its DNA, is capable of picking up, storing and broadcasting information (that is to say order and neguentropy) about the environment.

This suggests, among other things, that living matter organizes its environment, an idea which recalls the Gaia hypothesis of James Lovelock (1989), who demonstrated that cells communicate with one another, coherently, by exchange of photon quanta.

The Order and Coherence In Matter

Neguentropy, or neg-entropy, is a negative entropy, without which no living system would be viable. By opposition to entropy, which expresses an increase of disorder in the universe, neg-entropy is an impregnation of order and coherence into the structure of matter. In other terms, neguentropy is a force of information that organizes the structures and functions of living systems and participates in inter-cellular bio-communication.

Jacotte Chollet, former television documentary film producer, has met with many remarkable men, including Krishnamurti, Karl Pribram, David Bohm, Fritjof Capra, Paul MacLean, and other wise though lesser-known people, such as the Papuans of New Guinea, the aborigines of Australia, the medicine-men of North America and the Caribbean. These encounters inspired her to make the attempt to expand her cerebral faculties.

Her quest led to a period of intense research that was to last over 10 years, investigating the acoustical phenomena beyond the limits of human perception. During this research, her path crossed that of Lydie Ries, a biologist, and Pr. Regis Dutheil, doctor and professor, co-director of the Louis de Broglie Foundation, who was working specifically on phonons, the particles that Albert Einstein had posited in his Theory of Relativity.

Jacotte has spent the last 17 years in her studio creating what she calls "multidimensional music." Her experiences with the sound were extraordinary, to say the least. In 1985 Jacotte started to test the effect of her music killing cancer on willing participants to see what healing properties the music contained, if it did indeed kill cancer cells.

Blood samples were taken immediately before and after listening to multidimensional music for one to one-and-one-half hours in private sessions or workshops. These tests repeatedly showed a spectacular increase of up to one gram in the hemoglobin level of the blood samples. Resonance with the expanded consciousness field present in the music was inducing physiological, somatic transformations in blood makeup.

The rebalancing of potentials along the meridians of acupuncture is also noted. The effects are physical, psychic, and holistic .The phenomenon, originating with cellular perception of vibrations, is translated in part by increasingly specific sensations that correspond to a holistic self awareness.

Reference
1. Maman, Fabien (1997), *The Role of Music in the Twenty-First Century*, Redondo Beach, CA.

WHAT DOCTORS DON'T TELL YOU... ABOUT THE WAR ON CANCER
The Forces of Evil & Darkness on the Move, Yet Again

My friend Lynne McTaggart is at the center of a storm once again. Forces that don't want the public to read good news on cancer alternatives tried to shut down her magazine *What Doctors Don't Tell You* (known affectionately as WDDTY).

It's all reminiscent of the storm I found myself in last summer, when Marcus Freudenmann and I were threatened by anonymous government heavies, for daring to talk openly to the public about cancer!*

I've known Lynne for over 20 years. I gave her some advice on her daughter's health. I was one of the early medical advisors for WDDTY.

I worked a "naughty" for her by allowing her to clandestinely use my reader's card for the Royal Society Of Medicine. The library there is one of the finest in Europe and she or her minions were able to do a lot of research among medical journals, at no cost, on the pretense they were working for me!

When her first book came out, I was asked for a comment for the cover and described her as "a thorn in the side of conventional medicine." That was an understatement!

These days, of course, Lynne is best-known for her spiritual books, starting with the amazing, inspiring, and well-researched *The Field*, and has gone off in a rather different direction.

But WDDTY flourishes as always and continues to be reviled by the self-appointed guardians of what the public ought to be allowed to know. And with the November 2013 issue, things got very nasty in what I call the *"War About Cancer"* (not the war against cancer, the war about the right to personal choices and to circulate knowledge on this hoary topic).

Clearly, the ugly forces that control public information on cancer in the UK did not want that issue to be circulated and read. It contained, among other things, a gripping article about the successful use of homeopathy in treating deadly cancers, like brain tumors (glioma).

In the process, it made conventional cancer therapy seem very poor indeed; which it is, of course.

Probably because Lynne and her co-editor/husband Bryan Hubbard had announced they were going to publish a special cancer alternatives issue, the forces of greed and evil were up in arms, ready.

They tried to pressurize shops not to sell the magazine, using threats and bully-boys tactics. "They" stage-managed an attack in *The Times* newspaper, which contained malicious falsehoods, published on Oct. 1.

The so-called "charity," Sense About Science (actually a front group for Big Pharma), assembled what was claimed to be a group of experts, including doctors, scientists, and patients, who condemned the "disinformation" that WDDTY was putting out.

They bombarded stores selling the magazine with emails; took it higher, to the Advertising Standards Association, with complaints about WDDTY advertisers (in an attempt to scare them off and bring down the magazine financially); and called for WDDTY to be "banned."

The disinformation about Lynne and her team was wild, aggressive, and evil.

It got into *The Times* (a sorry shame to that ancient paper, now a filthy rag under Murdoch's aegis). Without even bothering to check the accusations, the paper went ahead and printed. What was obvious, says Hubbard, is that not one of the journalists had actually read the article they were complaining about.

The next thing, it's escalated to TV and "The Wright Stuff," a seedy Channel 5 (UK) show with failed journalist Matthew Wright. No one from the program bothered to check the story or the facts with WDDTY! It's unbelievable.

Instead, a picture of Lynne was flashed on the screen and then they tore into her, with no right of reply, parroting the same ugly claims circulated by Sense and Science and *The Times*. It was open season on WDDTY.

All this—please note—before the issue was even written, never mind in print!

Why? You can read this fascinating issue yourself and find out: the editors have generously decided to circulate it free, all round the world.

So this is just to say that it reveals fascinating work showing that homeopathy is MORE successful than chemo and, of course, less dangerous and not distressing like the "proper" treatment. So much so that 6 out of 7 glioma patients had complete regression. That's unheard of.

More: it turns out that the MD Anderson Cancer Center (MDACC) in Houston, Texas, got involved in researching homeopathic remedies and were so impressed by the results, that MDACC is now offering homeopathic treatment. The US National Cancer Institute is also impressed and has called for more research. Homeopathy (carcinominum, phytolacca, thuja, and conium) are already written up in my book, *Cancer Research Secrets*, (visit: http://www.www.alternative-doctor.com/stopcancer) which you simply MUST get, if you want to know the latest cures that work and have GOOD science.

References
1. New Scientist, 22 January 2014, p. 10. by Catherine Brahic
2. PNAS, DOI: 10.1073/pnas.1320115111

THIS BIOACTIVE COMPOUND STALLS MELANOMA

An international team of scientists led by Gary Goldberg, PhD, of the University of Medicine and Dentistry of the New Jersey School of Osteopathic Medicine (UMDNJ-SOM), has found that a protein from the seeds of a plant used for centuries in traditional medicines may be able to halt the spread of melanoma, a lethal form of skin cancer.

On average, melanoma kills one person nearly every hour in the USA, and many more in other countries. The American Cancer Society, with its usual breathtaking lies, claims the overall 5-year survival rate for melanoma is 91%. For localized melanoma, the 5-year survival rate is 98%.

Now there may be a solution; a very simple solution at that.

In fact, this new remedy kills or blocks the growth of many other cancers too.

But melanoma is particularly dismal because it kills very fast and, apart from maybe Abnoba's homeopathics (Quercus), there is no specific treatment, only the general anti-cancer measures I give in my book *Cancer Research Secrets*. (visit: http://www.www.alternative-doctor.com/stopcancer)

The remedy in question comes from the seeds of a legume tree — *Maackia amurensis* — that is native to parts of Asia.

References to *Maackia* being used medicinally can be found in ancient Chinese documents that date back more than 400 years. Dr. Goldberg and his colleagues believe that MASL, a specific component found in the plant's seeds, interacts with a receptor called podoplanin (PDPN) that is carried by many types of cancer cells.

This is wild, because the PDPN receptor is what promotes tumor invasion and metastasis to other parts of the body! PDPN allows tumor cells to break out of their microenvironment, invade new areas and metastasize. (Metastasis is what causes the vast majority of cancer deaths.)

In other words, MASL from the *Maackia* seeds **blocks cancers from doing what cancers do that is most dangerous: spreading to other parts of the body.**

But according to Dr. Goldberg, that's not all. MASL not only significantly reduces cell migration and metastasis, it also inhibits cancer cell growth.

MASL can effectively suppress the growth of lung, breast, prostate, colon, and brain cancer cells that are often resistant to current therapies.

Amazingly, MASL works at non-toxic doses and had no noticeable side effects at doses necessary to inhibit cancer cell growth and migration. Moreover, it can be taken orally. This is good news indeed.

The findings appear in the July 23, 2012, edition of *PLoS ONE*.

WHEN IS A CANCER DIAGNOSIS REALLY NOT CANCER?

When it is over-diagnosed and over-treated for the doctor's financial benefit, not for the patient's health and safety.

And that happens a great deal, especially in the USA.

Now a working group sanctioned by the National Cancer Institute has come up with a position statement, making it pretty clear that no one accepts this current situation as ethical. In fact it's criminal.

Very dramatically, the working group has stated that a number of pre-malignant conditions, including ductal carcinoma in situ and high-grade prostatic intraepithelial neoplasia (means iffy-looking growth but not cancerous changes), should no longer be called "cancer." Instead, the conditions should be labeled something more appropriate, such as indolent lesions of epithelial origin (IDLE).

Indolent means slow to heal, grow, or develop; inactive or relatively benign; an indolent ulcer [http://www.thefreedictionary.com/indolent].

The report was published online July 29, 2013, in *JAMA*.[1]

"Use of the term 'cancer' should be reserved for describing lesions with a reasonable likelihood of lethal progression if left untreated," write the three people who make up the working group.

This will create a furor the like of which we have never heard before (either that or it will just be buried), because over-diagnosis of non-malignant "cancers" is where the industry gets most of its figures for supposed success. They want non-cancers in the net, so they get more money…and can claim more success, because these phony tumors would never kill anyone anyway.

It only looks like a "cure."

It's going to be a hard slog and the NCI work group has wisely suggested the convening of an independent group (if there can be such a thing, in the corrupt medical world of the USA), charged with the task of revising the naming of lesions now called cancer and creating a new classification system that includes explicit recognition of the indolent slow-growing non-malignant lesions now falsely labeled cancer.

No need to worry: tests that can accurately identify these slow-growing, relatively harmless lesions are well established and proven (but of course they are kept from the public by corrupt clinicians and the cancer industry).

These proposed reforms are needed because, over the past 30 years or so, cancer screening in the United States has become highly problematic, the group explains.

The most shocking part of this whole fiasco is that–contrary to industry propaganda–there is NO significant improvement in survival of late-stage cancer.

Orthodox therapies are more or less worthless. So they have padded out the statistics with these harmless or slow-growing early "tumors," to make it look like they are getting some traction.

Take away the IDLE inclusions and the miserable truth emerges: SURVIVAL RATES FOR LATE-STAGE CANCER ARE UNCHANGED OVER MANY DECADES.

In other words, while national data demonstrate significant increases in early-stage disease, there is no proportional decline in later-stage disease. Wouldn't you expect that, if catching the cancers early led to better treatment and longer survival, the late-stage cases should drop?

Well they don't. All that is happening is that screening procedures are identifying more cancers that are "potentially clinically insignificant" (the working party's own wording). They are still missing and failing on the clinically dangerous cancers.

Let's look at the figures:

- Over a 35-year period, from 1975 to 2010, the incidence rate of thyroid cancers jumped 185% - from 5 to 14 per 100,000. However, the mortality rate remained at roughly 0.5 per 100,000.

- In addition, the incidence rate of melanoma rocketed up 199% - from about 8 to 23 per 100,000. But the mortality rate did not drop; it actually increased from 2.07 to 2.74 per 100,000!

- In 1975, before mammography screening was prevalent, the incidence rate for breast cancer was 105 cases per 100,000 population. In 2010, the rate was 126 cases per 100,000 - an increase of 20%. Over that time period, there was a related 30% mortality decrease - from 31 to 21 deaths per 100,000. However, "at least two thirds of the mortality reduction is believed attributable to adjuvant therapy," the working party note.

The position of the working party mirrors, in a number of key ways, a 2009 essay by Drs. Esserman and Thompson that called for a "rethinking" of prostate and breast cancer screening, in part because of the over-treatment of indolent and low-risk lesions.[2]

That essay prompted the chief medical officer of the American Cancer Society to famously declare, in an interview with a major news outlet, that "the advantages to screening have been exaggerated," which triggered a firestorm of controversy.

See, the industry doesn't want their dirty game leaking out and becoming known. Screening for the majority of oncologists is not a health measure; as I have famously said on many occasions, it's a marketing measure. It sells scare tactics and brings patients to their knees with fright, so they opt for chemotherapy.

It's totally unjustifiable, based on the real figures buried in this report. In fact, as we know, chemotherapy and radiation, and/or surgery are completely unjustified, with the results currently being achieved.

Whereas I recognize the right of every patient to choose for themselves–and knowing many will opt for chemo, maybe through fear–it cannot be seriously recommended as effective.

The Other Proposals

This remarkable position paper, or "viewpoint" as they call it, had other things to say about serious flaws in the existing system.

The first is a public relations effort. "Physicians, patients, and the general public must recognize that over-cancer diagnosis is common and occurs more frequently with cancer screening," the working group writes.

Another proposal is to create observational registries for lesions with low malignant potential. This would improve information about related disease progression, which would help in the uptake of "alternative treatment strategies, such as active surveillance," the group explains.

They propose a range of strategies, designed to "mitigate over-diagnosis" — which includes ways to reduce the detection of indolent disease, such as reducing low-yield diagnostic evaluations (that means worthless tests!) appropriately; reducing the frequency of screening examinations; focusing screening on high-risk populations; and raising thresholds for recall and biopsy.

Currently, far too many patients are recalled (and terrified) by lesions that are described as "suspicious."

These changes will not be popular, among the greedy, insane, and criminally inclined oncologists. However, it's nice that a few voices do see the need. Remember, not all oncologists are crooks (just misguided!)

Moreover, there are good findings to be gleaned. In a number of cancers, screening has significantly helped, WITHOUT this inclusion of fake or indolent tumors. There is a real trend of success. It usually occurs where there are clearly identifiable pre-cancerous lesions.

Colon and cervical cancer are the best examples of this. The incidence rate of colon cancer dropped 31% from 1975 to 2010 — from about 41 to 29 per 100,000. The mortality rate dropped 45% — from 28 to 15 per 100,000.

The improvement in cervical cancer was even more dramatic. The incidence rate dropped 55% over the study period — from about 15 to 7 per 100,000. The mortality rate dropped 59% — from 5.5 to 2.2 per 100,000.

Basically, the group's recommendations amount to tying screening procedures to the cancer's growth rate. If a cancer is fast-growing, screening is "rarely" effective. However, if a cancer is slow-growing but progressive, with a long latency and a precancerous lesion such as colonic polyps or cervical transitional changes, "screening is ideal."

But it has to be less (e.g., 10 years for colonoscopy, not the current fad for annually).

The really exciting thing about this position paper to me is that at least the scamming and the misuse of oncology tools is being recognized and talked about by orthodox doctors and scientists.

Whether that will lead to any significant improvement in ethical standards remains to be seen.

References
1. *JAMA*. Published online July 29, 2013.
2. *JAMA*. 2009;302:1685-1692

A FINAL WORD ON CANCER...
We are all battling cancer, here's why...

1 in 2 men and almost as many women will develop cancer in their lives.
It affects everyone in one way or another.

Here's the shocking part…it's a modern-day disease.

It was virtually unseen in Victorian times. *So what has changed?* Well, two things: diet and lifestyle.

In my groundbreaking book **Cancer Research Secrets**, I help you understand how to prevent cancer with nurture by nature. I explain my three pillars of healing: diet, emotions, and chemical clean-up, all backed up with solid science.

You need to get your copy NOW of my powerful and comprehensive 259-page book of cancer cures that work and those that don't.

Visit: http://www.www.alternative-doctor.com/stopcancer

SECTION 6

UNLOCKING THE FOOD CODE

Sidebar

LET'S TALK ABOUT WEIGHT LOSS!

WHY WE NEED SALT

IT'S NOT JUST FAT; IT'S FAT AND STRESS

FOOD FRAUD: WHAT ARE YOU REALLY EATING?

IS CAFFEINE MORE TOXIC THAN DRUGS?

THE TRUTH ABOUT GENETICALLY MODIFIED ORGANISMS (GMO'S)

THE SLIPPERY SCIENCE OF FATS AND OILS

A SIMPLE WEIGHT-LOSS MIND STRATEGY

YET AGAIN THEY ATTACK "RED MEAT"

THE BLOOD FATS STORY SCREWED UP

VINEGAR MAY AID IN FAT LOSS

CHOLESTEROL IS GOOD

A BIG BUM PROTECTS

BEWARE OF THOSE BATHROOM SCALES - THEY LIE!

IF YOU WANT LASTING WEIGHT LOSS, KEEP A FOOD DIARY

You know, science can be tricky. Even with the best intentions and complete honesty, facts emerge that make it look like someone has been fudging all along.

Take obesity. There could be said to be a "science of obesity" today. We know a lot about it; including the metabolic syndrome, the dangers of belly fat, the inflammatory nature of visceral fat, and how all this can lead to degenerative liver disease (fatty liver causes over 50% of cases of cirrhosis; alcohol abuse only 6% of cases).

Fat ages us fast. It also causes progressively earlier death. Obesity is a killer…

Deaths From Obesity Almost Quadruple What Was Thought

No surprise there. Insurance actuaries have known for over half a century that obesity will shorten your life. They don't wanna pay up so they study the odds in microscopic detail.

But for me, now living in the USA, I'm astonished at how little this has been regarded and how estimates of the risk have been consistently lower than they should be.

Obesity-related deaths stood at 5%; that was the official figure–till today! Now it's 18%, according to a new study published online Aug. 15, 2013, in the *American Journal of Public Health*. That's almost quadruple the previous estimate and much more believable.

Researchers analyzed 19 years' worth of annual U.S. National Health Interview Surveys from 1986 through 2004 and compared those findings to individual mortality records from the National Death Index. They focused on ages 40 to 85 to exclude deaths caused by accidents, homicides, and congenital conditions, which are the leading causes of mortality for younger people.

Earlier estimates of the dangers of obesity erred by overlooking generational differences. Because younger generations have been exposed longer to risk factors for obesity, they are at even greater risk of becoming overweight or obese and suffering all the health problems that accompany the extra pounds.

So, for example, obesity accounted for about 3.5% of deaths for those born between 1915 and 1919, but it accounted for about 5% of deaths for those born 10 years later; obesity killed off around 7% of those born another 10 years later; and so on.

"A 5-year-old growing up today is living in an environment where obesity is much more the norm than was the case for a 5-year-old a generation or two ago. Drink sizes are bigger, clothes are bigger, and greater numbers of a child's peers are obese," study co-author Bruce Link, a professor of epidemiology and sociomedical sciences at Columbia, said in a statement. "And once someone is obese, it is very difficult to undo. So, it stands to reason that we won't see the worst of the epidemic until the current generation of children grows old."

But wait a minute! It's not all like that; lots of holes have appeared in the old story. In fact scientists have now started to refer to "metabolically healthy" fat or healthy obesity (really!). It seems that not all obesity is the same. we are stardust obesity

The concept of "metabolically healthy obesity"—that is, individuals with a body mass index (BMI) above 30 who do not have metabolic-syndrome factors that put them at risk for cardiovascular disease events—is not new, but is only now being more widely recognized by experts.[1]

Metabolically healthy obese individuals have smaller waist circumference (pear vs. apple shape), high insulin resistance, and are "fat and fit," but there are no standardized cutoff points to identify metabolically healthy vs. unhealthy obese individuals.

So, without any helpful test (as yet), it's difficult to spot these different individuals, for whom the normal advice might be wrong. Not that anyone is saying it's OK for them to remain overweight; just that they are not subject to the same "rules" as other overweight individuals.

A Far Better Measure Than Body Mass Index

Part of the problem is the definite confusion caused by the so-called BMI measure (body mass index). According to this test, Michael Jordan, one of the world's greatest athletes (National Basketball Association), is technically obese!

A better measure by far is waist circumference, especially in normal or moderately obese individuals; if yours is over 40 inches (male) or 35 inches (female), that's bad news. Blood tests shed light on the probable risk factors of obesity far more than simply weighing one's self on the bathroom scales.

For example, insulin levels are revealing. When insulin resistance sets in, the tissues cannot metabolize glucose properly; the result is glucose is turned to fat and dumped in the tissues. Insulin resistance is shown by sampling blood levels after a sugar-loading challenge test.

Other problem issues include inflammation, which is the number one aging phenomenon in our bodies. Markers for widespread inflammation include c-reactive protein (CRP), adipokines, interleukin-6 and TNF-alpha (all this is in my book *Fire in the Belly*, incidentally).

Eye-Catching Twin Study

What caught my eye this week is a study of identical twins, published online Oct. 6 (2013) in *Diabetologia,* in which each pair had one lean twin and one obese twin (so that gets rid of the genes issue!)

The identical twin pairs were aged 22 to 35 years old with a mean difference in weight between twin pairs of approximately 17 kg (37 lbs.), in other words, quite a lot.

The researchers examined detailed characteristics of metabolic health, including subcutaneous, intra-abdominal, and liver fat (as measured by magnetic resonance imaging or spectroscopy), plus oral glucose tolerance, lipids, adipokines, and C-reactive protein. They also assessed mitochondrial function and inflammation in subcutaneous adipose tissue.

In half the twin pairs, the obese twins turned out to be as metabolically healthy as their lean counterpart, with low levels of liver fat, good glucose and insulin-sensitivity profiles, and little sign of chronic inflammation in their adipose tissue.

But the remaining eight obese twins had the classic hallmarks of unhealthy obesity, with marked insulin resistance, dyslipidemia, and a fatty liver (more than a seven-fold increase in liver fat compared with their lean twin), as well as up regulation of chronic inflammation in their fat tissue.

That's very dangerous.

These obese metabolically unhealthy twins also had significantly greater insulin production in response to an oral glucose tolerance test, greater levels of C-reactive protein (CRP), higher levels of LDL (bad) cholesterol, and lower levels of HDL (good) cholesterol than their lean twin, PLUS a tendency toward hypertension.[2]

What Was the Difference?
Not totally clear, but the results suggest that metabolically healthy obesity is characterized by an adipose tissue that maintains normally functioning mitochondria, does not exhibit inflammation, and is able to handle the excess energy by making more fat cells and not just bigger fat cells.

That's according to lead author Jussi Naukkarinen, MD, PhD, from the Obesity Research Unit, University of Helsinki, Finland.

More fat cells for the same amount of fat means less fat per cell (adipose). That could be significant.

Then the study goes off the rails: according to the authors, no medication currently exists for the specific purpose of preventing adipose tissue inflammation or to promote mitochondrial health for efficient processing of food into energy, but it is possible that such treatments could be developed, the researchers say.

This is wrong. You can beat down inflammation, using a host of herbs like curcumin and using omega-3 fatty acids. They don't even think of these things because they are not "medication." But the result will be valuable to you. Keep reading to find out how we can beat obesity and win the battle for good!

LET'S TALK ABOUT WEIGHT LOSS!
It's one of the biggest industries in the world!

There is a never-ending stream of weight-loss books, magazine articles, diet aids, and propaganda. It's not just a stream; it's actually a tidal wave.

I've seen just about every claim that has been made: eat more of X, eat less of X, eat more of Y, eat less of Y, any diet will make you gain weight, fat is beautiful anyway (it isn't, it's unhealthy), and so on. It's a jungle of predatory lions trying to get at your money. People with whacky opinions have found they can make a fortune out of this desperate market; they write books; they pretend expertise. If you're a sucker for it, then there is not much we can do to protect you.

However, there are one or two guiding principles, based on decades of experience that will help you to choose. We are not trying to sell you anything, so at least it is unbiased opinion.

First, the ultimate weight-loss plan is to eat less! It sounds simple, but it's amazing how many people, if they are honest, are searching for ways to lose weight without giving up their guzzling addictions.

Eat less does not mean be a supermodel and quit food. Less can mean just cut down by 10%. Look, if your weight is a steady 80 pounds over the ideal, you only need to reduce your intake by 10% and it will start to fall. Logical? If you are on a maintenance food intake, yes, it's logical. If you are gaining steadily, however, you may need to cut down more than that. One of the simplest regimes I know is to cut out one meal a day and eat only two-thirds of the portions you normally eat.

The second vital fact you need to know is that carbohydrates make you hungry. The famous "RAF Diet" of the forties was just a low-carb plan. The famous Scarsdale diet was also low-carb and worked wonderfully well. People were not hungry! Nowadays Atkins is the big name in low-carb eating.

It happens that carbohydrates (flour, starch, sugar etc) are highly addictive.

For decades, the orthodox medical profession has been telling people to eat carbohydrates. That's got them all hooked on sugar drinks, cookies, tortillas, pizza, and the like. **The result is an epidemic of obesity**. It's advice that kills!

Recently, Atkins was proved right. I think the shock of the medical profession beginning to come around killed the poor guy!

Thirdly, nobody needs a schlock product, berries, pills, or anything else to lose weight (especially beware of those that contain Chinese ma huang or ephedrine; it's an amphetamine-like substances and will send you spinning). I've seen lot of these over the years and studied them.

They all come down to this: take our product, follow this eating plan in the "handy guide," and you are guaranteed to lose weight. It's perfectly obvious that if you just followed the eating plan and threw away the product, you'd lose weight anyway. To me, this is fraud under the guise of pseudo-science. Where glob and goo products might help is in creating the sense of being on a plan. A reminder you should not be doing what you always do at mealtimes. But it's an expensive way to buy your determination of mind!

Finally, the question of exercise.

It has been said that a slice of pizza is about equivalent to an hour of hard tennis. It's easier to give up the pizza than sweat away like that! It's true to a degree. But after following that line for years with my patients I have gradually come to realize the true value of exercise.

It isn't for working off calories at all. It's about feeling good (endorphins perhaps), boosting the immune system (a *New England Journal of Medicine* study showed that exercise boosts white cells in the peripheral blood), keeping up cardiac efficiency, reducing stress, staying supple and youthful, rhythm, and a host of other health factors that can't be tabulated as just calories.

So, putting the two sides together, one can say that you can eat a bit more liberally if you exercise regularly and, if you want to stay young and feel good, make sure you do between 20 and 30 minutes of some exercise, at least three times a week. You don't have to be a gym junkie.

WHY WE NEED SALT

The low-salt diet is a scientific nonsense that has gripped the medical fraternity for years. **We NEED salt.** When the weather gets really hot out here in the deserts of the West, guess who are the first to die of heat stroke?

Patients on a low-salt diet go down like flies. Yet the dogma is never questioned.

Doctors go on recommending low-salt diets and refuse, absolutely, to keep an open mind on whether this is wise.

You'd probably lose your post if, as a doctor, you suggested caution in this. Well, some individuals have been brave enough to challenge orthodoxy and investigate the truth.

What they found was that lower sodium intake-- as measured by the *"gold standard"* of 24-hour sodium excretion--was **associated with higher cardiovascular mortality.** That's the opposite of what doctors are told.

"What our study basically shows is that it might not be right to impose a general reduction on sodium intake," said senior study author Dr. Jan A. Staessen (University of Leuven, Belgium).

We are not negating previous studies, and I think sodium restriction is meaningful for patients who already have hypertension and perhaps for patients with heart failure, but there are very few arguments showing that reducing salt intake in the general population would result in substantial benefit.

However the study did also show that **salt increases blood pressure slightly**. We've known that for years (so deal with the cause of hypertension, don't use aggressive low-salt diets!)

Of course there are the naysayers. "Doesn't make sense," says one US expert, adding he suspects, "the bias of the authors." He, of course, doesn't have any bias whatever; odd, isn't it?

He even attacks the integrity of the scientists in Belgium, accusing them of "Trying to create a stir. This is clever, but it's harmful in my view. It's like saying we don't think cigarettes are harmful so we shouldn't do anything about smoking."

It may, of course, be something to do with the fact they are not Americans and therefore can't be right. But of course the smoking dangers are PROVEN, the benefits of low-salt diet are by NO MEANS settled. So he's just blowing smoke and trying to evoke an unpleasant emotional response, instead of using a scientific argument (he didn't give one).

The blunt truth is that those in the lowest 33% of salt intake were 50% less likely to die. Or, put more scientifically, mortality was 50% higher in the lowest tertile of sodium excretion (excretors are not retaining sodium, remember).

IT'S NOT JUST FAT; IT'S FAT AND STRESS

According to a study published in the journal *Obesity* (Aug 2009), monkeys fed an American diet get fat, but those under chronic stress put on much more belly fat.

I did a double take on that. It seems counter-intuitive. Fat is just fat—calories—*right*? What has stress got to do with it?

Well, apparently the stressed monkeys (lower on the social pecking order) not only put on more fat but it was the deadly belly fat. That's far more serious from the point of view of blocked arteries, metabolic syndrome, diabetes, and heart disease.

In previous studies, socially stressed monkeys—those at the bottom of the pecking order in a monkey colony—get blocked arteries far faster than other monkeys fed the same high-fat diet. That's reasonable. In human terms; this is reflected by the famous "Whitehall Study", showing that workers lower in the civil service hierarchy die sooner.

But why do stressed monkeys get more belly fat?

Over a two-year period, the researchers collected a vast array of data on stressed and unstressed female cynomolgus monkeys. They used a CT scan to detect visceral fat -- abdominal fat that often (but not always) protrudes as a "beer belly" on the outside. On the inside, it wraps around the organs.

Even compared to other monkeys with the same body mass index and weight, CT scans showed that the stressed monkeys had a great deal more belly fat. And when the researchers looked at the animals' arteries, they found plaque clogging the arteries of the stressed monkeys.

During the years of the study, the low-status monkeys had high levels of a stress hormone called cortisol. Over time, high cortisol levels cause belly fat to accumulate. It also makes individual fat cells get larger.

This is basically *"sick fat."* Your fat cells are getting bigger and your fat tissue is getting bigger and neither the cells nor the tissues work as well as they should. The fat is sick.

End of gender difference: All of the monkeys in the study were female. One way monkeys are like humans is that females are less likely to get heart disease than males. Yet stressed female monkeys that put on belly fat are at least as likely to get heart disease as are male monkeys.

And, in fact, this may even be a worse disease for women than men, because they get complications and die faster when they have heart disease.

The researchers found that the stressed monkeys had abnormal menstrual cycles. Compared to the unstressed monkeys, they were much less likely to ovulate. This was linked to abdominal fat -- but not to body mass index or other kinds of fat.

There's something else that wasn't discussed, but I'd like to point out that no ovulation means less (or no) estrogen. That could speed osteoporosis in a post-menopausal woman.

FOOD FRAUD: WHAT ARE YOU REALLY EATING?

Some years ago I read something startling. Oil used to wash syphilitic sores was reused and sold for cooking purposes (in Africa). In the same book, it told of corpses being cut up and sold as antelope meat. It wasn't the cannibalism that made my flesh creep; it was the fact these were humans who died of leprosy!

Since that time, I have never been squeamish about what food manufacturers do to our food. As a bunch, they are cynical beyond belief, despicable, and totally untrustworthy. Ask my wife and she'll tell you I'm even suspicious of farmer's markets and where all that supposedly fresh produce comes from!

If I don't know the grower and the farm or orchard, I'm not impressed.

Nothing has changed. In the 21st century, lies about food and outright fraud are as rampant as ever. It seems that Monsanto is not the only hoaxter to worry about.

Recent stories have pinpointed the adulteration of milk, olive oil, honey, sheep's milk cheese, Sturgeon caviar, maple syrup, vinegar, and wine. Britain was in a furor a few weeks back, when it was revealed that "beef" was being sold in supermarkets that consisted of quite a lot of horsemeat; the Brits are horse lovers and that went down like a lead balloon!

Much of this is coming to light today because of DNA testing. It's something that was not an option a few years ago and traders in fake foodstuffs could get away with lies. Now the truth is coming out—and it's pretty ugly.

DNA testing reveals that more than 20% of fish sold in stores and cooked in restaurants are not the species claimed. In fact a survey by ConsumerReports.org in the USA found the following startling facts:

- Only four of the 14 types of fish the researchers bought—Chilean sea bass, Coho salmon, and bluefin and ahi tuna—were always identified correctly.

- Eighteen% of study samples didn't match the names on placards, labels, or menus. Fish were incorrectly passed off as catfish, grey sole, grouper, halibut, king salmon, lemon sole, red snapper, sockeye salmon, and yellowfin tuna.

- All 10 of the "lemon soles" and 12 of the 22 "red snappers" bought weren't the claimed species.

- One sample, labeled as grouper, was actually tilefish, which averages three times as much mercury as grouper (the Food and Drug Administration advises women of childbearing age and children to avoid tilefish entirely).

See, that's one of the hazards; you may be buying certain fish for health reasons and you are not getting the true healthy species but some substitute that may give you a real problem.

This List Goes On...

"Food fraud" has been documented in fruit juice, olive oil, spices, vinegar, wine, spirits, and maple syrup, and appears to pose a significant problem in the seafood industry. Victims range from the shopper at the local supermarket to multimillion companies, including E&J Gallo (wines) and Heinz USA.

A crabmeat seller on the Chesapeake Bay imports cheap crab and repackages it as Chesapeake blue crab, a different species that can be sold for twice or three times the price.

Some honey-makers dilute their honey with sugar beets or corn syrup, their competitors say, but still market it as 100% pure and at a high price.

An expensive "sheep's milk" cheese in a Manhattan market was really made from cow's milk. A jar of "sturgeon caviar" was, in fact, Mississippi paddlefish.

And last year, a Fairfax man was convicted of selling 10 million pounds of cheap, frozen catfish fillets from Vietnam as much more expensive grouper, red snapper, and flounder. The fish was bought by national chain retailers, wholesalers and food service companies, and ended up on dinner plates across the country.

Peter Xuong Lam, president of Virginia Star Seafood Corporation of Fairfax, was convicted last year of selling the mislabeled catfish. Ten other individuals and companies were also charged. Lam was sentenced to five years in prison and is barred from importing food into the United States for the next 20 years.

The Assistant US Attorney Joseph Johns, who prosecuted the Fairfax fish importers, said, "It was the rare exception, not the norm." But he's talking baloney (I mean real baloney, not the falsely labeled stuff!) How can he know what he doesn't know? Other agency officers are more realistic: we just don't know the scale of this crime but it's right to suggest that it is vast, indeed.

The recent development of high-tech tools, including DNA testing, has made it easier to detect fraud that might have gone unnoticed a decade ago. DNA can be extracted from cells of fish and meat and from other foods, such as rice and even coffee. Technicians then identify the species by comparing the DNA to a database of samples.

Another tool, isotope ratio analysis, can determine subtle differences between food - whether a fish was farmed or wild, for example, or whether caviar came from Finland or a US stream.

New techniques are easy to administer and high school students, working with scientists at the Rockefeller University and the American Museum of Natural History last year, discovered after analyzing DNA that 11 of 66 foods - including the sheep's milk cheese and caviar - bought randomly at markets in Manhattan were mislabeled.

It's Not the Big Guys

Just for once, it isn't the major conglomerates that are to blame. They get suckered too.

Heinz USA and Kraft Foods, two giant food-makers with well-established internal controls, nevertheless fell victim to "Operation Rotten Tomato," a conspiracy in which the son of a California farming dynasty disguised millions of pounds of moldy tomato paste as a higher-grade product.

And E&J Gallo, the nation's largest wine seller, sold 18 million bottles of Red Bicyclette Pinot Noir between 2006 and 2008 that had been filled in France with wine made from cheaper merlot and syrah grapes, according to a French court that last month indicted a dozen of its citizens in a scam dubbed Pinotgate.

This Is Dangerous Stuff

800 people died and 20,000 more were hospitalized, many with irreversible neurological and auto-immune damage, in the so-called "toxic oil syndrome" incident in Madrid, Spain in 1981.

In November 2008, China reported an estimated 300,000 victims of milk contaminated with melamine, with six infants dying from kidney stones and other kidney damage, and an estimated 54,000 babies being hospitalized.

The issue raised concerns about food safety and political corruption in China, and damaged the reputation of China's food exports, with at least 11 countries stopping all imports of Chinese dairy products.

A number of criminal prosecutions occurred, with two people being executed, and another given a suspended death penalty, but this bureaucratic bloodletting hardly allays fears of serious corruption in China where, to use a tainted expression, *everyone is on the take*.

Food Intolerance Reaction

Those of you who know me well will realize that I care most about people who are trying to keep inflammatory foods out of their diet. It can be bad enough to suspect milk allergy, wheat and grain intolerance, allergy to fish, whatever… only to find that the reaction was not due to the foodstuff at all but the adulterated version.

Or, in the reverse, it's even more deadly to have found a "safe" food and then eat it and become VERY sick, because it was the wrong food or a contaminated version of it, falsely labeled as "organic" (yes, I'm cynical about most "organic" labeling too).

It's extraordinary the effect of good pure food on our system (since over 70% of what we eat is not "natural": grains, dairy, sugar, tea, coffee, alcohol) plus all the naturally toxic chemical compounds in foodstuffs anyway. As I reported in my book *Diet Wise*, it is only with the development of fire that we were able to render enough foods safe to eat that, as a result, Mankind swept all over the planet.

Be very, very careful what you buy and eat. Always choose whole foods where you can; that way you can identify it. Use your nose and tongue too! Animals will sniff and slightly taste food and if for any reason it's suspect, they will go hungry, rather than eat it. The typical human will wolf it down and then groan, "I don't feel good!"

If you want the REAL science of good food choices, it's all in my book *Diet Wise (visit: www.alternative-doctor.com/dietwise)*. You'll be asking your body to choose, "What's right for me?"

Never mind all the propaganda.

IS CAFFEINE MORE TOXIC THAN DRUGS?
Spiders Blown Away!

Look at the effect of different drugs on the performance of spiders spinning their webs, according to NASA research reported in *New Scientist*, April 27, 1995.

Spiders on marijuana are too laid back to finish the job, while those dosed with the sedative chloral hydrate drop off to sleep before they can lay down more than a few silky filaments, although the web is OK as far as it goes.

On an "upper," such as benzedrine, the spider demonstrates great gusto but not much planning, leaving large holes in the structure. But caffeine seems to have had by far the worst effect and the web is a very chaotic affair. In fact, it's a disaster!

Ask yourself: do you really want to drink this stuff?

Many reported allergies to tea and coffee are not allergies in the true sense of the word but simply caffeine poisoning. Doses above 250 mg a day are toxic and potentially harmful. Children are more prone to caffeine's negative effects. You might think children aren't consuming a lot of caffeine, or at least not as much as their Starbucks-guzzling parents.

In fact, a 2010 study, published in the *Journal of Pediatrics*, found that 75% of children surveyed consumed caffeine on a daily basis and, the more caffeine the children consumed, the less they slept.

Cola drinks may legally contain up to 60 mg of caffeine per portion. Parents actually encourage kids with cola drinks, on the daft notion that it "energizes" them. The American Association of Poison Control Centers has reported roughly 1,200 cases a year of caffeine toxicity in children younger than age 6!

We all drink too much tea and coffee. Trouble is, you see, caffeine makes you pass more water through the kidneys. So you lose fluid, feel thirsty as a result and want to drink all over again! It's a vicious circle. Great for the tea and coffee companies but not good for your brain and kidneys.

A typical cup of coffee contains 90 to 100 mg of caffeine. So-called de-caffeinated coffee has about 2 mg. A 5-oz cup of tea contains about 50 mg caffeine and 1 mg theophylline. Cocoa and most chocolates have significant amounts of caffeine, a fact that is often overlooked.

People have been drinking caffinaceous drinks since the dawn of time. Maté, still drunk by 20 million South Americans, was known to Paleolithic man. Tea from the bush *Camellia chinensis* has been drunk in China for 2,000 years.

Coffee, taken from the *Coffeia arabica* plant, was established more recently, because without the fermentation, extraction, and roasting processes, which must have taken some ingenuity to discover, its taste is unpleasant.

The distinctive aroma of coffee comes from over 500 compounds that arise during roasting. Almost none of these compounds have been properly evaluated for toxicity; they include thiopenes, thiazoles, oxazoles, furans, pyrroles, pyridines, quinolines, quinoxalines and indoles. There are others.

Remarkably, coffee has some terrific health benefits, scientifically documented. But I have to warn you that almost all these positive studies were from Europe, where coffee is a different affair than in the New World.

Over there we drink a very small espresso (half to one ounce per serving, no cream and no sweetener). That's a far cry from the 20-ounce and 32-ounce cream and sugar-shlock guzzlers served over here in the typical coffee shop!

I suggest you find your own small local artisan coffee shop—one that knows how to make real espresso—and patronize them. They need all the help they can get under the onslaught of giants like Starbucks and Coffee Bean.

THE TRUTH ABOUT GENETICALLY MODIFIED ORGANISMS (GMO'S)

GM foods don't just make you fat; they will inflame your tissues and shorten your life and they definitely cause cancer.

My wife Vivien pointed out that on television we are drenched with a saturation coverage of the problems in Syria, with a few hundred people dead from chemicals and a few thousand likely to be affected. That's nothing compared to the death of millions I am going to explain to you, also caused by the chemical industry.

When you have absorbed the full impact of what I am saying here, you might even wonder, as Viv suggested, whether the TV obsession with far-flung wars might be little more than a diversion, to keep your attention off the real "chemical warfare" we are being subjected to!

First, the Weight Gain Issue...

A study published in a peer-reviewed journal, *Food and Chemical Toxicology,* shows that eating GM food is almost certainly contributing to the obesity epidemic. GM foods cause inflammation and I have been at pains to repeatedly remind you that inflammation leads to obesity problems.

But I'm not just limiting my warnings to the weight gain issue. The test animals also showed increases in circulating glucose and triglycerides, plus significant damage to major organs.

Effects were mostly associated with the kidney and liver, the dietary-detoxifying organs, but other effects were also noticed in the heart, adrenal glands, spleen, and hematopoietic (blood making) system.[1]

Now learn this: in another shocking study, pigs fed a diet of genetically engineered soy and corn showed a 267% increase in severe stomach inflammation compared to those fed non-GM diets.

In males, the difference was even more pronounced: a 400% increase. So the fact that GM foods are inflammatory in character is now beyond question. The study was carried out over a 23-week period by eight researchers across Australia and the USA and was published in the *Journal of Organic Systems*, a peer-reviewed science journal.[2]

Of course the study was quickly attacked by the food industry; that's quite standard. They put their shill scientists on it, to try and find details to criticize. For them there must never be any acknowledgement of possible dangers from GM foods…never, never, never.

To keep up their standpoint, all they have to do is ignore the gathering tide of evidence or lie about it. They do both very well.

The usual bluster and denial tactics were used against another powerful and disturbing report published in 2012, also in a peer-reviewed journal, *Food and Chemical Toxicology,* by Gilles-Eric Seralini.3 The world was shocked by hideous photographs of rats fed on grains engineered to be tolerant of Monsanto's infamous "Roundup" pesticide, bearing grotesque tumors that had grown in just a matter of a few months.

The implications for humans are appalling.

With GM foods deliberately hidden in our supply chain, we face the likelihood of eating them for many years to come, maybe generations to come, and growing similar cancers.

The trouble is, it will take a long time for the truth to emerge and by then millions of individuals will have been doomed to a miserable death just for corporate profits.

But yet again, the study was cynically and systematically attacked. The trouble is, some unknowing souls might have believed some of the criticisms. But Seralini's own website counters every single twisted and dishonest objection.[4]

10 Points on Which Industry Criticisms Are False:

1. That Séralini's study was a badly designed cancer study. It wasn't. It was a chronic toxicity study – and a well-designed and well-conducted one. The cancers were what showed up.

2. Séralini's study is the only long-term study on the commercialized GM maize NK603 and the pesticide (Roundup) it is designed to be grown with.

3. Séralini used the same strain of rat (Sprague-Dawley, SD) that Monsanto used in its 90-day studies of GM foods and its long-term studies of glyphosate, the chemical ingredient of Roundup, conducted for regulatory approval.

4. Despite wild claims to the contrary, the SD rat is about as prone to tumors as humans are. As with humans, the SD rat's tendency to cancer increases with age.

5. Compared with industry tests on GM foods, Séralini's study analyzed the same number of rats but over a longer period (two years instead of 90 days), measured more effects more often, and was uniquely able to distinguish the effects of the GM food from the pesticide it is grown with.

6. If we argue that Séralini's study does not prove that the GM food tested is dangerous, then we must also accept that industry studies on GM foods cannot prove they are safe.

7. Séralini's study showed that 90-day tests commonly done on GM foods are not long enough to see long-term effects such as cancer, organ damage, and premature death. The first tumors only appeared four to seven months into the study.

8. Séralini's study showed that industry and regulators are wrong to dismiss toxic effects seen in 90-day studies on GM foods as "not biologically meaningful." Signs of toxicity found in Monsanto's 90-day studies were found to eventually develop into organ damage, cancer, and premature death in Séralini's two-year study.

9. Long-term tests on GM foods are not required by regulators anywhere in the world.

10. 1GM foods have been found to have toxic effects on laboratory and farm animals in a number of other studies. This is not a "one-off" finding.

The truth is that we and our governments are being tricked and manipulated and science is being ill-served by fake short-term reports and studies and, frankly, a wall of lies to cover up quite serious crimes against humanity.

It's the biotech industry versus the human race.

Keep your eye on the alternative press and activist websites like InfoWars.com and NaturalNews.com — they fight hard to make public the hidden lies, corruption and deceitful agenda of the biotech industry.

Otherwise you risk being left in the dark.

Bet You Didn't Know You Are Already Eating This Stuff!
You could be eating GM foods and not even know it. A new USDA-funded survey, reported by WebMD, shows you're not alone.5 Researchers from the Food Policy Institute at Rutgers' Cook College found that only 52% of Americans realized that genetically modified foods have already entered the supply chain and are being sold in grocery stores.

The **USA is the largest producer of genetically modified crops**. But more than a dozen other countries around the world have latched on to the technology, including Argentina, Canada, China, Australia, India, and Mexico.

The Europeans are in an enviable position, where their governments are fighting hard to stem the GM tide. But the shocking truth is that as much as 70% of processed foods in the U.S. contain GM ingredients.

The FDA effects not to be concerned and holds to the line that these foods are safe. The recommendation that GM food be labeled for what it is, so people could make an informed choice, is rejected: "Genetically modified is an inappropriate term, in that all crop varieties have been modified by plant breeders."

According to a WebMD feature article, the most common genetically modified foods are soybeans, maize (corn), cotton, and rapeseed oil.6 That means that many foods made in the U.S. containing corn or high-fructose corn syrup, such as many breakfast cereals, snack foods, and the last soda you drank; foods made with soybeans (including some baby foods); and foods made with cottonseed and canola oils could likely have genetically modified ingredients.

Then there are secondary foods. Chocolate, for instance, could contain at least a few GM ingredients: high fructose corn syrup from GM corn, sugar from GM beets, and soy lecithin from GM soy.

Soy lecithin is an emulsifier that keeps the chocolate solid and gives it a longer shelf life.

Meat is indirectly contaminated. Chicken, pigs, and cows that eat unnatural GM feed become GM themselves. To make matters worse, a study out of Italy shows that the GM feed that animals eat even affects the milk they produce. According to the study, GM corn DNA was present in 25% of milk samples. Even if you steer clear of GM foods, your animal products may be passing their synthetic diet along to you.

How to Avoid GM Foods

In the USA, you can't; it's too late. The supply line is already irretrievably contaminated. Even supposed GM-free crops by now have become contaminated by cross-pollination with DNA from adjacent GM fields. Short of blowing every insect out of the atmosphere, this cross-contamination process will continue relentlessly.

We have been screwed and screwed good. Maybe this GM invasion is a big reason why some of you are having weight problems? Many scientists think it could be so. But it makes sense to fight the process and slow down the damage to your body.

Try to buy only quality organic, raw, grass-fed, or naturally pastured foods.

Buy the best you can with "certified organic," which can itself be a scam. But it's important to understand that even when you think you're eating "all natural," that food is probably as far from natural as you can get. And it may be full of GM ingredients.

Buying organic may cost more. But the higher price tag often comes with a greater peace of mind. Just don't think you are totally safe, is all.

References:

1. de Vendômois JS, Roullier F, Cellier D, Séralini GE. A Comparison of the Effects of Three GM Corn Varieties on Mammalian Health. *Int J Biol Sci* 2009; 5(7):706-726. doi:10.7150/ijbs.5.706.
2. Judy A. Carman, Howard R. Vlieger, Larry J. Ver Steeg, Verlyn E. Sneller, Garth W. Robinson, Catherine A. Clinch-Jones, Julie I. Haynes, John W. Edwards (2013). A long-term toxicology study on pigs fed a combined genetically modified (GM) soy and GM maize diet. *Journal of Organic Systems* 8 (1): 38-54. Open access full text: http://www.organic-systems.org/journal/81/8106.pdf
3. Gilles-Eric Séralini et al., Long term toxicity of a Roundup herbicide and a Roundup-tolerant genetically modified maize; *Food and Chemical Toxicology* 50 (2012) 4221–4231.
4. http://GMseralini.org/ten-things-you-need-to-know-about-the-seralini-study/ accessed Oct 16 2013, 7.00 am BST.
5. http://www.webmd.com/food-recipes/features/are-biotech-foods-safe-to-eat, accessed Sep 16, 2013, 9.00 am BST.
6. Ibid.

THE SLIPPERY SCIENCE OF FATS AND OILS

There is probably nothing more misunderstood in medicine and nutrition than fats. In fact, if I use the term lipids, it's all-encompassing and takes into account blood fats too.

Never has there been a subject so hedged about out with lies, ignorance, stupidity, disinformation, and dangerous incompetence as this topic.

It kills—yes, KILLS—hundreds of millions of people a year. Doctors, dieticians, and government meddlers murder uncountable numbers, due to getting the science wrong.

But AT LAST, the wheel is beginning to turn around.

Let's grab some quick facts, so you are armed like a nutri-pirate for bloodthirsty hand-to-hand combat!

1. Heart disease as we know it since the early 20th century did not exist prior to the introduction of artificial fats, in the form of margarine. This is despite the fact that the population ate nothing but milk, butter, cheese, cream, and curds.

2. Eskimo populations traditionally ate diets up of to 50% fat, yet cancer and heart disease were unknown until they moved into the bases and started consuming the standard carbohydrate and trans fat-loaded diet.

3. Key vitamins like A, D and E are fat-soluble and are not absorbed, or hardly at all, if the diet is fat deficient.

4. Robert Atkins showed that you can eat a diet loaded with fats and lose weight dramatically. "Experts" still say this diet is "dangerous." Why? Because it's high in fats. Why is that dangerous? Because we say so, not because there is any evidence whatsoever.

5. Even successful low-fat plans work because they take people off dangerous fats (trans fats) not because they take people off saturated fats. All "experts" agree that saturated fats are dangerous and every single one who does is a dangerous nincompoop. There is no evidence for such a claim but LOTS of evidence that saturated fats are essential to us.

6. The recommended alternatives are dangerous. Polyunsaturates, so-called, are KILLERS, despite endless media propaganda for "heart-healthy" margarine and cooking oils. It's elementary nutrition and a kid of 10 years old could figure this out: we need essential fatty acids (EFAs) like EPA, polyunsaturates are essential fatty acids, they squeeze out the EPA by competing with it, we get rampant inflammation. I rest my case: inflammation is the cause of diabetes, Alzheimer's, coronary artery disease, all the problems of aging, which have… what? Gone up astronomically since the introduction of low-fat dietary recommendations. It's elementary, my dear Watson (yes, Arthur Conan Doyle, who wrote Sherlock Holmes, was a doctor, remember!).

7. So-called "trans fats" or hydrogenated oils are completely unnatural, beloved of the food industry and totally backed by "official" heart-health campaigns. In the decades since the attack on saturated fats and the promotion of margarine, hydrogenated oils, and vegetable fats, heart disease rates have soared. The more the message is hammered in that fats are the cause, the worse the health of the nations who propagandize this garbage.

Science Has Been There All the Time

Now get this: it's not a case of science going down the wrong road and finally realizing the mistake. It's the story of very stupid and criminally dishonest people, working for the food industry, wrapping up pseudo-science and disguising it, for other ends than health of the population.

There hasn't been a year go by, while I have been watching the scientific literature, when the dangers of low-fat plans, polyunsaturated substitutes, artificial fats and oils or the health value of healthy saturated fat has not been published.

IT'S JUST ALL BEEN TOTALLY IGNORED.

The advertising and media machine goes on grinding out the same old message; *"everyone knows"* that fats are bad for us, right?

It's hammered so much and so hard that medical students are taught to believe it, doctors believe it, each country's own heart health charity campaign bashes it out, TV anchors are experts and repeat this message as glibly as if they were professors of physiology…

It's an international chorus of "the Earth is flat, not round!"

To suggest that fats are good for you is considered a heresy as unthinkable as religious dissension in the days of The Inquisition.

Indeed, we have medical inquisitions sitting all over the world today, and revoking the licenses of any doctors who do not toe the party line (would make everyone else look pretty stupid if the dissenters turned out to be correct, right? So crush them, rather than figure out where the truth lies).

New Science

I hinted that the wheel is finally turning and huge cracks are appearing in the classic picture. For example:

A paper published in the *Canadian Medical Association Journal* in November 2013 mounts a credible challenge to the claim that that polyunsaturated fats could reduce the risk of heart disease through their ability to lower blood cholesterol levels.

The research showed that omega-3 fatty acids significantly reduced the dangers of heart disease, but had no effect whatever on lowering cholesterol levels (well, it wouldn't, would it, since cholesterol has absolutely nothing to do with heart disease).[1]

In the so-called Sydney Diet Heart Study, about 220 men aged 30-59 were instructed to reduce saturated fat intake and increase polyunsaturated fat intake.

The men were supplied with safflower oil and safflower oil-based margarine (rich in the omega-6 fat known as "linoleic acid," but very low in the omega-3 fat found in plants and known as "alpha-linoleic acid"). A similar number of men got no dietary instruction and acted as controls.

In the men eating the "heart-healthy" diet, risk of death was elevated by 62 percent. Risk of death from cardiovascular disease was increased by 70%.[2] In other words, lowering cholesterol levels leads to early death. I'm sorry to say "I told 'em!" but all my old-time subscribers will recognize this war cry I use often!

On Nov. 7, 2013, the US Food and Drug Administration (FDA) announced that it is now considering removing partially hydrogenated oils—the primary source of trans fats—from the list of "generally recognized as safe" (GRAS) ingredients.[3]

According to the FDA, 12% of all processed foods contain at least one partially hydrogenated oil, aka trans fat.

Numerous studies have shown that consumption of trans fats can have "lots of adverse health events, including raising bad cholesterol and lowering good cholesterol," said Penny Kris-Etherton, a professor of nutrition at Penn State University in University Park, Pa.

"There really is no safe level of consumption of trans fat," FDA commissioner Margaret Hamburg said.[4]

Cynics would jump to the conclusion that this turnaround was because the FDA was being sued for failing to point out the evidence showing the dangers of trans fats! Joe Mercola tells us that Dr. Fred Kummerow, a 99-year-old heart disease researcher, has been studying heart disease for about 60 years. He first wrote about the health hazards of trans fats all the way back in 1957.

Finally, Dr. Kummerow filed a citizen petition with the FDA in August of 2009 to have trans fats banned, based on the scientific evidence of harm. The agency is legally required to respond within 180 days. Four years later, no response had been issued, so Dr. Kummerow resorted to suing the agency.

Suddenly they are questioning the safety of trans fats, after all these years! A coincidence? Who cares…

But it comes down to this: you have to research and learn for yourself about health and nutrition. No government agency is going to protect you from the lies and cunning of the food industry or the stupid/wicked scientists who work for them!

My Advice…
Eat lots of fat; don't worry about saturated. Cook in coconut oil (get used to the flavor). Try to find lard and cook in that; collect your own lard from roast meats (but not chicken). Dump all margarine and re-introduce butter (Yum!)

References
1. Bazinet RP, et al. Omega-6 polyunsaturated fatty acids: Is a broad cholesterol-lowering health claim appropriate. CMAJ online before print 11 November 2013
2. Ramsden CE, et al. Use of dietary linoleic acid for secondary prevention of coronary heart disease and death: evaluation of recovered data from the Sydney Diet Heart Study and updated meta-analysis BMJ 2013;346:e8707
3. http://www.theatlantic.com/health/archive/2013/11/the-trans-fat-ban-as-a-model-of-slow-health-policy/281299/
4. http://www.usatoday.com/story/news/nation/2013/11/07/fda-remove-trans-fat/3458465/

A SIMPLE WEIGHT-LOSS MIND STRATEGY

Connirae Andreas, PhD, an internationally known trainer and researcher in NLP, coauthor of the marvelous book *Heart of the Mind*, gives a very simple technique, which I have tried, taught others, and found to be valuable.

She calls it the "Naturally-Slender Eating Strategy"! We all do different things in our minds, when we think about work, love, pleasure, and eating. These structured sequences of thought are what NLP practitioners call mind "strategies."

Connirae points out that people who are slim, eat well and stay healthy must be doing something different when they think about food. Since she is a naturally slim person, she asked herself *"What goes on in my mind when I start to think about food?"*

Her answer goes something like this:

1. I check how my stomach feels now.
2. I ask myself "What would feel good in my stomach?"
3. I imagine a portion of food: a sandwich, a bowl of soup, etc.
4. I visualize eating this food and get the feeling of how this amount of food will feel in my stomach over time, if I eat it now and it stays in my system for some hours to come.
5. If I like this feeling better than the feeling of not eating at all, I keep this food item as a possibility.
6. She repeats this for several food options and then, when she has enough choices, she finally picks the one that she knows will feel best over time.
7. She feels good after eating that food because she spent a lot of thought making sure she would!

That's a "no-guilt" strategy, as you can readily see. Unfortunately, for most obese people, their mental strategy is rather like this:

1. I think about food.
2. I realize I feel hungry.
3. I like pizza pie.
4. I'll eat pizza pie, probably a second helping because I really LIKE pizza pie.
5. I give no thought for how this will make me feel over time.
6. I eat the food and maybe another helping.
7. About half an hour after eating, I start to feel yuck in my stomach
8. I start wishing I hadn't eaten that. I tell myself to feel guilty.
9. Soon I start thinking about food all over again and fall into the same dumb strategy, even though it doesn't work.

Contrast this last thought with Connirae's own food strategy. Her thoughts will help you realize why she's thin.

You can simply try the same Naturally-Slender Eating Strategy technique she uses when you start to think about food too help watch your weight.

YET AGAIN THEY ATTACK "RED MEAT"

That's "red meat" in quotes because they didn't test red meat—they tested red meat AND processed meat junk. Then they tell us red meat is bad. Duh!

You'll hear incessant bleatings that red meat is bad and we shouldn't eat it; it leads to heart disease, strokes, etc. This is all NONSENSE. You put poison with good food, feed it to people, and say, "Don't eat this, it hurts people." That just condemns good food.

We NEED meat. It's our ancestral food (Neanderthal and Cro-Magnon man were big meat eaters). Red meat, such as beef, contains important food substances we need, such as carnitine and omega-3s. Yes, believe it or not, grass-fed beef is the richest source of omega-3s we have (this does not apply to grain-fed beef, of course, even though grains are technically grass).

This is where it gets stupid, because carnitine is used as a treatment for vascular disease. Several clinical trials show that L-carnitine and propionyl-L-carnitine can be used along with conventional treatment for angina to reduce medication needs and improve the ability of those with angina to exercise without chest pain.

"This study adds to a large and growing body of literature on the relationship between red meat and chronic disease," study author Adam M. Bernstein, MD, research director of the Wellness Institute at the Cleveland Clinic, Ohio, told *Medscape Medical News*.

No it doesn't! Hello!... professor of nutrition here, are you listening to me?

All these silly studies show is that processed meats are toxic junk. Listen, you only have to watch it being made to know that. I once worked as the duty doctor for a sausage manufacturing company. There was stuff put in the sausages that would burn and blister the skin of workers, if they spilled it!

Where there is data incriminating red meat, they never address secondary issues, like maybe the food is fried. Or meats in the USA are commonly eaten with fries and rarely with vegetables. We know fried food is bad. Fried ANYTHING will shorten your life considerably. It so happens that meats get fried (or roasted, same thing). That doesn't mean meat is bad.

I always fall back on quoting the Inuit (Eskimo) diet. Their traditional food is over 90% fat meats and fish; no carbohydrates. Eskimos do NOT get strokes and heart disease—not until they adopt the modern diet and start eating burgers and fries.

Protein Substitutions

Although there was no significant association between increasing intakes of fish, dairy, or legumes and the risk for stroke, there was an association when some of these protein sources took the place of what they called red meat.

For example, by substituting one serving of red meat with a serving of nuts or fish, the stroke risk was reduced by 17%, and by replacing the red meat with low-fat dairy, the risk went down by 11%. Substituting one serving of red meat with a serving of poultry resulted in a 27% reduction in stroke risk.

When substituting these foods, it is possible to maintain energy balance by, for example, eating nuts or yogurt instead of bacon at breakfast, or yogurt or nuts in a salad instead of a hamburger at lunch or dinner, said the authors.

The message is clear: **DON'T EAT MANUFACTURED MEATS!**

[SOURCE: Stroke. Published online December 29, 2011. Abstract]

THE BLOOD FATS STORY SCREWED UP

So, we all know the model: **cholesterol is the problem, too much is a bad thing and it kills you, right?**

Well, no; evidence is emerging for what I have never wavered from over the years, which is that you need more cholesterol than is currently allowed. It may even be healthier to have cholesterol over 200. I have never wavered from this in over 40 years and I watch the papers coming out regularly, showing that **we need saturated fats to be healthy**.

But, you say, HDL is the "good cholesterol" and it protects you, right? Wrong. Apparently it's not that simple at all.

But the bad cholesterol, low density lipoproteins (LDL), those are bad, definitely, right? No, that's probably not true either.

All the old myths are collapsing; they were only myths anyway and good scientific trials, looking for the right things, are showing a different story.

My attention was caught recently by a trial in which there were dramatic improvements in patient HDL (increase of 72%) and significant reduction in LDL (25% reduction), yet patients still had 60% excess cardiovascular morbidity and mortality. The outcomes were so bad in fact, the trial had to be stopped, before they killed any more patients![1]

Don't you find this confusing? It's not what all the press releases and propaganda say, is it? For years we've been told the problem is these blood fats and we should ALL be taking statins, even children; stop eating eggs and red meats; use polyunsaturates instead of saturated fats. Fat-free; fat-free; and fat-free for good measure. It's a litany. A litany that sold a lot of drugs, killed a lot of people and still holds center stage in the minds of most clinicians. Hardly ever was there a stronger case of ignorance killing.

Insights from Phase III Trials of Torcetrapib and Dalcetrapib

The simple idea that that more HDL is better was unequivocally refuted by the failure of the drugs, torcetrapib and dalcetrapib, intended to prevent cardiovascular events. Subjects taking torcetrapib had a 72% increase in HDL and a 25% decrease in LDL (due to concurrent statin therapy). They should have lived dramatically longer. But instead, the patients died faster than ever, resulting in premature termination of the study.

The study involving dalcetrapib was also halted early because it was determined that there was virtually no chance of a positive outcome, despite increasing serum HDL by 31% to 40%.

So now they are coming up with a patch of sorts: not that their theories are wrong, but that this must have been some "dud" HDL that didn't have any protective benefit, resulting from the absence of some undetermined function of normal HDL, or because of development of "large dysfunctional HDL molecules."1

Seriously! They call this science.[2]

Don't follow the statistical data and clear evidence showing your theory is wrong; instead, twist the story a bit, till you can ignore the inconvenient findings.

I ask you! If this faulty HDL existed, why did it never show up before? Because it doesn't exist. It's a theoretical patch and they are claiming this "solution" as science!

Here's the Truth on Finding Ways to Lower Cholesterol

HDL molecules increase blood viscosity and increasing HDL levels deliberately has been shown to leads to a big increase in blood clotting, stroke, and heart attack (myocardial infarction, so-called). Bad idea.

LDL is known to stick red blood cells together and so naturally increases the likelihood of clotting. Normally, HDL (which is a small molecule) doesn't do that. But increase the HDL abnormally and it too will clump red bloods cells, causing disastrous sludging of blood flow and the tendency to clot.

The bonds that form these aggregates are reversible and weak, forming in areas of slow blood flow. For an analogy that is easy to understand, a similar phenomenon is seen with a ketchup bottle.

While ketchup is still, intermolecular bonds form and its viscosity increases. However, shake the bottle, and the viscosity of the ketchup decreases and it flows more quickly.

I've written before that blood viscosity is a far more crucial measurement of blood health than fats (blood lipids). This study seems to prove that is correct.[3]

Cancer and Other Diseases

It's not just about heart disease. **Almost all diseases depend on blood flow; the more poorly provided are oxygen and nutrients, the less the body's ability to fight back.**

It even impacts cancer. If the body can't get its troops to the site, in the form of nutrient ammunition in sufficient quantity, the cancer will flourish. We know, for example, that cancer thrives on low oxygen levels. In which case sluggish blood flow is a disaster!

Not surprising then, that torcetrapib therapy, leading to this HDL sludging effect, was also associated with increased non-cardiovascular mortality. In particular, mortality from cancer and infections were increased, despite there being no increase in the number of cancers or infections.

Indeed, increased blood viscosity and decreased blood flow are fundamental defects that would increase mortality from any disease.

Position Paper

As a result, the National Lipid Association has had to do a complete about-face (2013):

For four decades it has been recognized that elevated serum levels of high-density lipoprotein cholesterol are associated with reduced risk of cardiovascular disease (CVD) and its sequelae… Consequently, it was assumed that, by extension, raising HDL through lifestyle modification and pharmacologic intervention would reduce risk of CVD… However, a number of recent randomized studies putatively designed to test the "HDL hypothesis" have failed to show benefit… In response to the many questions and uncertainties raised by the results of these trials, the National Lipid Association convened an expert panel to evaluate the current status of HDL as a therapeutic target… The expert panel concludes that… HDL is not a therapeutic target at the present time.[4]

This is testament to the appeal of the over-simplistic and incorrect notion that the accumulation of lipids in arteries causes atherosclerosis.

This is also really incredibly arrogant and typifies the fact that doctors always "know best" and seem to think they might need to correct the way Nature does things. As if!

Eat Lard to Help Your Heart

Lard. Once, it was the great cooking fat of Europe, from Shetland to Gibraltar and east beyond the Caucasus, in China, Mexico, in South America.

In Ukraine they have a festival devoted to it. Polish immigrants caused a UK shortage in 2004. Most of our ancestors ate it and not many of them died of obesity. For thousands of years there has been lard wherever there were pigs, and there were pigs, broadly speaking, wherever there weren't Muslims.

It's a supremely versatile fat. Because it smokes so little when it's hot it's perfect for bringing a golden shatter to a chip or a fritter – only dripping (beef fat) does a better job.

But is it healthy? You decide: gram for gram, it contains 20% less saturated fat than butter, and it's higher in the monounsaturated fats. It's one of nature's best sources of vitamin D. Unlike shortening, it contains no trans fats, probably the most dangerous fats of all.

Disillusioned by decades of conflicting advice and food company propaganda, many people are returning to diets unsullied by fads and dogma. That lard is both "healthier" than butter and yet so despised shows the empty logic of the standard position. The fat amply qualifies as "real food," which Michael Pollan defined as *"the sort of food our great grandmothers would recognize as food"*.[5]

Enjoy! And don't feel guilty.

References:

1. http://www.bloodflowonline.com/editorial/high-density-lipoprotein-protects-against-cardiovascular-disease-decreasing-blood
2. http://www.bloodflowonline.com/editorial/high-density-lipoprotein-protects-against-cardiovascular-disease-decreasing-blood
3. http://www.alternative-doctor.com/newsletter/medicineoutsidethebox-28.html
4. *J Clin Lipidol.* 2013 Sep-Oct;7(5):484-525. doi: 10.1016/j.jacl.2013.08.001. Epub 2013 Aug 11.
5. http://www.theguardian.com/lifeandstyle/wordofmouth/2011/feb/15/consider-lard

VINEGAR MAY AID IN FAT LOSS

Would you feel happy if you weighed 10% less? Here's some good news for you then...

Ordinary household vinegar appears to turn on genes that help fight fat. Well, they would say that, since they are obsessed with genes. Of course it may just be a metabolic effect. But it works!

Vinegar, especially cider vinegar, has long been touted as a cure-all for many ills. The substance has been used as a folk medicine remedy since ancient times. Modern medical evidence is slowly adding credence to some of the claims. In recent years, research has suggested that the main chemical in vinegar, called acetic acid, can help control blood pressure and blood sugar.

The current findings suggest that vinegar might help a person lose weight or fight obesity. Researchers in Japan gave acetic acid or water to mice via a stomach tube. All were provided a high-fat diet to eat normally.

Researchers found that the mice developed a lot less body fat (up to 10% less) than mice who didn't receive the vinegar compound. The amount of food eaten by the mice was not affected. OK, it was mice not humans, but that certainly rules out any psychological or placebo effect. The two groups of mice lived identical lives, except for the vinegar.

It's believed that acetic acid turns on genes that produce proteins that help the body break down fats. Such an action helps prevent fat buildup in body, and offsets weight gain. The findings are scheduled to be published in the July 8, 2009, issue of *Journal of Agricultural and Food Chemistry*.

So, out with the vinegar. I like Balsamic, myself. Brits use lashings of malt vinegar on "fish and chips" (fish and fries). But we can all add it healthily, to make oil-and-vinegar salad dressings. Maybe some pickles, too?

CHOLESTEROL IS GOOD

We are all taught to fear cholesterol. Any cholesterol is bad, *right*?

Well, did you know that cholesterol is a good free-radical scavenger (antioxidant)? Probably not. In fact, cholesterol is an extremely abundant substance, widely distributed throughout the body of a healthy person. Doesn't that alone make you suspect the drug industry story? Why would Nature put all the stuff there if it was bad?

Sorry: I'm not buying it.

Cholesterol has a purpose. **It is GOOD for us.** Cholesterol is the precursor to lots of good hormones; the steroid group, including testosterone, estrogen, and cortisol. Too much cortisol is bad for us but, with no cortisol, you die.

Cholesterol is needed for bile secretion; that aids digestion and is also a very crucial detox pathway for heavy metals.

It's an important "lipid" molecule that shows up in cell walls and membranes.

Cholesterol is part of neuron cells in the brain, forming the insulating myelin sheath. Without it, our brains would not be able to transmit electrical signals. In fact, brain cholesterol is not removed from the brain by metabolism, so the amount and condition of brain cholesterol is a good marker for free-radical damage.

Never mind the "good" and "bad" cholesterol. It's all good! It's just the proportions that matter. LDL isn't "bad," it's just we don't need too much: HDL isn't "good," it's just that more seems better and it's not healthy for it to be below a certain level.

Yet everyone is taught that LDL cholesterol is bad and we must lower it at all costs. That's not what science really shows, actually. With the release of ENHANCE in 2008, a study showing that reductions in LDL cholesterol did not translate into improvements in atherosclerosis as measured by carotid IMT, it's time we let go of the "bad" LDL theory. Dr. Rodney Hayward (University of Michigan, Ann Arbor), has stated categorically that the "current evidence supports ignoring LDL cholesterol altogether."

Of course the die-hards will go on mouthing the old myths for many years to come, attacking anyone who steps out of line.

What we do need to be concerned about is that oxidized cholesterol, especially the LDL faction, is quite toxic and pro-inflammatory. Only oxidized cholesterol is dangerous. You can have LOTS of cholesterol safely, if it is "pure." What we have to do is clean up our diet and lifestyle and get the protection of real antioxidants to stop from damaging cholesterol.

Protect your cholesterol: it's precious!

A BIG BUM PROTECTS

I want you to take a tape measure and measure your waist. Don't cheat or breathe in! Let it hang out. Then measure the largest circumference of your hips and note down the two figures. Your waist should be LESS than your hips. Preferably a couple of inches less.

The reason is that yet another study has suggested that waist-to-hip ratio is much more sensitive than body mass index (BMI) at predicting risk of subsequent coronary disease.

Writing in an early online edition of *Circulation*, Dr. Dexter Canoy (University of Cambridge, UK) and colleagues report that increased abdominal obesity, measured in terms of waist-to-hip ratio, was more "consistently and strongly" predictive of coronary heart disease (CHD) than BMI among men and women participating in the European Prospective Investigation into Cancer and Nutrition in Norfolk (EPIC-NORFOLK) study.

"In our study, in men who were obese and had lower waist-to-hip ratios, their rates of CHD tended to be slightly lower than if they had high waist-to-hip ratios," Coney said. "But in women, at all levels of BMI, waist-to-hip ratios were *strongly predictive of heart disease*" [my italics, KS-M].

The study showed that, even if we take into account habits like smoking, alcohol intake, or sedentary lifestyle, and we take into account what we already know are important predictors of CHD, such as hypertension and dyslipidemia, you will still have an excess risk of a heart attack if you have a higher than 1.0 waist-to-hip ratio.

Waist circumference alone was also a fair predictor of CHD events, but not nearly as accurate as taking the ratio of waist and hips together. Other recent studies have also shown that this is the best predictive measure we have.

Basically, for every increase of roughly 6.5 cm (2.5 inches) in hip circumference for men, and for roughly 9 cm (3.5 inches) in women, risk of developing CHD was reduced by 20%.

That's not to say people should develop a big hip circumference to protect themselves from risk but, for any body size, those with bigger hips tended to be associated with lower risk.

The importance of this new direction in health is this: we know that being overweight and obesity are risk factors. But, if the overweight individual has larger hips than waist, the risk is actually somewhat attenuated. Conversely, if you are of a normal weight or maybe only mildly overweight, you should not be smug. Formerly, doctors would pat you on the head and say "Don't worry; you're fine."

Well now we know that **if your waist-to-hip ratio is bad, you are in danger, even if your weight is a healthy average.**

That's different from what you have learned over the years, I'm sure. But you need to let it sink in. I want you to live much longer than average and now I can no longer say just keep your weight in trim.

I have to say keep that waistline inside your hipline! To be very exact (if you have a calculator handy), your risk can be assessed as follows:

MEN	**WOMEN**
0.95 or less (low)	0.80 or less (low)
0.96- 1.0 (moderate risk)	0.81- 0.85 (moderate risk)
over 1.0 (high)	over 0.85 (high)

[SOURCE: Canoy D, Boekholdt SM, Wareham N, et al. Body fat distribution and risk of coronary heart disease in men and women in the European Prospective Investigation Into Cancer and Nutrition in Norfolk Cohort. A population-based prospective study. *Circulation* 2007; DOI: 10.1161/CIRCULATIONAHA.106.673756. Available at: http://www.circ.ahajournals.org.]

BEWARE OF THOSE BATHROOM SCALES - THEY LIE!

A recent trip to a doctor to have my ears syringed resulted in a routine weighing on a balance scale—you know, the kind where you are balanced against weights that slide along a beam. These are accurate to within 0.5% or less.

This is very different from the spring-loaded bathroom scales. As metal springs age, they go stiffer. What does that mean? They stretch more reluctantly and won't let the needle on the dial get right around to your true weight.

In other words, they lie and tell you that you are lighter than you really are.

I found with a shock I was 12 pounds heavier than I thought (hastily instigated more time in the gym and changed my evening diet routine).

So, let me warn you of this. You probably weigh more than you think you do. Get a proper weight on a balance scale (make sure the doctor's office has the right scales—the nurse will probably do it for you for no cost). Check this against your bathroom scales on the same day and if the difference is more than 5 or 6 lbs, junk them.

Junk them anyway after about two years max.

Simple spring-loaded bathroom scales are fine for following change of weight, such as when you are determinedly dieting. But you must still check your true weight from time to time.

In any case, know that your weight is NOT the most critical health measure. Muscle weighs more than fat so you can go heavier as you exercise and replace fat with muscle.

What's the most important measure for health? Waist-to-hip ratio. Measure yourself round the widest part of your abdomen (let it out, no cheating!) Then do the same round your hips. Men should be 1:1 maximum (waist same as hips). Women should be 0.85 (waist at least 1- 2 inches LESS than the hips).

This supersedes the old discredited measure of body mass index (Michael Jordan, a superb athlete, is obese according to BMI).

And gals, waist to hip is what attracts guys the most!

IF YOU WANT LASTING WEIGHT LOSS KEEP A FOOD DIARY

If you want to lose weight, you need to eat less - and if you want to eat less, it helps to write it down.

When researchers studied the eating behaviors of female dieters, they found that the most important tool linked to successful weight loss was a pen and notebook. It's called a "food diary."

Women who kept food journals and consistently wrote down the foods they ate lost more weight than women who didn't.

What's more, researchers found that skipping meals and eating out frequently, especially at lunch, led to less weight loss.

That's according to a study that appeared in the latest issue of the *Journal of the Academy of Nutrition and Dietetics*.

Over the course of a year, the women followed a restricted-calorie diet with the goal of achieving a 10% reduction in weight in six months. Half the women were put on an exercise program and the other half were not.

All the participants were asked to record the foods they ate daily in seven-day diaries provided weekly by dietician counselors.

At the end of the year, both the diet-alone and diet-and-exercise groups had lost an average of 10% of their starting weight.

But… here's the kicker: women who consistently filled out a food journal lost about 6 pounds more than those who didn't.

Those who skipped meals lost an average of 8 fewer pounds than those who didn't.

Women who ate in restaurants at lunch at least once a week lost an average of 5 pounds less than those who ate out less.

Why should keeping a food journal help? Seems straightforward: it helps to prevent mindless eating.

This isn't a one-off study, either: a 2008 study found that dieters who kept food diaries at least six days a week lost twice as much weight as those who kept the journals one day a week or less.

Most experts recommend writing down the foods you eat as soon as you eat them, rather than waiting until the end of the day.

[SOURCE: Kong, A. *Journal of the Academy of Nutrition and Dietetics*, July 13, 2012]

SECTION 7

HIDDEN CAUSES OF ALLERGIES & HOW TO GET ALLERGY RELIEF

Sidebar

FOOD ALLERGY: WHAT'S ALL THE FUSS?

MECHANISMS OF ALLERGY – CHEMICAL SENSITIVITY

TOTAL BODY LOAD – THE MOST IMPORTANT OF ALL HEALING PRINCIPLES

SYMPTOMS OF ALLERGY

CHEMICAL CLEAN UP - CHEMICAL INTOLERANCE & HYPERSENSITIVITY

TREATMENT FOR ALLERGIES

It's a discovery and health secret that I put on a par with anesthetics and antibiotics, not for the measure of it, but just the sheer NUMBERS of people it affects.

It's so common that it virtually affects everyone! It's the unsuspected enemy that gets missed in the field of health and nutrition.

I am sure you are thinking, what can this possibly be?

It is actually a **"hidden food allergy."**

It's not a normal food allergy, like the drama of a peanut allergy emergency that threatens lives. By "hidden" I mean it's buried deep and almost impossible to detect, unless you know the secret code I will teach you.

I'm talking about the everyday foods you eat that are making you sick in countless ways. Even foods that are good for you!

This "hidden or masked allergy" effect also underpins many serious diseases, such as diabetes, even cancer, psychological disorders, earning, and behavior problems… raw fruits and vegetables

In fact, the sheer number of effects evening speeding up the aging process is what has prevented a proper understanding and acknowledgement of the hidden allergy effect.

Most doctors can't believe it.

Not Just a Food Allergy…

In modern times, we think beyond just food allergy, into the realm of genetic food incompatibility (DNA disruptions).

I'm talking about specific and unique food reactions. If it attacks your brain you could get a migraine; if it attacks your skin, you could get a rash; and so on…

It's a sort of secret "food code," which I am willing to share with you. It's unique to you and every other person. Keep reading and I will show you to unlock this code.

FOOD ALLERGY: WHAT'S ALL THE FUSS?

I almost invariably recommend that a patient with a high score from the inventory of symptoms start by **trying to any identify food allergies and intolerances**.

This is not to say that everything is a food allergy. But diet adjustments are a great place to start because there is usually some kind of beneficial result and they are relatively easy to do. If you can feel much better just avoiding, say, milk or wheat, that is far easier than battling against multiple environmental shocks and stressors.

The reason is simple if you understand the overload principle: avoiding one stressor, especially if it is an important one, may free your body defenses up enough so that it can cope with the rest, without your help!

Even if you feel no better after eliminating certain foods, that doesn't mean that you don't have allergies, but it may mean that you have simultaneous non-food or, as we term them, environmental allergies.

Even that may not be the whole story. You may have concomitant vitamin and mineral deficiencies, hormone disorders, and disturbed bowel bacteria, but more of that in later chapters.

Symptoms Suggesting Food Allergy
- Bloating and flatulence
- Food binges
- Food cravings
- Overweight, underweight or wildly fluctuating weight (gain a few pounds in a day)
- Symptoms actually come on while eating
- Symptoms after food (falling asleep, chills, sudden rapid heartbeat)
- Feeling unwell without food (food addiction)
- Feeling tired, crabby or very lethargic on waking (usually due to addiction maladaptation)

The last may seem strange: most everybody wakes up feeling bad, *don't they*?

True, but as I revealed in my first book about food allergies, that's because almost everyone is suffering the addiction effects of allergy (*The Food Allergy Plan*, Unwins, London, 1985 and CRCS, Reno, 1985).

Think about this: by the time we wake in the morning, we may not have eaten for 10 to 14 hours; that's more than enough time to set up withdrawal symptoms. With breakfast, we get our first "fix" of wheat, sugar, caffeine, or whatever and the symptoms start to clear right away. *You don't believe me?*

Wait until you have followed the instruction in this section and you'll see the truth of what I say.

The Secret of Food Allergy Test Dieting
The secret of successful identification of food allergies is to give up sufficient foods to be able to feel well, then to re-introduce these foods one at a time, so that detecting a reaction is relatively easy.

We call this elimination and challenge dieting.

It rarely works to give up just one food at a time because anyone who is ill is almost certain to have more than one allergy. If it was simply one major allergen, the person would have spotted it eventually, as indeed some lucky people do. Dr. Doris Rapp of New York coined an instructive term: the *"eight nails in the shoe trap."*

She points out that if you have eight nails sticking out in your shoe, and then pull just one of these nails, you will still not be comfortable – because of the other seven. It can be the same with multiple allergies. You have to work at it just that little bit harder.

Make no mistake; elimination diets can be tough; *they should be*. But it is important to remember that I am talking here of a trial diet, an experimental procedure. You do not need to stay on a tough diet long-term; indeed you are specifically cautioned not to do so, otherwise you run into problems caused by inadequate nutritional sources.

The purpose of the strict diet is to isolate the culprits. Once you know these, you can eat most anything else. This means you shift into a maintenance diet, solely avoiding these offending foods, something you stay on for months or years. Almost anyone who feels much better by avoiding one or two foods has the will power to continue; the rewards are high!

Please don't mix up these two grades of diet. You'll suffer needlessly.

Three-Tiered Allergy Diet Plan
The rest of this section is given over to discussing three-tiered dieting, from which you can choose the most appropriate approach for you or your family.

In following the instructions, it is vital that in all cases you also avoid manufactured foods. This is not because food additives are a common problem (they are surprisingly uncommon, in fact) but because manufactured foods contain numerous foodstuffs that are hidden and disguised, such as corn starch, wheat, sugar, egg, and other notable allergens. Don't trust to labeling, it may throw off the whole test. Just eat only fresh whole versions of the foods allowed, in other words nothing from tins, packets, bottles, or jars. Don't even trust to foods cooked and packages by supermarkets and stores.

It may cost you the results you are looking for.

Special note: people often ask me about using organic foods in an elimination diet. The answer is YES, it is always better to eat organic, if you can. But that may not be easy and it is not really necessary. Almost everyone will feel better by eating ordinary commercial food supplies, providing they are fresh. Only if you are very sensitive or very poorly, is it recommended that you go the whole nine yards and eat fully organic foods.

A Word About Drugs
Drug allergies are not rare and it may be wise to discontinue medications that are unnecessary. However, certain drugs are essential and should not be stopped, such as anti-epileptics, some cardiac drugs (such as digoxin), insulin and thyroxin. Some medications, such as cortisone derivatives, need to be phased out gradually.

To be certain, it is better to discuss the implications with your doctor and ask his or her advice on stopping your treatment. Don't be put off by the high-handedness that some doctors, sadly, are prone to when their prescriptions are questioned. You are entitled to know the effect of any drug you are taking and also precisely why you are taking it, and it may be that your doctor will not even understand the workings and side effects of drugs being used.

The key question that you want answered is, *'Will I come to harm if I stop this drug?'*

Nine times out of ten the answer is, "No."

Don't forget, tobacco is a drug. You must **stop smoking** if you are serious about getting well.

Now, let's start with the easiest level diet as an entry.

An Easy Elimination Diet (14-21 days)

It is logical to start by eliminating only the common likely food allergies. This leaves plenty of foods to eat and you should not find this diet too onerous. It is especially suitable for a child and consists basically of fresh meat, fish, fruit and vegetables, with juice and water to drink. We call it the "Stone-Age" or "Caveman" diet. (my first nickname with the UK press was "The Stone Age Doctor"; I used to joke this was an unfair exaggeration, I had only a few grey hairs at the time!).

FOODS YOU ARE ALLOWED TO EAT:

- Any meat (not processed or smoked)
- Any vegetables (fresh or frozen, not tinned)
- Any fruit, except the citrus family (lemon etc.)
- Any fish (not processed or smoked)
- Quinoa (grain substitute)
- All fresh unsweetened fruit juices, except citrus
- Herb teas (careful: some contain citrus peel)
- Spring water, preferably bottled in glass
- Fresh whole herbs
- Salt and pepper to taste

FOODS YOU ARE **NOT** ALLOWED TO EAT:

- No stimulant drinks – no tea, coffee, or alcohol
- No sugar, honey, additives, or sweeteners
- No grains: absolutely no wheat, corn, rye, rice, barley, oats, or millet. That means no bread, cakes, muffins, biscuits, granola, pastry, flour, or farina
- No milk or dairy produce: no skimmed milk, cream, butter, margarines, or spreads, not even goat's milk
- NO MANUFACTURED FOOD: nothing from tins, packets, bottles or jars. If somebody labeled it, they likely added to it.

Here are some important points to keep in mind:

It is vital to understand that you must not cheat on this or any other exclusion diet. This is not a slimming diet, where you can sneak a piece of chocolate cake and still lose weight. Remember that it takes several days for food to clear your bowel and eating it as little as twice a week will prevent you clearing it from your system. If you do slip up, you will need to extend the avoidance period for several more days. Later on, when the detective work is complete, the occasional indiscretion won't matter. In the meantime… follow the instructions exactly.

Don't forget about addictions. It is quite likely that you will get withdrawal symptoms during the first few days. This is good news because it means you have given up something important. Usually the effects are mild and amount to nothing more than feeling irritable, tired, or perhaps having a headache, but be warned - it could put you in bed for a couple of days. I have seen wheat "cold turkey" that was just as grim as narcotics.

Please also note that it is possible to be allergic even to the allowed foods - they are chosen simply because reaction to them is less common. If you are in this minority, you might even feel worse on this diet, but at least it proves you have a food allergy. In that case, try eliminating, also, the foods you are eating more of (potato is a common offender) and see if you then begin to improve If not, you should switch to the Eight Foods Diet, or a fast as described below.

While on the elimination diet, try to avoid hanging on to a few favorite foods and eating only those. You must eat with variety, otherwise you will risk creating reactions to the foods you are eating repeatedly. It is senseless to go on with old habits. The whole point of exclusion dieting is to make you change what you are doing - it could be making you ill.

Don't worry about special recipes or substitutes at this stage. By the time you have fried, baked, steamed and grilled everything once, the two weeks will almost have passed! If, in the long term, it transpires that you need to keep off a food, then you can begin searching for an alternative.

Patients usually ask: What about my vitamin and mineral supplements while on an elimination diet, do I need to take those? The answer is NO. Most vitamin and mineral tablets contain hidden food ingredients, such as cornstarch.

Even those that say "allergy-free" formulas are misleading. They may not be made up with common allergens, such as wheat, corn, or soya derivatives; but nevertheless, vegetable ingredients are present, such as rice polishings and potato starch. To call this "allergy-safe," or even hypoallergenic, is in my view dishonest.

Don't take the risk, you won't come to any harm without supplements for a short period.

This leads on to another major **Dr. Scott-Mumby Rule**:

The biggest and commonest health hazard by far today is not what you are lacking that you should be having, but what you are already taking that you shouldn't! In other words, giving up allergens, toxic or overload items has far more dramatic results in terms of health recovery than supplementing stuff you are deficient in.

How Did You Get On?
If you felt a whole lot better, you can skip the on food challenge testing.

DO NOT, simply because you do not improve or feel any different, make the erroneous assumption that you could not then be allergic to milk, wheat, or other banned foods. Remember the eight nails in the shoe? This would be a serious mistake, which could bar your road to recovery. You might like to try an alternative exclusion diet. Several are suggested here.

You can, in any case, carry out useful challenge tests, taking a careful note of what happens when you re-introduce a food. Careful! You do not want to hammer a pointed nail back in that shoe!

The Eight Foods Diet (7-14 days)

Not as severe as a fast but tougher than the previous regime, is what can be called the "Few Foods Diet"; I prefer to use an eight-food plan. Obviously it is more likely to succeed than the previous plan, since you are giving up more foods. Any determined adult could cope with it, but on no account should you subject a child to this diet without his, or her, full and voluntary cooperation. It could produce a severe emotional trauma otherwise (factually, there is rarely a problem -- most children don't want to be ill and will assist you, providing they understand what you are trying to do).

The basic idea is to produce one or two relatively safe foods for each different category we eat. Everyday foods are avoided, since these include the common allergens. Thus we would choose fruits such as mango and papaya, not apple and banana; flesh such as duck and rabbit, not beef and pork; quail and ostrich, not chicken. The diet below contains my suggestions. You can vary it somewhat according to what is available to you locally.

The Few Foods Diet

In addition to the stipulated foods, you are allowed salt to taste but not pepper, spring water, but not herb teas or juices. Even herbs and pepper must be challenged correctly on introduction. Note that neither of the starch foods is in the grains family.

The main problem with such a restricted plan is boredom. However, there is enough variety here for adequate nourishment over the suggested period of 7 to 10 days, provided you eat a balance of all eight foods. Exotic fruits can be expensive, but you won't need to eat them for long and, in any case, few people would deny that feeling well is worth any expense.

- **Meat, protein**
  - Rabbit, venison
  - Fowl
  - Ostrich or quail
- **Fruit**
  - Mango, kiwi fruit
- **Vegetables**
  - Spinach, turnip
- **Starch**
  - Buckwheat, quinoa

The chances are that, on a diet like this, you will feel well within a week, but for some conditions, such as eczema and arthritis, you will need to allow a little longer. Be prepared to go the full 10 days before deciding that it isn't working.

A variation of this diet is the exotic food diet. Don't worry how many foods you can round up to eat, choose as many as you can find; just make sure they are all unusual, you personally have never eaten them, and they are not related to any common food category. You will need to learn about food families (groups of foodstuffs that are related).

The Fast (5-7 days)

Although a fast is the ultimate approach in tracking down hidden food allergies, I don't recommend it lightly. It is quick (fast!), inexpensive, and an absolute yes-no statement on whether your illness really is caused by food allergy. Although it can be tough at first, by the morning of the fifth day you can expect to feel wonderful! That's why fasting is popular as a religious exercise and why sometimes people with a severe attack of gastro-enteritis, who expel almost all the food content of the bowel by diarrhea and vomiting, are suddenly "cured" of some other health condition.

The real problem is that sometimes it can then be difficult to get back on to any safe foods. Everything is unmasked at once and the patient seems to react to everything he or she tries to eat. This can cause great distress.

Undertake a fast only if you are very determined or you still suspect food allergy and the other two approaches have failed.

Fasting is emphatically not suitable for certain categories of patients:

- Pregnant women
- Children
- Diabetics
- Epileptics
- Anyone seriously weakened or debilitated by chronic illness
- Anyone who has been subject to severe emotional disturbance (especially those prone to violent outbursts, or those who have tried to commit suicide)

The fast itself is simple enough - just don't eat for four or five days. You must stop smoking. Drink only bottled spring water. The whole point is to empty your bowels entirely of foodstuffs. Thus, if you have any tendency to constipation, take Epsom salts to begin with. If in doubt try an enema! Otherwise the effort may be wasted.

It may help to do what I call a grape-day step-down. This means eating grapes only for a day, as an easy-in step towards fasting.

Special note: A variation, which I call the 'half fast', is to eat only two foods, such as lamb and pears. This means taking a gamble that neither lamb nor pears are allergenic, and it is not as sure-fire as the fast proper. It is permissible to carry this out for seven days, but on no account go on for longer than this.

Food Challenge Testing
As soon as you feel well on an elimination regime, you can begin testing, although you must not do so before the four-day unmasking period has elapsed. Allow longer if you have been constipated.

Of course, you may never improve on an elimination diet. The problem may be something else, not a food. In that case, when three weeks (maximum) have elapsed on the simple elimination diet, two weeks on the Eight Foods Diet, or seven days on a fast, then you must begin re-introducing foods. This is vital. It is not enough to feel well on a very restricted diet; we want to know why. What are the culprits? These are the foods you must avoid long-term, not all those which are banned at the beginning.

Even if you don't feel well, as already pointed out, this does not prove you have no allergies amongst the foods you gave up. Test the foods as you re-introduce them, anyway - you may be in for a surprise

My recommended procedure is as follows, except for those coming off a fast:

Eat a substantial helping of the food, preferably on its own for the first exposure. Lunch is the ideal meal for this.

Choose only whole, single foods, not mixtures and recipes. Try to get supplies that have not been chemically treated in any way.

Wait several hours to see if there is an immediate reaction, and if not, eat some more of the food along with a typical ordinary evening meal.

You may eat a third or fourth portion if you want, to be sure.

Take your resting pulse (sit still for two minutes) before, and several times during the first 90 minutes alter the first exposure to the food. A rise of ten or more beats in the RESTING pulse is a fairly reliable sign of an allergy. However no change in the pulse does not mean the food is safe, unless symptoms are absent also.

Alkali Salts

If you do experience an unpleasant reaction, take Epsom salts. Also, alkali salts (a mixture of two parts sodium bicarbonate to one part potassium bicarbonate: one teaspoonful in a few ounces of lukewarm water) should help. Discontinue further tests until symptoms have abated once more. This is very important, as you cannot properly test when symptoms are already present; you are looking for foods that trigger symptoms.

Using the above approach, you should be able to reliably test one food a day, minimum. Go rapidly if all is well, because the longer you stay off a food, the more the allergy (if there is one) will tend to die down and you may miss it.

Occasionally, patients experience a "buildup" that causes confusion and sometimes failure Suspect this if you felt better on an exclusion diet, but you gradually became ill again when re-introducing foods, and can't really say why. Perhaps there were no noticeable reactions.

In that case, eliminate all the foods you have re-introduced until your symptoms clear again, then re-introduce them more slowly. This time, eat the foods steadily, several times a day for three to four days before making up your mind. It is unlikely that one will slip the net with this approach.

Once you have accepted a food as safe, of course you must then stop eating it so frequently, otherwise it may become an allergy. Eat it once a day at most - only every four days when you have enough 'safe' foods to accomplish this.

Special Instructions for Those Coming off a Fast…

Begin only with exotic foods, which you don't normally eat; do not be tempted to grab for that coffee or cake! The last thing you want to happen is to get a reaction when beginning to re-introduce foods – it will mean you cannot carry on adding foods until the symptoms settle down once again.

Instead, for the first few days, you want to build up a minimum range of "safe" foods that you can fall back on. Papaya, rabbit, artichoke, and dogfish are the kind of thing to aim for - do the best you can with what is available, depending to your resources.

The other important point is that you cannot afford the luxury of bringing in one new food a day: you need to go faster than this. When avoided even for as little as two weeks, a cyclical food allergy can die down and you may miss the proof of allergy you are looking for. It is possible to test two or even three foods a day when coming off a fast. Pay particular attention to the pulse rate before and after each test meal and keep notes. It is important to grasp that some symptoms, even if not very striking, usually occur within the first 60 minutes when coming off a fast. You need to be alert to this, or you will miss items and fail to improve without understanding why.

If the worst happens and you are ill by the end of the day and can't say why, condemn all that day's new foods.

The buildup of foods is cumulative: that is, you start with Food A. If it is OK then the next meal is Food A + Food B, then A + B + C and so on. An example table of foods tests might be:

days 1-4	no food
day 5	**breakfast** - poached salmon **lunch** - mango (plus salmon) **dinner** - steamed spinach (plus salmon and mango)
day 6	**breakfast** - baked pheasant, quail or partridge + day 5 **lunch** - kiwi fruit + day 5 **dinner** - steamed marrow or zucchini (courgette) + day 5
day 7	**breakfast** - lamb chop (plus any of the above) + days 5, 6 **lunch** - baked potato (do not eat the skin) + days 5, 6 **dinner** - banana + days 5, 6

Grape is not allowed on Day 5 if you used a grape-day step-down.

All safe foods are kept up after an allergic reaction. Therefore, if Food F causes a reaction, while you are waiting for it to clear up, you can go on eating foods A-E, until symptoms clear.

Within a few days, you should have plenty to eat, albeit monotonous. From then on, you can proceed as for those on elimination diets if you wish.

Your Personal Exclusion Program
Whichever program you chose, once you have carried out the challenge tests you will have a list of items that you are intolerant of. You must now avoid these, if you are serious about your health. You have, in effect, designed your own personal diet plan for health. Use it as something you return to in times of trouble or stress, a safe platform.

There should be no rush to try and re-introduce any of these items, if at all. Design your living and eating plan without them, long-term. However, the good news is that allergies do settle down, sometimes quite rapidly, especially if you pay attention to everything else I have explained in this book. If you develop and practice a newer, safer ecological lifestyle, you may have surprisingly little further trouble. You may feel better than you have felt in years. Many patients feel and act younger, so much so that friends and relatives often comment. I noticed this over 30 years ago and that is one of the reasons I now find myself part of the anti-aging movement.

Another **Dr. Scott-Mumby maxim**: a low-allergy diet is the finest possible cosmetic agent for a woman's skin! She glows!

If you find your personal diet plan oppressive because you discovered quite a few reacting foods, then consider desensitization.

Food Diary
It is a good idea to keep a food diary during your experiments with food. Write down everything you eat at each meal, or between meals, and also mark in any symptoms, that you experience, with the time of onset in relation to meals. It is often possible to spot a pattern that recurs time and time again but which is not evident when relying only on short-term memory.

Warning: a food diary does tend to make you very conscious of food, which is probably a good thing in the short term. However, taking the long view, try to avoid the exercise making you too introverted about feelings and symptoms, otherwise it can start becoming an obsession. Many allergy patients become so consumed by anxiety about what they are eating that they cannot eat or socialize normally. Food allergy investigations, as described here, are merely a tool, not an end, and should not become a way of life, otherwise family and friends will feel excluded and that, in turn, leads to rejection.

Many "amateur" gung-ho food allergy books actually tend to create this major social incompetence, because the authors do not have sufficient experience to be aware of the dangers (and likely because they too are obsessive). Make no mistake, food allergy restrictions can ruin relationships and break up marriages, if they are taken to extremes, as many know to their cost. I do not automatically take the patient's side, but I sympathize with both points of view (because ultimately I see this as in the patient's broader interests).

Eating can become a psychological burden on the patient and an intolerable nuisance to family and friends, if you go too far. True health does not mean isolation from society, it means full social well-being included in the deal.

The food diary is merely a tool and should be discontinued as soon as practicable.

SPECIAL NOTE: A fetus in the womb may have food allergies! Crazy as it sounds, I learned long ago that certain babies in the womb are already hyperactive. They show it by kicking a great deal and being restless at times, but not continuously. Mother may carry out allergy and sensitivity testing indirectly. She goes on an elimination diet; if the baby settles down, this is good evidence your unborn child will be hyperactive soon after birth if you do not take steps to prevent it.

You can carry out food challenge testing, exactly as here described, keeping a food diary, and work out which foods upset your baby and cause restless kicking. You will have more restful nights before birth and many more happy days after the birth, if you take this seriously. Of course, all babies should kick vigorously. That's their way of saying "Hello!" Only if it becomes excessive or seems to be triggered after meals should you suspect food allergy *in utero*.

Alternative Allergy Exclusion Diets
If the simple exclusion diet has not worked, you might like to consider alternative eliminations.

For example, you could try following a meat-free diet. Some people do feel better as vegetarians, certainly; but probably more feel ill because of the high incidence of grain and dairy allergies, as grains and dairy products are staple foods for vegetarians.

Organic Food
Some people (only a few) are better avoiding food treated with chemicals. A diet avoiding this sort of commercial produce is called "organic." It is easier nowadays to follow such an eating regime than formerly. Try it if you have reason to suspect you may be reacting to chemicals, but

don't go overboard; many people are convinced that pesticides on food make them ill but fail to detect them when challenged double-blind.

Organic food suppliers belong to various bodies to help promote themselves and their ideas. Try to make contact with these organizations and find out about your local suppliers. The Henry Doubleday Research organization is a good place to start (see the Useful Addresses section). They have been pioneers in organic farming methods for decades. They can usually supply a list of vendors. The Soil Association even goes so far as to vet produce showing the label "organic." Look for their sign of approval but be warned: this is not a legal requirement and anyone can call their wares "organic," whether they have used chemicals or not.

Your local health food shop should also be able to help find locally-grown supplies.

To reduce your pesticide intake, avoid the 10 "dirtiest" foods from the Environmental Working Group's Shopper's Guide to Pesticides in Produce

Eating the 12 most contaminated fruits and vegetables will expose a person to about 15 pesticides a day, on average. Eating the 12 least contaminated will expose a person to fewer than two pesticides a day.

"Federal produce tests tell us that some fruits and vegetables are so likely to be contaminated with pesticides that you should always buy them organic," said Richard Wiles, EWG's senior vice president. "Others are so consistently clean that you can eat them with less concern. With the Shopper's Guide in your pocket, it's easy to tell which is which."

The "Dirty Dozen" (starting with the worst)
- peaches
- apples
- sweet bell peppers
- celery
- nectarines
- strawberries
- cherries
- pears
- grapes (imported)
- spinach
- lettuce
- potatoes

The "Cleanest 12" (starting with the best)
- onions
- avocados
- sweet corn (frozen)
- pineapples
- mangoes
- asparagus
- sweet peas (frozen)
- kiwi fruit
- bananas
- cabbage
- broccoli

- papaya

Nut- and Pip-Free

A very useful exclusion diet is the nut- and pip-free diet. This is a wide group of foods and includes a number of common allergens. Some members of this group can come as a surprise: for example, coffee is a nut.

It is an ambitious diet: it is recommended that you don't go on it until you have established a number of alternative safe foods, such as rice, rye, millet or quinoa.

Otherwise you may find yourself with very little to eat. The following foods must be strictly avoided for a short test period:

- Tomatoes, sauce, purees
- Apples, pears, plums, damsons, cherries, apricots, peaches
- Strawberries, raspberries, gooseberries, blackcurrants
- Oranges, lemons, other citrus fruits, marmalade and all fruit juices, squash, fruit-flavored drinks
- All varieties of fizzy drinks, including cola
- Jellies, instant puddings
- Chocolate, cocoa, coffee, and coffee "creamers"
- Grapes, sultanas, raisins, currants, prunes, figs, dates
- Nuts, coconut, marzipan, macaroons
- Peas, beans, lentils, soya, peanuts
- Melon, cucumber, marrow
- Spices, pepper, mustard, curry
- Cooking oils of all kinds and soft margarines
- All herbs (including mint)
- Bananas, pineapple

Gluten-Free

Probably the oldest established allergy to food is hypersensitivity to gluten. It is a sticky protein that is found in wheat, rye, oats, and barley and gives rise to the special gluey cooking texture these foods have.

The result of a gluten allergy used to be a very serious wasting condition known as celiac disease or sprue; the patient simply starved with malnutrition, despite eating adequately. It was eventually discovered that gluten allergy was damaging the lining of the intestine so that it couldn't perform as it should. This meant that food was not being digested and absorbed properly.

Another condition known to have a definite connection width gluten sensitivity is dermatitis herpetiformis. This is a blistering, intensely itchy

PHYSICAL FACTORS	Heat Cold Electromagnetic radiation Oxidative stress
CHEMICAL FACTORS	Pollution Alcohol Recreation drugs Medicines
BIOLOGICAL FACTORS	Micro-organisms (virus, bacteria, parasites) Endocrine dysfunction Allergy Nutritional deficiency Fatigue
PSYCHOLOGICAL FACTORS	Stress Work load Personality disorder

rash that usually affects the outer surface of the elbows, buttocks, and knees but can occur on any part of the body.

Personally, I think that a lot of the people who get well on a gluten-free diet do so because they are wheat-allergic. They can tolerate rye, oats, or barley with impunity, so gluten cannot be the offender.

Try a gluten-free diet if you are suspicious, but you must be prepared to stick at it for a minimum of six to eight weeks to be sure of feeling any benefit.

Special Dieting Cases

For most people, the problems of exclusion diets are few. Withdrawal symptoms, extra expense, or the sloth encountered in changing the habits of a lifetime are the main difficulties. However, two situations require extra comment:

CHILDREN

Children have more food allergy problems than adults. Yet food is vital to them; their growth will be stunted if nutrition is inadequate. Consider the size of a newborn infant in relation to that of an adult and you will see at once the wisdom in the old adage, "You are what you eat."

Whatever dietary experiment are undertaken with children, it is therefore vital to see they get adequate substitutes. Milk is a problem food. It is by far the most common allergen in children. The important ingredient in milk, I believe, is not really calcium but vitamin D. Fish oils are a good alternative source. Iodine is also vital to prevent stunting and poor mental development. Since most of our supply comes from milk, alternative provision needs to be made for this element also. Kelp or iodized salt should suffice.

If you are faced with complex or long-term eliminations for your child, it is important to weigh him or her regularly (at least once a week) and keep a record of growth. Body size can be compared with charts showing average ranges for males and female youngsters and also percentiles for those who are clearly above or below average, showing how fast they too should be gaining weight. If weight gain is affected, you must get help or discontinue what you are doing. Almost no condition (the possible exception being retarded mental growth occurring because of a food allergy) is worth stunting your child's growth. It is better to defer treatment until the child is older.

Remember that withdrawal symptoms can be experienced by children, too. Be very tolerant for the first few days. He or she may crave favorite foods: just say "No" firmly and offer an alternative, Eventually, hunger will be on your side.

It's remarkable to watch how a youngster who is a faddy eater (a reliable sign of food allergy) suddenly finds his or her appetite and begins to eat heartily.

DIABETICS

For diabetic patients managed by drugs and diet alone, there should be little problem with an elimination diet. Those on insulin, however, must be very careful about embarking on a low-carbohydrate diet and should not do so without medical supervision.

The simplest modification of the basic exclusion diet is to eat rice as a source of carbohydrate. Quinoa is a good food in this context also, if you can obtain it. Better still is to cut down your insulin gradually and reduce your starch intake similarly – under the supervision of your doctor.

The best challenge test to perform (if you have a glucometer and can use it) is to monitor which foods increase your blood glucose. If you haven't a glucometer, just carry out the challenge tests in the normal way.

PSYCHIATRIC PATIENTS

Some care needs to be taken when the patient has pronounced mental problems; that is to say, severe enough to have been admitted to a psychiatric ward or hospital. Psychiatrists and psychologists have a pronounced blind spot when it comes to physical causes of mental illness. Many reject this possibility outright, yet doctors who practice my kind of medicine have seen many, many people helped by a simple change of diet and lifestyle. Food reactions can be so severe as to precipitate mania and psychotic delusion; this sometimes has to be seen to be believed. The common diagnosis of "depression" very often means that the patient feels miserable, due to the hidden allergy, and no one has solved the problem. That is enough to make anyone feel depressed.

Which all means that it is not only permissible but desirable to investigate any psychiatric state in this way. But caution is required: In my book Dietwise (visit: www.alternative-doctor.com/dietwise) I have referred to a young Irish patient who went on a murderous rampage when he ate certain foods. I am pleased to say that the law courts were willing to accept my evidence that this was not only possible but demonstrated it for the entire nation on prime-time TV. Obviously if this individual had been put on an elimination diet and then challenged with the danger foods, without skilled supervision, someone could have been hurt very badly or even paid with their lives.

Equally serious, is the possibility that the patient may try to injure himself or herself, or even try to commit suicide, when challenged in this way.

The best recommendation is to avoid food challenge tests but to use some other approach. I made most of my startling discoveries in the field of mind states and allergy by using Miller's Method (found in DietWise Book). Never leave such a patient unattended, even if the response appears mild at first.

MECHANISMS OF ALLERGY – CHEMICAL SENSITIVITY

In time it became obvious that **some individuals were sensitive to environmental chemicals.** It is hard to describe this as an allergy; probably the term "low-grade poisoning" would be better, since many of these chemicals would make anyone exposed to them in sufficient concentration feel ill. The problem is just that certain individuals react to smaller doses. We are all subject to a barrage of alien chemicals in our bodies (Greek word: *xenobiotics*, meaning alien to life. We have chemical pathways in our bodies designed to remove toxic substances: a process called detoxication or biotransformation.

The trouble is that these new man-made chemicals have no equivalent in nature and so we do not have the right systems in our body to fully eliminate the toxicity. In fact, in its attempts to deal with the problem the body sometimes, by mistake, actually coverts these xenobiotics into something even more toxic.[1]

It's a self-perpetuating problem, since the alien chemicals can poison the enzyme pathways that are there to remove them. The result is that sick and sensitive people get sicker and sicker. Pioneer UK psychiatrist Richard Mackarness christened these patients "chemical victims."[2]

The media used extreme phrases like "allergic to the 20th century" but there is no doubt that, for these sufferers, our modern techno-chemical society is a nightmare. The phenomenon of chemical overload and the chemical-sensitive patient is one that we have created for ourselves with our advanced lifestyle. Toxic chemicals, such as benzene, formaldehyde, methacrylate, tetrachloroethylene, toluene, zylene, naphthalene, phthalates, and styrene, can come from many sources in the home (this particular list of substances are all given off by new carpets). Then there are more chemicals at work; some are recognized occupational hazards and strictly controlled, but the majority are not considered "occupational": photocopy fluid, glues, plastics, paper treatments, inks, dyes, fabrics, and so on.

Then there are numerous chemicals sprayed onto or added to our food supplies, which we are constantly assured is safe.

Most doctors don't believe these low ambient levels of chemicals can make you ill. But they are grievously in error, through ignorance. First, most doctors don't know any toxicology; it's another sad case of one discipline being completely isolated from another. All toxicologists know that present ambient levels of chemicals are more than capable of making individuals ill; there are tens of thousands of scientific papers attesting to this fact.

The second major black hole in medical practitioners' knowledge is that, although they admit occupational chemical exposures and diseases to their mindset, they do not believe in home exposure. Yet repeated tests show that levels of toxic chemicals in the average home are way above those encountered at work and, in many cases, well above the legal safety limits that are imposed in the workplace.

That much ignorance causes much unnecessary suffering and may cost lives.

This problem, of course, can co-exist with other mechanisms and often does.

Indeed, multiple chemical sensitivity seems to provoke intolerance of others substances (and probably vice versa). Integrate this knowledge with reading about other ways allergies and overload cause symptoms.

References

1. Casarett and Doull's *Toxicology. Basic Science of Poisons*. Third Ed. Klaasen CD, Amdur MO, Doull J, (eds.) Macmillan, New York, 1986.

2. Mackarness R., *Chemical Victims*, Pan Books, London, 1980.

TOTAL BODY LOAD – THE MOST IMPORTANT OF ALL HEALING PRINCIPLES

Let us now introduce one of the most important of all healing principles, if not the most important: that of total body load. It is the key to all recoveries and overcoming all disease processes. No doctor really cures anything; Nature does that. All that the successful physician can do is to reduce body load to allow this process to take place. Unfortunately, modern medicine with its pharmacology arsenal often adds to the biological burden instead of relieving it.

Along with all living creatures, we are endowed with a number of key regulatory mechanisms. One can only be amazed that they rarely seem to break down, rather than being surprised and disconcerted when they do. The skin protects us from temperature variation and dehydration, the immune system wards off micro-organisms, the kidneys eliminate poison waste, the liver detoxifies an ever-increasing amount of xenobiotic chemicals, and other factors regulate the acid-base balance within the body.

Every day, every minute, trouble is nipped in the bud before it gets started and we remain unaware of what is taking place: we feel OK. It is only when the defenses are overworked that we actually experience any health problems at all. By the time we are aware of a symptom, any symptom, the defenses have already broken down and matters are really quite serious.

Overload
Overloading the system is thus asking for trouble.

The commonly used metaphor image for the overload phenomenon is that of the overflowing barrel. If we imagine the barrel to be the body's ability to cope with exterior stressors and the moment of overflow to be the onset of symptoms, then it is obvious that anything that adds to the liquid in the barrel will potentially precipitate disease.

The actual overload process isn't specific. Any one of a number of etiological factors could cause it to occur, such as an allergy, lack of sleep, poor nutrition, a sudden shock, overwork, stress, or an acute viral episode. It may seem superfluous to point out that several of these factors can work in combination, bringing an almost infinite diversity of symptom and disease possibilities. Mental breakdown, heart disease, ulcers and cancer are just some of the possibilities. There are many ways to overload – the table below summarizes most of these. A mere glance will tell you that this list is also a summary of clinical ecology to date.

A word of warning: Much confusion can result from the fact that the last overload factor introduced may seem to be the (only) one that causes symptoms. This is very misleading. One stressor alone is unlikely to overwhelm the body's considerable defense resources. It is a cumulative thing, so an individual may be living an entirely unhealthy lifestyle, eating and drinking stress foods, not taking adequate rest, feeling disoriented and depressed due to brain allergies and then, when made redundant at work, suddenly "flips," as people say, and guns down a bunch of innocent people in the neighborhood.

Much may be made in court of this person's unhappy reaction to the fact that his wife just walked out. But it is not the cause of the violent outburst, it is the last overload factor to operate against this person's ability to balance and cope with life. Other factors may have been operative for years: unhappy childhood, financial stresses, poor diet, hypoglycemia, a wheat allergy that makes him feel aggressive, lack of magnesium (which soothes and calms), a smoldering virus that makes him feel ill most days, and toxic chemical overload that spaces him out, like a Mickey Finn. Looked at in this light, mental rage is only one aspect of a much greater situation of compounded overload.

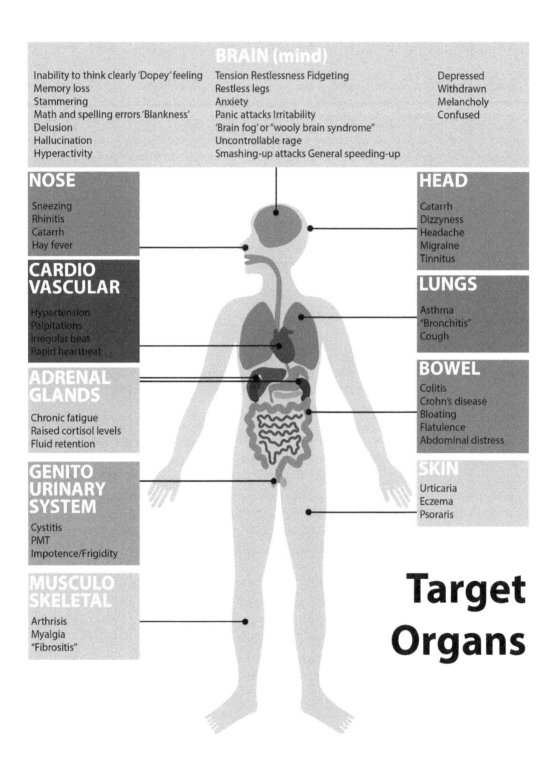

Target Organs

Reducing the Load

The opposite side of the equation works just as effectively and can be turned to good use by a physician. Any legitimate means of reducing body load helps, directly or indirectly, with any illness: better nutrition will aid the fight against cancer; clearing up hidden infections such as *Candida* will reduce PMT; eliminating hairsprays and perfumes may improve catarrh (even though dust may be the main cause); stopping smoking aids fertility and moving away from geopathic stress will help alleviate almost any disease process. Eating fewer stress foods definitely helps. Stress foods include allergenic and difficult-to-tolerate foods, refined carbohydrates, and food additives (chemical burden).

I am famous, or perhaps I should say notorious, for saying on the BBC that even a divorce might help your allergy problem!

Now you may understand why you can eat a food you are normally allergic to while on holiday (where your mental stress and, probably, the amount of chemical pollution is far less) with no ill effects but why, when you are upset, all your food cravings return with a vengeance!

If you understand overload and work to avoid it, this very important principle will serve you well. I believe emphatically in Hippocrates' key holistic health principle: that we must all take responsibility for our own health and strive to maintain balance, avoiding the risk of overload.

SYMPTOMS OF ALLERGY

Probably no recent development in the study of allergy has caused more confusion than the recognition of the multiplicity of symptoms it can produce.

No doubt this has hampered progress, since the traditional medical view of patients with many and variable symptoms has always been that they were somehow neurotic and "putting it all on."

This dismissive tendency is made worse if the patient suffers psychological disturbances, yet few doctors have ever thought to question whether such personality changes could also be caused by an allergy. Even if they were not, if you had a chronic disease or symptoms that came and went in a baffling way – headache one week, sore throat the next, diarrhea the next, and so on – wouldn't you expect to feel bad mentally? Some doctors now like to use the term "pseudo-food allergy syndrome," which does not help patients at all. One of the sacred texts of this disagreeable trend appeared in The Lancet in an article by D. J. Pearson, K. J. N. Rix and S. J. Bentley entitled "Food Allergy: How Much Is in the Mind?" (*Lancet* i: 1259-61, 1983).

The trouble is, there researchers made no allowance for the fact that their tests might be at fault and assumed, because they got no reaction, that the patient was deluded (their tests were the equivalent of evincing the effect of eating a beef steak by allowing the patient only two capsules of beef). This is not to say that there are no neurotic individuals whose symptoms are an attempt to win sympathy from a world they find too hostile; merely that such people are in a small minority.

How do such changeable and mysterious symptoms come about? The modern allergist thinks in terms of **target organs** or shock organs.

The concept is really very simple: an allergic reaction is, of course, a manifestation of the whole person, but some part of the body, or a particular organ (for reasons which are not clear) receives more of the trauma than the rest. Symptoms will depend largely on the function of this organ.

Five Key Symptoms of Allergy

The range of potential symptoms caused by an allergy is vast. Nevertheless, Dr. Richard Mackarness gives five key symptoms that point the way to allergic illness and that have special importance. He believes that, without one of the following symptoms, diagnosis is unlikely:

- Over or underweight, or fluctuating weight
- Persistent fatigue that isn't help by rest
- Occasional swellings around the eyes, hands, abdomen, ankles, etc.
- Palpitations or speeded heart rate, particulary after meals
- Excessive sweating, not related to exercise

It needs mentioning that there should be no other obvious explanation for these symptoms!

Symptoms that May Be Attributable to Allergies and Maladaptation

ORGAN	COMMONLY ATTRIBUTABLE SYMPTOMS
eye	**redness, itching,** blurred vision, 'sandy' or gritty feeling in the eyes, seeing spots, heavy eyes, seeing flashing lights, dark rings under the eyes, double vision (comes and goes), unnatural 'sparkle' to the eyes, watering
ear	ringing in the ears, hearing loss, itching and redness of pinna (outer ear), recurring infections (especially if the sufferer is a child), earache
cardio-vascular	rapid or irregular pulse, chest pain, palpitations, especially after eating, tight chest, pain on exercise (angina), raised blood-pressure
lungs	tightness in chest, wwheezing, hyperventilation (over-breathing) coughing, poor respiratory function
nose, throat and mouth	metallic taste, post-nasal drip, mouth ulcers, stuffed up nose, frequent sore throats, sinusitis, stiffness of throat or tongue, sneezing
gastro-intestinal	nausea, diarrhoea, dyspepsia, constipation, variability of bowel function, abdominal bloating, flatulence, hunger pangs, acidity, pain in the stomach, abdominal distress
skin	eczema, urticaria (hives), rash that isn't eczema, excessive sweating, itching, blotches, chilblains
musculo-skeletal	swollen, painful joints, aching muscles, muscular spasm, shaking (especially on waking), cramps, fibrositis, pseudo-paralysis
genito-urinary	PMT, menstrual difficulties, frequency of urination, genital itch, bedwetting, urgency, burning urination
head	mild or moderate headache, migraine, sick headaches, solid feeling, pressure, throbbing, stiff neck, stabbing
nervous system	inability to think clearly, memory loss, 'dopey' feeling, stammering (attacks), terrible thoughts on waking, insomnia, maths and spelling errors, blankness, delusion, crabby on waking, hallucination, difficulty waking up, desire to injure self, convulsions, light-headedness, twitching
stimulated overative mental state	silliness, anxiety, intoxication, panic attacks, hyperactivity, irritability, uncontrollable rage, tenseness, restlessness, smashing-up-attacks, fidgeting, general speeding up, restless legs
depressed underactive mental state	'brain fag', depression, feeling withdrawn, lack of confidence, melancholy, low mood, unreal or depersonalized feeling, confused, tearful
other very revealing symptoms	Sudden tiredness after eating, sudden chills after eating, vertigo, abrupt changes from feeling well to unwell, feeling unwell all over

The table below lists symptoms commonly encountered with allergies and maladaptation syndrome. The list is far from complete.

It is important to say that most of the symptoms could be caused by some other illness, although several – such as sneezing attacks – are peculiar to allergies. What really matters are the spread of symptoms – the more of these you have, the more likely it is that your illness is allergic in origin.

Some are quite obvious; those denoting digestive disturbance would point particularly to a food allergy in the absence of any other pathology. Those affecting the brain show up clearly as mood changes, altered feelings, etc. Abrupt changes from being well to unwell (well one minute, sick a few hours later) are also pretty characteristic of allergic reactions.

What often surprises people are those symptoms of feeling bad first thing in the morning. This is so common that most people can't accept that it is even a disorder, never mind an allergy. It's almost considered normal to feel that way! The key is food addiction. By the time a person wakes up in the morning, he or she has often been off food for 12 to 14 hours: that's enough to start up withdrawal symptoms. He or she then has breakfast, which acts like a "fix" and symptoms start to clear. Certainly these feelings are common, but that's only because masked food allergies are very common.

Another surprise is the "four–day flu," which isn't really flu at all – it's a food allergy. Dr. Arthur Coca, a pioneer of allergy detection and treatment, said, "You don't catch colds, you eat them." He had a point: a person eats a food, symptoms are centered on the nose and muscles so he or she experiences headache, runny nose, aches and pains, may even have a temperature, but a few days later, when the food leaves the bowel, the symptoms disappear. That's too quick for the natural course of a viral disease.

CHEMICAL CLEAN UP - CHEMICAL INTOLERANCE & HYPERSENSITIVITY

We spoke a few chapters ago about a BIG topic, albeit a highly controversial one: the question of chemical "allergy" or intolerance. I am not talking here merely about chemical "pollution" in the atmosphere, but contact with substances that are common in the home and that release fumes which we breathe on a daily basis.

Some of this chemical exposure is deliberate and part of our modern living style: cosmetics, detergents, aerosols, and even medical drugs are all intentional chemical exposures. I particularly object to the concept of spoofily-named "air fresheners," when all they do is add more chemicals to the air, in an attempt to disguise existing contaminants. It is rather like taking dirty trench water to wash away stains --- "Not logical," as Mr. Spock (Leonard Nimoy, not the pediatrician) would have said.

It is surprising to most people to learn that indoor chemical pollution is often many times the allowed safety limits allowed at work. A five-year-study carried out by the US Environmental Protection Agency (EPA) found that peak concentrations of 20 toxic compounds monitored were 200-500 times higher inside some homes than those outdoors.

Formaldehyde and toluene (from paints and varnish) are good examples of dangerous indoor pollutants. Formaldehyde, given off by many home substances, from PVC to particleboard, is a known carcinogen. Toluene, released by fresh paint, dissolves brain tissue and causes permanent brain damage. There is a move to ban it in industry as a health hazard, but homes have no such protective legislation. In the di-isocyanate form (tdi = toluene di-isocyanate), released by wet varnish, it is notorious for sensitizing people to allergens. Pronounced exposure to this latter chemical has been the start of a descent into Allergy Hell for many individuals.

[SPECIAL NOTE: sometimes the products which harm us are not initially present in the product and may not appear on the label, so the danger is overlooked. For example diethanolamine (DEA), triethanolamine (TEA) and monoethanolamine (MEA) are relatively non-toxic substances added to soap and personal hygiene products. Who can object? Well, everyone should! In the presence of nitrates, which are present in many manufactured food products, these "innocent" compounds form dangerous nitrosamines. Most nitrosamines are known to be carcinogenic.]

Human Canaries

Increasing numbers of people simply cannot accommodate the everyday load of ambient chemicals and it begins to undermine their health in many unsuspected ways. In my radical 1986 book, *Allergies: What Everyone Should Know* (London, Unwins) I introduced the term "human canaries." The phrase seems to have caught on. This likens chemically sensitive people to the canaries taken down mines in olden days. If the bird fell dead, it meant that the air was dangerous and a warning to humans to get out fast. It seems to me that we have many human canaries today but few people are heeding the warnings.

Something like 6 million new chemicals have been manufactured since the 1960s, when the chemical boom got under way worldwide. Of these, upwards of 100,000 are in production or have been until recent years. We call these synthetics xenobiotics (foreign to life). This is not an idle word: it implies that our bodies do not know how to deal with these substances. Nature did not endow us with the necessary enzyme equipment to safely detox them, because they are not naturally occurring compounds. This increases their danger considerably.

In my view it is unarguable that we will all go under if we don't soon start to reduce the total chemical load in our environment. This is not merely green politics but an out-and-out survival issue. There is dirty work afoot and that, of course, means Big Business dollars getting in on the act and perverting truth. We are told we need most of this chemical junk, that pesticides save lives and help grow more crops, which we need to feed the planet, and so on. I am not in the agribusiness, I'm a doctor. My take on this is very simple and very blunt:

The word "pesticide" is a con trick. Plant and animal physiology does not recognize human value judgments, such as "useful" and "nuisance" life forms. The correct word is biocide, which means that it kills any life, not just pests.

The idea of "responsible" or "controlled use" of toxic substances and talk of "reducing" usage levels is meaningless and dishonest: chemicals in the environment persist. Last year's output is added to that of the year before, to this year's, next year's, and so on. It's cumulative.

There are already enough xenobiotic substances in our environment, working their way through the water table and ecosystem to keep us all ill for decades, even if output was curtailed tomorrow, which is a pretty unlikely event in any case.

Now that's said, let's get back to chemical sensitivity:

Arguments I have heard against this phenomenon are frankly absurd:

Many otherwise sound clinicians refuse to accept that small traces of chemical substances can make an individual ill. Yet the toxicologists, who have very precise and quantitative scientific techniques, know it and have written tens of thousands of papers on what I have termed "low-grade poisoning" – susceptible individuals who feel the ill effects at doses that are supposed to be safe in normal circumstances. Confusion may stem from the fact that it may be long-term exposure which causes the trouble, as the chemical accumulates in the tissues (especially the brain). Allegedly safe levels don't count if you are storing the toxin.

That small, simple molecules don't command an antibody response, is another ridiculous assertion. We all know that people can be highly sensitized to nickel: that's just one atom! You can't get simpler than that. But experts should know also about haptens. These are small molecules that plug into an antigen-antibody pair and excite a reaction which might not otherwise have happened.

Overload

The key to chemical intolerance of this type is the matter of individual biological variation. It is no good measuring averages or the mean when it comes down to the fact that most people are not at all average and some individuals are very far from average. Is it right to condemn and ignore individuals who are extremely poorly tolerant, or accusing them of making it up, when we know (for sure) that there are individuals equally far from average in the opposite direction, who can tolerate very large exposures apparently without harm? An enlightened and compassionate medical science must include everyone and not dismiss those who don't fit the reductionist demographic formula.

Dr. Theron Randolph, who first pioneered chemical susceptibility in a massive seminal book, *Human Ecology and Susceptibility to the Chemical Environment* (Springfield, IL, Charles C Tuttle, 1962), points to this major difference between conventional medicine and the allergy/ecology approach: the one is for the mass, the other is for the individual. He called these two approaches endogenous and exogenous medicine. It is worth tabulating the key differences.

ENDOGENOUS MEDICINE	EXOGENOUS MEDICINE
Treats the average	Treats the individual
Blames the patient	Blames the exterior causes
Symptom-oriented	Cause-oriented
Sees averages	Sees uniqueness
Over-rides nature in the cure	Seeks to enlist nature in curing
Treatment adds burden	Treatment by reducing burden

The point is that, sooner or later, everyone reaches their threshold limit and, from then on, symptoms escalate. It matters not whether we call it susceptibility or overload; the result is the same.

Suspect chemical intolerance or overloading when you develop the following signs:
- Symptoms worse in closed spaces (shopping malls, long car journeys)

- Symptoms worse on weekdays (chemicals at work)
- Symptoms better on holiday (fresh air!)
- Worse in an urban environment
- Gasoline or gloss paint gives you a headache
- Acute sense of smell to chemicals
- Sense of smell lost or it comes and goes
- You get a "lift" or liking for certain chemical odors
- Intolerant of synthetic fabrics (sneezing, skin rash, irritation)
- Others similarly ill in the home or workplace
- Illness began after moving to present location or current employment

Does the idea of a "lift" or buzz from chemicals sound crazy? Why should it? Think about glue and solvent sniffers. They do it on purpose – but just because they are too stupid to realize the dangers, that doesn't mean it is not pleasurable brain stimulation.

Note that, with exposure at work, symptoms may not begin till Tuesday or Wednesday, as the cumulative effect builds up. Similarly, symptoms may not clear by Saturday morning but could linger through till later. Yet you may get the worst reaction on Monday and Tuesday, as your body is challenged by chemicals, which have gassed out over the weekend.

Why would someone develop chemical intolerance?

I have learned of at least four reasons a person becomes chemically sensitive. Others may come to light in time:

- Chronic over-exposure (as in the workplace)
- Sudden massive over-exposure (as in a contamination incident)
- Metabolic (enzyme) deficiency
- Overload

Once intolerance to one chemical substance is established, it tends to spread rapidly to other substances. We call this the spreading effect.

Causes of Chemical Exposure: What to Look For
SCOTT-MUMBY'S RULE OF THE NOSE: I have a maxim, based on decades of experience, which is that if there is enough substance present to cause an odor, there is enough to cause symptoms. Some chemical substances, of course, have no odor.

There are many other chemical contacts, of course: plastics, urban atmospheric pollution, perfumes and cosmetics, cleaners, solvents, aerosol sprays, paints, and food additives, to name but a few. Most of these are derived, ultimately, from petroleum and the whole group we call "hydrocarbons" from their chemical structure. Interestingly, all petroleum (and coal) products originated as pine trees in carboniferous forests millions of years ago. Yet we find pine and its terpene derivatives today are quite potent allergens! Is there a connection?

Chemicals at Work & School
Don't forget the work environment as a source of chemical exposure. In some trades there are specific hazards and the monitoring of these exposures since the Health and Safety at Work Act of 1974 has come under the control of the Environmental Safety Officer (ESO) in the Environmental Medical Advisory Service (EMAS).

However, to pretend this system is working efficiently and protecting workers properly is to be foolish and gullible in the extreme. Only a very small percentage of workers - those employed in larger factories and offices - effectively come under this sort of umbrella. Although the act supposedly covers all offices, factories and places of work, in actual fact it is impossible to monitor the countless small businesses that this represents. Only if the individual worker complains is any action likely to be taken in the event of a hazard and many workers are reluctant to report breaches of the codes for fear of losing their jobs, either as retribution or indirectly because the works are closed down due to not being able to afford all the safety procedures required.

It may be obvious to you that you are working with major chemical toxins. Elaborate precautions and safety instructions would tell you that. However, many chemical allergens at work are much more insidious and difficult to detect unless you consider the possibility. Problems can come from photocopier fluids, solvents, aerosol, powerful cleaning agents and detergents (common where contract cleaners are employed), air purifiers and, last but not least, the fabric of the building and its furnishings (formaldehyde particularly). If your office has that new "plastic" smell, this could be a problem. Air conditioning often makes matters far worse by circulating indoor pollution.

The Allergy Handbook
This problem can be so bad that we have begun to pinpoint what is called the *Sick Building Syndrome*. Some modern buildings have such a high internal accumulation of these obnoxious substances that almost everyone feels ill to some degree. Headaches, sore eyes and runny nose, fatigue, and inability to concentrate are almost the norm. The effect on work efficiency is disastrous and absenteeism runs sky-high.

Since it is costing industry money in lost man-hours, you may be sure (especially if you are cynical, like me) that a lot of money is now being spent on researching this problem.

In the meantime, the answer is simple. Open the windows! The problem is made far worse by the modem craze for energy efficiency. For allergy sufferers, at least, drafts are good news. They help to circulate air and keep down internal pollution. This applies in the home also - double glazing and draft-proofing may be disastrous to those who suffer within the home environment.

The list below gives pointers towards allergies in the work environment.

- The presence of any known hazards (e.g., toluene diisocyanate, formaldehyde)
- You feel better at weekends
- Symptoms clear up on holidays
- Co-workers affected ("sick" building syndrome)
- Reaction started when you started your present employment
- Worst on Monday and Tuesday
- Keep in mind potential physical factors e.g., VDU's and back or eyestrain (not necessarily an allergy)

Cleaning Up Your Chemical Environment
It makes good sense to clear your environment of as many unnecessary chemicals as possible. This will reduce your overall environmental burden. We choose the home for this because it is something you can control to a great extent. You can't do much about what is beyond your doors and windows (except move if you are downwind from a factory or such) but, unless you have a particularly unsympathetic and selfish family, you should be able to effect enough

changes indoors to produce a worthwhile improvement. Some substances you will be able to replace with safer substitutes. Many you will be able to dispense with altogether. Some you will need and no substitutes can be found. The answer is to recognize the danger, use them as infrequently as possible, preferably get someone else to carry out the task involved, and store these substances outside the house, for instance, in the garage

I usually get patients to comb the whole house, room by room, cupboard by cupboard and shelf by shelf, listing all the chemicals found. Sometimes, the list itself is a shock and this is salutary. To pinpoint all potential trouble, I get them to supplement what can be seen with what can be smelled. Most chemical allergics have a very sensitive sense of smell; others have none and will need to enlist the help of someone else - I call this a nose survey: if you can smell it, it can make you ill. That is, if there is enough to cause an odor, there is enough to cause symptoms.

The list of potential chemical allergens shown below will help you search out trouble. Store, replace, or throw out as much as possible of what you find.

Aerosols. We all know about the effect aerosol propellants (CFCs) have on the environment. What is more important and often forgotten is that they have a bad effect on humans too! Also, beware of so-called "ozone-friendly" products. These simply contain alternative chemicals. Remember that ozone-friendly doesn't mean "biofriendly."

- Air fresheners
- Tap water
- Cavity wall insulation

Urea-formaldehyde foam insulation (UFFI) is a cause of considerable health problems, so much so that it was banned some years ago in the US — although in the UK we are still being told it is safe..

Cleaning Materials

There are always simpler alternatives, even if they do call for a little more manual effort. Sodium bicarbonate or borax can often be made to serve where more powerful alkaline agents would be used. Avoid "biologicals" like the plague. Especially avoid fabric "conditioners," which seem to cause strong reactions in some.

For personal washing, use Simple, Castille, or Neutrogena soaps. For household duties, try soft green soap (that's its name!), obtainable from pharmacies or drug stores.

Cooking Utensils

Allergics should avoid using non-stick pans with Teflon type coatings. Nor is aluminum cookware recommended, due to toxicity problems. Glass and enamel are best.

Fabrics

Most people are better off in natural fabrics, such as wool and cotton. Man-made fabrics all give off fumes long after they are new. Of course, some people are allergic to natural fabrics, especially wool, and trial and error is required to find what suits you best.

Flues
Chimney flues may present problems, as they can leak and give off serious fumes. The only safe course is to have the flue lined with a modern flexible flue liner which, although expensive, can be passed up the chimney with the minimum disturbance and mess.

Better still, change to electrical radiators and eliminate gas or open fires.

Garages, integral
Gasoline fumes are a common concern; I find It is far better (and safer!) to park the car outside and to use the garage to grow mushrooms or for a model workshop.

Gas
All chemically sensitive patients should get rid of gas from their homes if it is at all practicable and economically viable to do so. Avoid open gas fires. Do not use gas for cooking, even if you have to retain it for heating purposes.

A final word of warning: under no circumstances whatever be tempted to use the free-standing butane gas heaters which can be wheeled from room to room. These give off very toxic fumes.

Heating
Avoid ducted air systems, fan heaters, and, to a certain extent, open bar electric fires. Best are central heating radiators or, for portable use, small oil-filled electric radiators, such as the Dimplex type.

Makeup
Cosmetics are generally biologically unfriendly. Try to get the hypoallergenic kind but remember there is no such thing as non-allergenic.

Paints
Paints can cause many unpleasant symptoms. There are a number of "organic" paints coming onto the market. These are water-soluble and free of the toxic solvent fumes. If you don't want to use water-based paints, latex paint is said to be best for allergics. Stir in sodium bicarbonate until the paint stops bubbling. Richard Mackarness suggests about 100 g to 5 liters of paint.

Toothpaste
Toothpaste may contain ammonia, ethanol, artificial colors and flavors, formaldehyde, mineral oil, saccharin, sugar, and carcinogenic PVP plastic.

Weleda makes a simple salt gel or plant gel paste, safer than any others. For the exquisitely sensitive, try oil of cloves.

Don't forget that car and upholstery are potential hazards. Nowadays, most are treated with complex stain-repellent and preservative chemicals. You may not want to throw out your nice new carpet or sofa but, if you can at least diagnose that's where the trouble is coming from, you will feel less distressed. Things will probably improve in time. However, for an unlucky few, the truth is simple, if bleak - they will never be well until the luxury wall-to-wall hazard is disposed of!

Organic Foods
It pays to avoid food additives and eat only whole foods, although it must be said there is some hysteria about "E numbers" at present. Only a very small percentage of the population can

never eat foods containing them. For the rest of us, it is a matter of prudence and it need not be magnified to become a fear of poisoning.

Probably the greatest hazard is from chemicals sprayed on our foods before harvesting. This can include fertilizers, weed killers, insecticides, fungicides, and others. According to official figures, 98 percent of green leaf crops, 94 percent of orchard crops ,and 95 percent of root crops are treated with chemicals. Sometimes foods are sprayed after gathering, to assist in storing. All of this poses a serious long-term health threat that has not been properly evaluated.

Foods grown without such chemicals are christened "organic" or "organically grown," and developments in this area are a welcome, fast-growing trend. Those with serious chemical allergies are advised to eat only organically grown food. However, it is difficult to get supplies and, fortunately, most people don't need to be strict in this regard.

A few weeks' experimentation with elimination and carefully judged challenge tests, comparing organic with non-organic ordinary commercial supplies, should settle the matter.

TREATMENT FOR ALLERGIES

All allergy management consists of two basic elements:

Avoidance and desensitization.

Avoidance is not always practical.

Desensitization is better.

Hypo-Sensitization

Unfortunately, this cannot be said of classical allergy desensitization or hypo-sensitization (means lowering of sensitivity). For decades it was practically the only desensitization method. The idea was to figure out what the patient was allergic to and then make up a cocktail formula of those substances and administer steadily increasing concentrations of it, until the patient learned to tolerate the offending substances.

It did have some validity; that is, it worked some of the time. The two main drawbacks were:

1. Testing was unreliable. Just because a substance reacts on a prick or scratch test does NOT mean it is a serious culprit (i.e., a person may be very allergic to cats but not be near any).
2. There were many instances of severe after-effects and deaths were quite common. That's a tough break if all you had was dermatitis or hay fever.

For the latter reason, hypo-sensitization is little used outside the USA, where business concerns try to maintain its status quo. Attacks on safer methods, like Miller's low-dose desensitization and homotoxicology, are vicious and based entirely on ignorance of the benefits and vest interest.

Other Treatments for Allergy

Some treatments are implicit in the method and have already been considered. For example, cytotoxic testing and Miller's method have an obvious related plan of treatment (exclusion diet for the former, administering neutralizing solutions for the latter).

Environmental control units are a testing/treatment element to themselves and are considered elsewhere.

Leaky gut and parasites would depend on what you found, but the treatment should follow logically.

It only remains to consider specific treatments, which might not be covered elsewhere.

Enzyme-Potentiated Desensitization
A bridge between conventional desensitization and low-dose neutralization is Dr. Len McEwen's method of enzyme-potentiated desensitization (EPD).

It is definitely a vaccine approach, whereas **Miller's method** of neutralization seems to be more akin to the antidote principle. Briefly, in EPD a cup is taped over the forearm (after the skin on the area has been scarified - scraped repeatedly - to remove the waterproof layers). Under this cup is placed a vaccine containing dozens of commonly encountered foods and environmental substances, along with an enzyme to make it work (hence the name). The cup is kept in place for 24 hours and then removed.

Antigens leak into the blood over several hours and this creates a favorable antibody response. Obviously the patient will not be desensitized to every ingredient, but since there are dozens of foodstuffs and most common environmental allergens in the mixture, even if only 20 percent of the items "take," this would mean a significant improvement to many patients.

The doses used are extremely small. In fact, more food appears in the blood after eating a meal than from this technique. It is vital, therefore, that the patient avoid most foods the day before, the day of, and the day after treatment.

The treatment takes up to 12 months to produce a worthwhile improvement in complex food allergies. **Environmental allergies,** such as grass, pollen, and house dust, respond much quicker.

McEwen estimates EPD is about 85 percent successful. It doesn't work for chemical sensitivity or insect bites.

Nowadays we dispense with the cup and administer the dose by intradermal injection, except in special cases.

EPD is a compound vaccine: the user-practitioner mixes the appropriate proportions immediately prior to administering the dose. The modern vaccine contains:

- 1-3 diol, a kind of alcohol that activates the enzyme
- beta glucuronidase, which appears to act as a lymphokine. It occurs naturally in human blood and is present in the vaccine in an amount equivalent to that normally present in 4 cc of blood. This enzyme, which gives the technique its name, is thought to be responsible for stimulating the Langerhan cells (immunologically active cells in the skin) to migrate to the local lymph glands and "reprogram" a new population of T-suppressor lymphocytes (those that switch off immune reactions). In the presence of antigen in the appropriate concentrations, this will result in a satisfactory desensitization. (Conversely, in the presence of antigen at a "wrong" concentration you may get a hypersensitization, probably by stirring up helper T-lymphocytes and B-lymphocytes.)

The following mixes are used most frequently:

1. "X" - mixed foods and additives, mixed moulds, mixed pollens, cat/dog, flock, fly mix, and bacterial mix.
2. "I" - inhalants alone. This is used to treat hay fever, cat, dog, horse allergies, pure mould, and house dust allergies.

Separate mixes of odds and ends, laboratory animal hair/dander, and sawdusts are also available. So far EPD has not provided any useful means of desensitizing for chemical reactions.

Hay fever and rhinitis usually respond to the first dose of inhalant mix. Two treatments are usually given in all. But doses of EPD are cumulative and a few of the more complex allergic patients will not start to improve until eight doses have been administered over two years.

Indications for EPD

A wide variety of conditions respond to EPD, including the following: asthma, eczema, rhinitis, chronic urticaria, angioneurotic edema, hyperkinetic syndrome, migraine and chronic headaches, irritable bowel syndrome, inflammatory bowel disease, food-induced psychological states - depression, anxiety - post-viral fatigue syndrome, and multiple food allergy.

McEwen draws attention to a combination syndrome of psychological disturbance, irritable bowel, and migraine, which he calls PIMS.

SETUP
Foods

Desensitization for foods demands that there are no circulating food antigens at the injection site. This means patients have to go on a diet of foods that have been found from experience rarely to upset EPD, such as lamb, sweet potato, buckwheat, carrot (cooked), celery (cooked), cabbage (cooked), sago, fructose, and rhubarb; chicory drink or spring water.

Alternatively, the patient may use one of a number of elemental or synthetic food supplements or replacements, such as Elemental-08, Vivonex (still available in some countries), Pregestimil, or Pregomin (Milupa). Dairy and grain-based meal replacers are not allowed.

Inhalants

Treatment for seasonal allergies should be given at least four weeks before the season begins. Desensitization to animal furs may not succeed if the patient returns straightaway to his or her pets. He or she will absorb pet antigen, which finds its way to the injection site in far greater concentration than that in the vaccine, and this may block desensitization. Fortunately, allergy to house dust and mites works well without patients having to leave home, but reasonable precautions against house dust and mites must be observed, especially prior to EPD.

Micro-Organisms

McEwen points out it is not uncommon to see patients who have become sensitized to their own gut flora. In these cases it is necessary to reduce the bowel antigen load, starting at least 10 days prior to a dose of EPD. The commonest problem is *Candida* allergy and this must be pre-treated with a suitable antifungal such as Nystatin. Allergy to gut bacteria often goes unnoticed and untreated. Preparatory treatment may be satisfactorily carried out with antibiotics such as tetracycline or nifuroxazide.

Failures

EPD can be blocked by a number of factors. If one or more of these factors is present, the physician must decide whether to defer treatment until conditions are more suitable:

1. excessive exposure to inhalants, foods, *Candida*, fumes, etc., close to the time of treatment
2. incidental infection such as a cold or flu
3. stress
4. nutritional agents: excess vitamin C, cod liver oil, evening primrose oil at treatment time (or large excess at other times)
5. drugs: paracetamol, aspirin, NSAIDs, high-dose estrogen (the Pill or HRT implants), progesterone-like drugs, H2 histamine antagonists (notably cimetidine or Tagamet), alpha and beta sympathomimetics (ventolin, bricanyl in large doses), cyclophosphamide, opiates, tri-methoprim, Septrin, and anti-malarials

Safety

Whenever antigenic material is injected into any person there is always the theoretical risk of anaphylaxis. Reactions to the "conventional" desensitizing injections are common, because large amounts of antigen are injected. In fact, deaths have occurred and this method of injecting large amounts of antigen is no longer considered justifiable.

With EPD, far smaller quantities of antigen are used, which greatly increases the safety margin. Over 30,000 treatments have been given by cup since 1966. No patient has been admitted to hospital to treat an emergency provoked by EPD. This includes patients who have severe asthma or who have previously suffered acute anaphylactic reactions to multiple foods.

EPD is now usually administered by intradermal injection, except for the high-dose inhalant vaccine, which must only be given by the cup method. However, the current practice is to retain the cup technique for patients who may be especially at risk of anaphylaxis, even for administering the low-dose vaccine. This bolsters the safety element greatly.

Insect bites have not been included in EPD for safety reasons.

Nutritional Supplements After EPD

Increasing the short-term availability of zinc appears to improve the effectiveness of EPD. So does the administration of folic acid and vitamin D3. The average response to treatment is accelerated by giving additional supplements of these substances for approximately three weeks after each dose.

Generally, these nutritional supplements are not used after hay fever treatments, although they may be added if the response to a first treatment has been poor. Inadequate patient nutrition must be tackled as a separate problem. As with any other approach, most patients benefit from multivitamin and mineral supplements.

Timing and Spacing of EPD Doses

EPD is a long-term project and this needs to be clearly understood by the patient. Treatment is begun at intervals of two months. Once the response is established, this can be increased to three months, then four, and so on. Usually, it is possible to get it down to once or twice a year. Some patients have been able to discontinue regular treatments altogether.

Patient response to EPD varies widely. Typically, nothing happens for about three weeks, then there is a sudden surge of improvement. This usually lasts a couple of weeks and then wears off. After the second dose, this improvement may last three to four weeks; then for longer and longer intervals until improvement is maintained right through to the next dose. This is the signal to start increasing the interval between treatments. Improvement, in this context, may mean either feeling better, or tolerating more foods, or (usually) both.

Homotoxicology

Perhaps one of the most important approaches is homotoxicology.

There are a number of HEEL remedies (German homeopathic manufacturer) that relate directly to allergies in two ways:

- treatments for specific symptoms and illnesses

- treatment for the allergic tendency

Both, of course, have a place in the physician's armory.

Symptom-Specific Homeopathic Remedies

The simplest way to put this material forward is to make a table and include suggested or recognized remedies, as examples. All are from HEEL, unless otherwise stated.

SYMPTOM	SUGGESTED REMEDIES
General, good for allergies	Schwef-Heel, Traumeel-S, Gallium-Heel, Apis-Homaccord
Asthma	Tartephedreel, Husteel, Drosera-Homaccord, Carbo veg
Chronic fatigue syndrome	Schwef-Heel, Lymphomysot, Engystol, Coenzyme comp.
Dermatitis	Belladonna-Homaccord, Psoriniheel, Graphites-Homaccord
Eczema	Schwef-Heel (strong!), Sulphur-Heel, Hepeel, Merc sol.
Hay fever	Luffa comp., Gallium-Heel, Nasol-Heel, Natrium-Homaccord
Migraine	Spigeol, Gelsernium-Hom, Chelidonium-Hom, Psoriniheel
Brain allergy	Ingnatia-Homaccord, Nervo-Heel, Valerian-Heel
Urticaria	Apis-Homaccord, Belladonna-Homaccord, Sulphur-Heel

Futureplex™ is worth a separate mention, because they have some really excellent formulas for many aspects of allergies, which I can say from experience work really well.

Eliminating the Allergic Tendency

This is a big subject, naturally, and I cannot teach anyone a science in just a few lines. The essence of it is removing toxins from the body (what we call drainage), stimulating the bodies' own defense mechanisms, and reducing other burdens. As always in good holistic care, treating any concurrent disease is treating the allergy!

I put forward the following suggestions:

Eliminating the after effects of past viral ilness and good "general allergy remedy". Good against vaccination damage.	Engystol
Lymphatic cleanser, great for drainage, helps clear out all toxins, "and restores" the overburdened immune system	Lymphomysot
Liver drainage and liver support. Vital when the body is overloaded with toxins and auto-pollution (such as diatary and enviromental damage)	Hepar compositum
Good kidney drainage. When the liver is overworked, the next place to get the shock of overload are the kidneys.	Populus compositum
Brilliant defence booster and zest giver. Specifically targets those childhood ear, nose and throat ilnesses that damage the immune system	Tonsilla compositum
General boost giver. I have gone on record saying if I were only allowed ever one remedy to treat all my patients, this would be it!	Coenzyme-comp.

You may be hard-pressed to find doctors who even know about these medicines, never mind how to use them. You may have to go it alone or seek help.

SECTION 8

ANTI-AGING SECRETS REVEALED

Sidebar

THOUGHTS ON AGING…

DO GENES DETERMINE YOUR DEATH?

HARMONIOUS BALANCE – THE KEY TO ANTI-AGING

ADVANCES IN ANTI-AGING

YOUR BRAIN & AGING

FOLIC ACID FOR A BETTER MEMORY

TOP 10 NON-HORMONAL ANTI-AGING SUPPLEMENTS

LIVE A YOUNGER LIFE

EXTEND YOUR LIFE WITH CARB CONTROL

HUMAN GROWTH HORMONE & DO WE NEED IT?

OXYGEN & WHY WE NEED ANTIOXIDANTS

THE MOTHER HORMONE: PREGNENOLONE

NO MORE WRINKLES!

THE ANTI-AGING VITAMIN

SOMETHING TO THINK ABOUT…

SENILITY IS INFLAMMATION

THOUGHTS ON AGING…

Most people think of aging as living too long and being a crumbly old ruin. *"I'd rather die young!"* is the cheerful reply (I doubt it very much, when the time comes). It actually misses the point entirely.

Being an old and crumbly is what happens when you DON'T take care of the anti-aging issues!

More and more people are living to a great age. Seventy odd years may be the life expectancy when you are born (varies in each country). But once you have reached retirement age, the average life expectancy goes up to 85 and beyond. That means a lot of people are going to live to ninety and beyond.

DID YOU KNOW THERE ARE ALMOST 10,000 PEOPLE NOW OVER 100 YEARS OLD IN THE UK ALONE? Most people think it's a few dozen or a few hundred at most. It's rising fast and many people alive today in their fifties will certainly make the century. Remember, the picture is changing fast, as the baby-boomer population comes through its fifties, and these conservative statistics will quickly become hopelessly out of date.

According to the American Academy of Anti-Aging Medicine and the World Health Organization, fully 55% of the baby boomers now in good health will reach the age of 100.

There will soon be hundreds of thousands, and eventually millions, over 100 years old. You could be centenarian, whether you choose to or not.

It's crazy not to prepare for age and try to prevent it being an unpleasant, unhealthy experience - as it is for some, though not, of course, everyone.

And this is a key point: if anyone is fit at age 100 years, it means anyone can be. Growing old does not harm you!! The sad and often overlooked truth is that it is disease that makes us unhealthy and ruins our bodies, as we grow older. If you care to remain fit and healthy, growing old can be a wonderful and fulfilling time.

The fact is that the major killers heart disease, stroke, diabetes, and most cancers are easily preventable if you go about it the right way. The appalling toll of deaths are simply a measure of the incompetence of a medical profession that is obsessed with drugs and treating only symptoms, instead of taking effective and proven action directed towards the known causes of these conditions.

It has been wisely said in a report in the prestigious journal *Science* that if we could eliminate heart disease, cancer, stroke, and diabetes as major causes of death, life expectancy would rise to 99.4 years!

Don't wait until it is too late. Sadly, most people will do that. But the smart ones, who can think ahead and plan intelligently, will realize that anti-aging is not really an option. You have to do it, or suffer unpleasant and maybe unbearable consequences.

It may help to picture this in terms of the aging of a motorcar. Typically, a well-used car will last 10 to 20 years and then fall apart, unsafe to be repaired. The better the maintenance, the longer it takes to crumble, naturally; if you omit routine oil changes and other vital tasks, the car will soon fail mechanically. But then some cars, so-called CLASSIC CARS, are in sweet running order and perform reliably when they are 80, 90 or even more than 100 years old. *Why is that*? The answer is so obvious, it screams at you: **they have been properly looked after.**

It's exactly the same with the human body. You have to ask yourself, do you want to be a classic car or an old "banger," rusting and clanking away? I doubt anyone in his or her right mind would choose to be a banger. Yet that is the outlook mentality of anyone who doesn't begin to take effective care of their health NOW.

We have one proven advantage over mechanical objects: our bodies can regenerate to a considerable degree.

It has been a medical hoax of long standing, to tell people they have to put up with miserable health conditions, just because the doctors don't know how to cure it. The fact is that if you turn to nature, instead of the drug industry, to look for answers, there are many exciting ways to gain back your health, even after many years of believing you were stuck with it. You probably already know of people curing themselves of arthritis, cancer, heart disease, and so on, without resorting to any further drastic medical intervention. These results show the way for us all: you can recover your health!

Add to this the many wonderful breakthroughs in the science of anti-aging, and there is really no good reason, other than self-neglect, to accept the breakdown of age. People routinely feel a sense of complete life renewal, increased vigor, mental clarity, and sexual pleasure. **You can turn back the clock.**

In the words of Dr. Walter Pierpaoli and Dr. William Regeleson:

Ours is the first generation that need not experience senescence, the dismal physical decline now associated with old age. We are the first generation that need not resign ourselves to accepting the fate that our later years will be filled with debility and disease. Ours is the first generation that has the capacity, by resetting our aging clocks, to actually prolong youthful health and vitality into our eighties, nineties, and possibly even our hundreds.

Do you want to grow old and sick or live a healthy zestful life to the very end? Do you want to be a classic car or on old crock? It's up to you!

DO GENES DETERMINE YOUR DEATH?

A common question about aging is whether or not genes have an important role to play; in other words, does it matter who your ancestors are and does that have much bearing on how long you will live?

Obviously, if you inherit a gene for a fatal illness it does. If you inherit a disorder that makes it difficult for your body to perform at optimum function, that too will play a part in how long you survive. Your family history will tell you this.

But the question remains: given a first rate set of genes, can you control when you will die, even in part, or is it already pre-programmed?

Obviously it is an important point because, if you can influence the outcome of an inherited health trait, or override it altogether, then truly your health and survival are in your own hands. The external or environmental factors that we bring to bear on issues can compensate for any destructive genetic material we have been provided with. The question is: can it be done?

The answer is slightly complicated but interesting. It's fashionable today, of course, to believe that everything is in the genes. But genes don't always show up. The gene for blue eyes, for instance, is subordinate to the gene for brown eyes. So if you get one of each (one from your mother and one from your father), the brown eyes will win. This is called a dominant gene (blue eyes are a recessive gene). But then it is found that sometimes even the dominant gene doesn't show up as it should. So scientists are beginning to talk of gene "expression" (whether it will come into play or not).

Many external factors will influence whether or not a gene expresses itself fully or partially. So really all this is saying that environmental factors are very important and genes are not the be-all-and-end-all, though science continues to peddle this silly story.

Let us make this clearer by inventing an example: supposing that mother eating a lot of garlic while pregnant will suppress the brown eye gene (this is not true, we made it up to illustrate a point!). Which then controls the eye color, genes or the garlic-rich diet? The answer is that it doesn't matter; because you can't change the genes, but you have the choice of eating garlic or not. So only the garlic is important. Do you see?

Where Does This Leave Us in Anti-Aging Science?

There are many genetic factors that are being studied right now. One is in relation to calorie-restricted diets. We have remarked elsewhere that calorie restriction (CR) is the only known way to increase maximum life span (as opposed to average life expectancy). Dr. Stephen R. Spindler, professor at the Department of Biochemistry at the University of California, Riverside, has studied the effect of long and short term CR diets on the expression of some 11,000 age-related genes in animals. He found something remarkable and published it in the *Proceedings of the National Academy of Sciences* (Sept. 11, 2001). Not only was the age-benefit effect of CR seen over and over again, but genetically determined age changes could be reversed.

Till then, science had assumed that the genes took effect but the resulting damaging changes were blocked by CR. What Dr. Spindler showed, using sophisticated microchip technology, was that the expression of many pro-aging genes was actually reversed.

The good news was that this occurred even in elderly animals. Because the effect was not merely blocking damage but undoing gene expression, they became younger animals, so to speak. Naturally, some genes decrease their expression due to aging; Spindler found 26. These are genes that protect against cancer, enable proper DNA maintenance, and several liver function genes. The best news of all was that even short-term calorie restriction could produce significant pro-survival health changes. Of the 46 liver function genes studied in mice, 27 benefited from a year or more of CR dieting, but 19 of this 27 (55%) changed for the better after just four weeks of CR.

It is interesting to note that Dr. Spindler found that 40% of the genes that increased expression with age were associated with inflammatory changes and 25% associated with oxidative stress. *Inflammation* is one of the key processes of aging; according to this finding, it's more critical than oxidative damage, which is supposed to head the list of aging causes. No wonder food restriction helps survival, if it reduces inflammation and other stresses. It would also explain the benefits of Luigi Cornaro's diet and indeed any detox (low-allergy) plan.

MY ADVICE: forget about genes and don't use them as an excuse to be lazy about your health. You can start reversing the expression of known and as yet unknown age-related genes right away. Read my book *Diet Wise* (visit: www.alternative-doctor.com/dietwise) fast, if you haven't already done so, and take your love of life seriously: do what we tell you!

HARMONIOUS BALANCE – THE KEY TO ANTI-AGING

"Youth is wasted on the young" - George Bernard Shaw

Attaining the optimum life of a human being, which should be our duty, our role - not a side-show issue - is to achieve wisdom, grace, beauty and health.

Often these only come to us with the years; they don't decline, as is sometimes perceived. You will know the saying that *"life begins at 40"* and, if you are beyond those years, you will have discovered this is true. In the main, we do not find ourselves or learn much about the process of living until we have had years of practice.

That's logical.

But the old way of looking at things was that, by then, it was too late; we had missed our chance.

Trash this belief at once! At 40, you have barely lived half your life - often the painful half. The remainder is the reward or pay-off. It's the part that brings about the reckoning or balance, if you like.

Now that's a contrived way of introducing the key anti-aging topic, which is BALANCE.

As in so many endeavors, bliss, success, or achievement only comes about from a harmonious balance of counterpoised forces. Buddha advocated the Middle Way; the Chinese introduced us to yin and yang; whereas we might talk of male and female virtues; nowadays we have the concept of right and left brain.

These are NOT competing elements. These are co-operative elements. Each plays its part. There is no good or bad side. It's the balance between the two that counts.

We need both, like night and day, sweet and sour, or fast and slow. Some combinations invent each other, like good and bad, high and low, or old and new; you need one to create the other (much advertising, for instance is to create the destructive unbalanced notion that "old" is bad, only "new" is good, but that's just to get you to part with your bucks).

Other combinations seem to exist in the nature of things. You can't have a left without a right, really; otherwise you would just walk around in circles. And that's a good way to think about this all-important issue. All left turns or all right turns is an idiot's way to get nowhere!

So it is that health and vitality, your main passports to a long and happy life, are built around many balances: **balanced nutrients, balanced energies, balanced hormones, and a balanced view of life.**

We'll be looking at ways of achieving all these desirable states in the following chapters. In the meantime, I suggest you make it your motto for the third age. Think it, speak it and act on it! You'll be calmer, happier, healthier, livelier and wiser.

That's a promise built into the fabric of life!

ADVANCES IN ANTI-AGING

Science is advancing so rapidly that we now understand many aspects of body chemistry that were unknown just over a decade ago. Modern medical discoveries have given us the knowledge to delay the process of aging for many decades and even, to a degree, reverse it. Whatever your span of years, we can now add quality and vitality, right to the very end.

One of the greatest advances in recent years has been the emergence of what we sometimes call **SUPERHORMONES**, that is, naturally occurring hormones and related compounds that can extend life energy far into the future.

Doctors have always portrayed growing old as an inevitable process. This lazy thinking is no longer acceptable. It is wrong to accept hormone levels that would be considered disease in a young person, just because the patient is in mid-life or beyond.

Superhormones are what William Regelson, MD, author of *The Superhormone Promise* calls the "biomarkers of age," that is. substances that are a true reflection of the aging process.

As the levels of these hormones decline, so do we, mentally and physically. The loss of these precious superhormones saps us of our energy and vitality, and shaves decades off our lives. By restoring these hormones to their youthful levels, it is possible to restore our youthful zeal and energy, and to strengthen and bolster both our bodies and our minds.

Regelson himself is a superb example of what he preaches, well into his 70s and busier than ever before writing, travelling and teaching the new gospel of regained sexual vigor and mental vitality.

One such superhormone is DHEA (dihydroepiandrosterone). It precedes testosterone, estrogen, and progesterone. Low levels of DHEA lead to fatigue, depression, loss of vitality, and decreased libido. Yet this important substance begins to decline in our bodies from the 20s onwards; by 40 we feel the effects of the loss, by 80 our DHEA could be as low as 15% of its "youth level."

Another common and important marker is thyroid hormone; if this declines, your metabolism slows down markedly.

Even more excitingly, human growth hormone (HGH) has been shown to actually turn back the clock. In a major study was published in the prestigious *New England Journal of Medicine* in 1990, Dr. Daniel Rudman showed that, in real terms, six months of adequate supplementation of HGH was capable of reversing the aging process by as much as 10 to 20 years; skin wrinkling was reduced significantly, lean muscle mass returned and excess fat melted away, resulting in weight loss even without dieting. While not exactly the elixir of life, it did mean that at last there was scientific proof of the possibility of not merely arresting the aging process, but reversing it.

The superhormone promise applies equally to men and women. Don't wait. Nature has given each of us a personal blueprint for age reversal - it is written in our hormones.

Other Factors

It would be foolish and misleading to suppose that only hormone supplementation was needed to ensure an active and enjoyable life right until the 9th and 10th decades. For most people, major changes need to be made in diet and lifestyle.

Proper nutrition builds and sustains health.

The biggest cause of premature death in Western society remains arterial degenerative disease (heart attacks and stroke).

Yet the sad irony is that this killer condition is almost entirely *avoidable*; it was very rare until the adoption of our modern way of life in the early 20th century.

Luckily, we now have a number of clearly understood biological markers that can point to increased risk. You can know where you stand right away. Not only that, but these are correctable measures - you can take the necessary steps to ensure that you don't join the appalling long list of casualties because of ignorance and folly.

Chelation therapy (a special intravenous infusion) is known to increase blood flow where hardening of the arteries has resulted in years of organ deterioration. It cleans and increases blood flow throughout the body and, at the same time, limits free radical activity by clawing misplaced toxic substances from sites where they have accumulated.

By adding brain-booster glutathione to the IV formula, we can make these important benefits into a powerful restorative package that can reverse brain aging, DNA cross-linkages, and tissue decay.

Renewed nutrient and oxygen supply for the tissues, especially the brain, can result in feeling years younger. Sexual organs can be revitalized, with obvious benefits. You don't need the new wonder drug, with its well-known side effects! You'll not only have the mechanism for satisfactory erection but enhanced vigor that requires it!

A Word About Cancer

The second biggest killer is cancer; almost one in two males and one in three women will develop it. Yet studies show over and over again that this too is an avoidable condition. A strong vigorous immune system is vital in your defense; our leading doctor is an internationally known expert in this matter. Chelation may also reduce the risk of cancer; one Swiss study showed that patients had a 90% less chance of developing cancer after undergoing this safe and simple treatment.

To repeat: almost all markers for early demise due to heart disease, stroke, and related factors are entirely reversible, given the necessary expertise. It makes no sense to wait until catastrophe has struck before acting. Don't let your body clock run down and reach the point where it is hard to correct the problems. You should take an interest in your 40s, at least to the point of having a check-up with a holistically oriented doctor. From your 50s onwards, you must take increasing care to ensure a long and happy life.

YOUR BRAIN & AGING

No organ is more critical than our brain, which means the wear and tear of aging will show up first in thought function; we begin to get slower in our movement and manners, easily muddled, more forgetful, and eventually a little silly.

Shakespeare summed up the final stage well in his "seven ages of man" speech: we go back to a kind of second childhood, where we are not fully capable mentally. This may be quite mild, where the patient is known to be a little dotty (short for dotage), or as severe as full-blown dementia. The "seventh age" applies to women also. In fact, women tend to suffer more from the dementias, a fact we attend to in the section of memory.

You do not want to enter this final stage, for sure. Many people dread losing their faculties as they get older and even, half jokingly, ask someone to put a bullet to their head, rather than allow this to happen, so great is the abhorrence of becoming mentally inept. We urge you to follow the advice given throughout this book and, with luck, you never will. Age-related deterioration of the brain is not inevitable, as many lucid centenarians prove, so don't buy into this mindset. Treasure yourself and be determined to go on and on, enjoying life to the full, right to the very end.

Facts You May Not Know

The human brain has been described as the 3-pound universe, meaning that all our thoughts, actions, perceptions, emotions, desires, and dreams are contained in an organ weighing no more than 50 ounces, lodged inside the skull!

There are approximately 100 billion brain cells (neurones), each making between 5,000 and 50,000 hard-wired connections or synapses. That means around 4 quadrillion connections!

This awesome power needs a great deal of energy (a total of 25 watts, for those who are technically minded). In fact our brain, which is only 2% of body weight, requires over 25% of our nutritional energy output. That makes the brain very vulnerable to damage and degeneration from lack of oxygen, poor nutrition, toxic overload, and chemical deposits, including drugs. It means we have to look after our brain with extra care.

At the age of 75, you still have 85% of the brain cells that you were born with, and the good news is that scientists at the Salk Institute in La Jolla, California have now proven that **brain cells can replace themselves**. Previously it was always thought that loss of brain cells was permanent, but we can now potentially regenerate and revitalize our brains. This is great news.

Therefore, the more we can look after our diet, take the right nutrients, and keep our minds active, the better our brains will work.

Your Brain: Use It or Lose It

The first point to grasp is that your brain thrives on activity! It's a use-it-or-lose-it thing. Science has shown that the number of connections in the brain can be increased, no matter the starting point, by simply making demands of the mind. More connections mean more brainpower. Any kind of stimulus is valid, be it crosswords, conversation, creative hobbies, sports or the arts, but doing what you love has the most benefits.

Which brings us to the point that smiles and laughter produce endorphins, which help raise our mood. Robert Holden, founder of *The Happiness Project,* gives a simple technique you can use every day: **smile at yourself in front of a mirror!**

It's amazing how gratifying and cheering the sight of yourself grinning with delight can be. Try on all kinds of happy facial expressions, until one makes you smile for real. It's the easiest and one of the best livelong techniques we've got for you!

Daily exercise is also important. It stimulates and tones up both body and mind. You know the old saying, *"Healthy body equals healthy mind."* We couldn't agree more.

Exercise releases endorphins and increases circulation, therefore increasing the oxygen supply to the brain. Endorphins are natural feel-good substances in our bodies. Don't just think in terms of swimming, jogging, or cycling. Walking is very good and non-stressful. Dancing is even better, since it has the added joy element, which reminds us we are young at heart and that life after all is great!

Balancing your hormones can return brain function to more youthful levels.

Foods to Feed Your Brain

Oily fish and flax seeds (linseeds) are rich in Omega 3 fats, which nourish nerve fibers. Eat oily fish at least twice weekly. Linseeds can be sprinkled over cereals and into desserts or blended with fresh juices.

Eat plenty of fresh fruits and vegetables, which are high in antioxidants that protect the brain from degeneration.

Dark blue foods, such as blackberries, blueberries, and bilberries, are rich in particularly powerful antioxidants called anthocyanins. Scientists at Tufts University in Boston recently found that eating a half a cup of fresh blueberries daily helps to reverse brain aging, thanks to their high antioxidant activity.

Green tea is also high in antioxidants but black tea also has plenty of catechins, which work as antioxidants. Recent studies have shown it has anti-cancer properties, too.

Foods to Eat Less of

Sugar over-excites brain cells until they become exhausted, at which point sweet foods no longer give you an energy boost but make you feel tired. This includes all sugars- maltose, dextrose, white and brown sugar, and honey.

Eliminate all refined white flour cakes, waffles, pancakes, breads, and junk take-away meals, most of which are high in sugar, fat, and salt (and sugar turns to a hard fat if not burned up during exercise.)

At all costs, eliminate sweeteners such as aspartame, which is found in 3500 foods and drinks. These substances over-stimulate the brain, which can trigger insomnia, anxiety and feelings of tension. They also place a strain on the liver, which can exacerbate weight gain in the long term.

Avoid or cut down on caffeine, which is a powerful brain toxin. Excess amounts can trigger headaches, insomnia, palpitations, and, in extreme cases, convulsions. We suggest adults should take no more than 300mg a day - this is equivalent to 3-4 cups of strong coffee. A can of cola contains 60-80mg of caffeine.

Reduce alcohol intake. In small quantities, it is a boon, increasing social contact and bonhomie, which is good for the brain and our emotions. But we must remind you, as always, excess alcohol can be very damaging.

Any foods which are bad for your arteries are bad for your brain, which depends on an efficient blood supply for essential nutrients.

Brain Supplements
The star nutrient is the antioxidant *glutathione*, a naturally occurring amino acid within the body. It is a powerful brain and liver food, which helps those organs detoxify and take care of themselves. But, as we age, glutathione levels fall, and toxins such as heavy metals and pesticides reduce levels even further. Glutathione is manufactured in our cells from a number of precursors such as alpha lipoic acid (ALA); acetyl L-carnitine and N-acetylcysteine (NAC).

In a published study, rats fed on extra ALA and acetyl L-carnitine lived 50% longer than normal rats and enjoyed greatly improved overall health. The animals were so vigorous that media headlines referred to the "dancing rats." The evidence is so convincing that the scientists concerned have patented the mixture, but there is nothing to stop you benefitting personally from this breakthrough. After the age of 50, we suggest you take 200mg of ALA, and 500mg of either NAC or acetyl L-carnitine on a daily basis.

Phosphatidyl serine and phosphatidyl choline help to protect nerve fibers and keep the brain fit and sleek - take a minimum of 50mg daily of either, or both. Lecithin ñ, derived from soya beans, is rich in phosphatidyl serine and choline. A teaspoon of the granules daily (make sure they contain at least 30% PS or PC) not only helps increase memory but also reduces LDL, the "bad" cholesterol.

Ginkgo biloba is a herb proven to improve memory, increase circulation, and act as a brain stimulant. Take 500mg of standardized extract daily. Remember that herbs are potent medicines and not always without side effects - take for six weeks, then stop for a month and then begin again.

Ginseng
This plant extract contains many good things to feed the brain. Special glycosides improve cerebral blood flow and work as stimulants for certain neurotransmitters, chemical messengers that the brain uses to send out signals.

Ginseng helps regulate blood sugar and so is of benefit in reducing the insulin resistance-diabetes progression. It also has benefits for the thymus gland and spleen, thus making it a great all-round anti-ager. Ginseng is taken as teas, powders, and capsules; the quality varies greatly.

Avoid its strong tone-up action if you already have blood pressure or heart disease (go for kava instead, which is a relaxant).

Vinpocetine

This substance is an extract of the wonder plant *Vinca minor* (periwinkle); from the same source, we also get two anti-cancer chemo-therapeutic agents (vinblastine and vincristine). In humans, vinpocetine has been shown to:

- dilate brain arteries (more nutrients)
- reduce the tendency of blood to clot (thus protecting against heart disease and stroke)
- speed up brain metabolism
- act as an antioxidant
- aid recovery after stroke

In a 1985 Japanese study, vinpocetine helped two-thirds of stroke patients recover rapidly, even when administered years after the original stroke. A 1987 study in the *Journal of the American Geriatric Society* showed unequivocally that vinpocetine protects against dementia and improves those who already have it. Good enough reasons for vinpocetine to be classed as a major anti-aging substance.

All health and recovery plans work better when there is general sound nutrition. Never forget to add a multi vitamin/mineral formula that contains at least 500mg of vitamin C, 25mg of B6, 25mg of B1, and 100mcg of B12.

Also 300mg of magnesium, which is also known as "Nature's tranquillizer." A deficiency of magnesium has a detrimental effect on a huge array of enzyme reactions, which take place in our bodies, many of them related to the energy-building cycle of metabolism that takes place in the mitochondria. The brain is one of the first organs to feel the lack.

Magnesium also helps prevent diabetes, blood pressure, irregular heart, headaches, osteoporosis, and many other conditions you would recognize simply as a catalogue of aging!

Is It Brain Fog or Early Dementia?

Alternative allergy doctors, who recognize food intolerance, multiple allergies, and chemical sensitivity have long known that the brain may be affected by these conditions. The result can be mania, violence, hallucinations, or even inappropriate sexual arousal when the brain is off key. But the most common reaction by far we call "woolly brain syndrome" or simply "brain fog." It is a mixture of fatigue and slow cloudy thinking, very distinctive to those who suffer it.

The point here is that it can seem very like the early stages of dementia.

Individuals who are accustomed to using their minds, such as entrepreneurs, professionals, or skilled people…suddenly find themselves *forgetting* simple everyday things, like phone numbers and people's names. It can be scary and often leads to fears of premature aging and loss of faculties. The good news is that this condition is almost entirely reversible.

Before you sink into melancholy and anxiety that your "mind is going," as people sometimes put it, make very sure you test and correct for this condition.

Professional help from a holistic doctor may be called for, but if you find yourself facing it alone, here is what you can do:

1. A short-term (10-day) detox diet, consisting only of fruit, vegetables, fish, meat, herb teas, and spring water. You can eat as much as you like but completely avoid grains and flour (bread, cakes, biscuits, pastry, pasta etc.), dairy produce (milk, cheese, cream, butter, yogurt), and stimulant drinks (tea, coffee, and alcohol), and absolutely no manufactured foods of any kind -- no packets, tins or jars of anything. No sugar is allowed, but then nothing on this diet plan needs sweetening. This a brief description of the so-called *Stone Age Diet*. You can work the rest out by imagining what a cavemen would have eaten and sticking only to that.

2. A chemical-free environment. This is impossible to achieve fully, but you must make sure you are not exposed to house gas, gasoline fumes, pesticides, strong cleaning agents, paints, cosmetics, and all other artificial chemicals in the home and at work. An amazing number of people react badly to these substances but never question it and so are unaware of where their foggy brain is coming from. Look out for gas leaks in the home and car exhaust fumes; get the problem fixed

3. Try to avoid as many drugs and medicines as possible. You will need to talk this over with your doctor, but it is important to realize that much of the pollution we face is medicinal in nature, from pills and potions, to antiseptics, creams, patches and inhalers. They could be making you groggy.

4. Stick to this program for a minimum of 10 days, even if you start feeling great sooner than that. You have shown it is reversible brain fag and *not* aging. Then try to reintroduce things, one at a time, and figure out which are the real culprits.

Chelation

Finally, we cannot close this section on the brain without reference to chelation. We recommend this safe and effective treatment unequivocally; both authors have experience of its effectiveness, despite any controversy you may encounter.

Basically, this technique requires intravenous infusions, in which are delivered multiple nutrients and a chelating substance known as EDTA (there are others). Chelation means grabbing the toxic metals and getting them out of the body. This, in turn, quenches damaging free radicals. Metals are among the most poisonous substances in our environment; almost none of them belong there and certainly not in the kind of quantities encountered in industrial society. Certain metals are already known to cause cancer. Aluminum and mercury have been implicated in Alzheimer's.

Getting rid of the toxic metal overload has a number of benefits, one of which is improving the condition of the arteries. This was formerly thought to be due to taking away calcium in atheroma plaque. Few doctors think that today but, whatever the mechanism, there is no denying the health benefits of chelation. We have seen strokes reversed and dementia patients come back into play. This is only logical, since brain performance is entirely dependent upon nutrient supply from the blood. Even a tiny degree of narrowing of the blood supply to the cranium can have adverse consequences and, like hardening of the arteries, this can creep up on one.

By adding intravenous glutathione, this can reach sometimes miraculous outcomes, in which Parkinson's patients can walk again, motor neuron disease and MS are bettered, and poor brain performance is reversed, at least in part. Remember also that glutathione is a powerful liver detox aid.

This is an exciting area and research is continuing apace. Hundreds of papers are being published every month on the importance of glutathione levels in the brain.

Predictably, mainstream medicine is slow in bringing the benefits into clinical practice, but some pioneer doctors have been forging ahead for years.

FOLIC ACID FOR A BETTER MEMORY

A study, published in *The Lancet* Jan. 20, 2007, has shown that daily folic acid significantly **improves cognitive performance in older adults** — specifically as it relates to memory and information processing.

A randomized, placebo-controlled trial, which included 818 subjects aged 50 to 70 years who were folate-deficient, showed that those who took 800 μg daily of oral folic acid for three years had significantly better memory and information processing speed than subjects in the placebo group.

Furthermore, serum folate concentrations increased by 576% and plasma total homocysteine concentrations decreased by 26% in participants taking folic acid, compared with those taking placebo.

The trial was really intended to study the effects of folic acid and arteries, a controversial subject, linked to whether or not homocysteine is a valid measure of risk for heart attack and stroke. These findings for cognitive function were quite incidental - but very welcome.

The trial took place between November 1999 and December 2004 in the Netherlands. A total of 818 patients were randomly assigned to receive 800 μg of daily oral folic acid or placebo for three years.

Baseline assessment of cognitive function included five separate tests, which measured vie cognitive domains — memory, sensorimotor speed, complex speed, information processing speed, and word fluency. In addition, patients also underwent the Mini-Mental State Examination (MMSE) to screen for possible dementia.

The authors report that participants in both groups were well matched, with similar baseline scores.

At the end of the study, the effect of folic acid on cognitive performance was measured as the difference in cognitive performance between the folic acid and placebo groups.

Among individuals in the placebo group, sensorimotor speed, information-processing speed, and complex speed declined significantly. In contrast, those in the folic acid group experienced a much slower rate of decline.

Furthermore, the three-year change in cognitive function was significantly better in the folic acid group in terms of information-processing speed. However, folic acid had no effect on complex speed or word fluency.

"The effect of folic acid might be restricted to basic aspects of speed and information processing, rather than high order information processing. Word fluency was not affected by folic acid supplementation, perhaps not surprisingly because encyclopedic memory is a component of crystallized intelligence that stays relatively intact as one grows older," the authors write.[1]

Another study, which followed 965 persons aged 65 or older, suggested that folate, B6, and B12 are all important.[2]

Scott-Mumby note: most folic acid supplements you are offered for sale are poor grade. Merck (the drug company) owns the patent on true natural folic acid (metafolin™, as they call it). Make sure you get the right stuff.

References
1. *Lancet.* 2007; 369:208-216.
2. *Arch Neurol.* 2007;64:86-92.

TOP 10 NON-HORMONAL ANTI-AGING SUPPLEMENTS

Remember, all good health measures are anti-aging! I've said it before… but **sugar** is particularly deadly for brain function and contributes to beta amyloid deposits.

Ronald Reagan's notorious sweet tooth may have led to his Alzheimer's. Also bad are excess alcohol, tobacco, saturated fats, and stress. I have put together a list of the following supplements that can be considered for a scientifically based anti-aging regime.

1. L-Carnosine

Although carnosine has been known for about a century, its anti-aging properties have only been extensively studied during the past few years.

It may turn out to be the greatest anti-ager of all. High concentrations of carnosine are present in long-lived cells, such as nerve tissues. The concentration of carnosine in muscles correlates with maximum lifespan, a fact that makes it a promising bio-marker of aging.

Unlike most antioxidants, which work by prevention, carnosine protects AFTER free radicals have been released. One of the cardinal anti-aging affects in the body is glycosylation, which leads to decay of protein function. Carnosine blocks this process. It also blocks amyloid production, the substance found in the brains of Alzheimer's patients. Other properties emerging are its apparent effects as an anti-cancer agent, toxic metal binder, and immune booster.

DOSE: 500 mg. daily. Best with vitamin E, 200- 400 IU daily.

2. Trimethyl Glycine (TMG)

TMG protects the youthful methylation process in our metabolism. Published research shows that TMG can lower dangerous plasma homocysteine levels, thus reducing the risk of heart disease and stroke. It helps the integrity of nerve fibers and so may improve Alzheimer's and Parkinson's disease. It protects against liver damage from alcohol and other dangers. Finally, it protects DNA and so may slow cell age.

DOSE: 500 - 2,000 mg daily. It works better with co-factors B6, B12, and folic acid.

3. Gingko Biloba

Extract of the tree *Gingko biloba* have been used by the Chinese for 2800 years. It is now well recognized as an important brain food and antioxidant and it improves mental function in people of all ages. It quenches free radicals and improves neurotransmission, thus protecting circulation and enhancing memory. Even the orthodox *Journal of the American Medical Association* reported it is well tolerated and effective. Protects against Parkinsonism, Alzheimer's, and other dementias.

DOSE: 50- 100 mg active ingredient. Look for products with less than 2 ppm of the toxic gingkolic acid (European limits set at 5 ppm maximum).

4. S-Adenosyl Methionine (SAMe, Pronounced Sammy)

A derivative of important methionine, SAMe is widely distributed in the tissues of young healthy adults. But with aging and sickness, it is depleted, leading to further deterioration. SAMe is needed for the body to metabolize efficiently, for neuronal regeneration and the synthesis of energy through ATP, the basic energy molecule. It may help prevent or reverse liver damage (from alcohol, viruses, and chemical pollution). It can help with ME and other fatigue states.

Additionally, SAMe may be the safest, fastest-acting anti-depressant available and is widely prescribed in Europe for that purpose, though not in Britain.

DOSE: 200- 800 mg daily. Best taken on an empty stomach, with water.

5. N Acetylcysteine (NAC)

L-cysteine is an important sulfur-containing amino acid. Others, taurine and methionine protect and nourish the liver. The form N-acetylcysteine is more readily absorbed and is a powerful antioxidant and anti-viral. This could be important when we recognize more and more the damaging effects of "stealth viruses." It also helps boost glutathione levels, which is one of the most important brain detox substances of all.

DOSE: 500 -1000 mg daily. Note: Take plenty of extra vitamin C at the same time, to prevent it being oxidized and rapidly destroyed in the body (three times as much vitamin C as N acetylcysteine is recommended).

6. Phosphatidyl Choline (and Phosphatidylserine)

No point in living to a great age if your brain doesn't travel along with you. Phosphatidyl choline, from lecithin, is an important protector for phospho-lipid cell membranes in the brain. These are the ones most easily damaged by free radicals.

We get it in our diet, in vegetables (especially cauliflower and lettuce), whole grains, liver, and soy. It also comes in lecithin (containing 10-20% phosphatidylcholine) in grains, legumes, meat and egg yolks. But we need more, to be on the safe side.

Most of these remarks apply also to phosphatidyl serine, a phospho-lipid. It is found in fish, green leafy vegetables, soybeans and rice. Over 3,000 published research papers and more than 60 clinical trials have established that phosphatidylserine can rejuvenate your brain cell membranes and cognitive function.

Both these compounds are valuable to memory and mood, mental clarity, concentration, alertness and focus. Got to keep those grey cells going!

DOSE: 500 mg daily of phosphatidyl choline/100 mg daily phosphatidyl serine.

7. Coenzyme-Q-10

This vitamin-like substance (also known as ubiquinone) was discovered in 1957. Since then, a deluge of scientific papers have attested to its ability to strengthen the immune system, lower blood pressure, prevent heart attacks, counter obesity, and slow aging. Studies in mice shows it increases their life span by 25%. CoQ10 is found in all cells, where it is responsible for the manufacture of ATP, the basic energy molecule. It is now being said that if CoQ10 levels drop by 25%, cancer is probable.

On a personal note, when I took co-Q-10 and selenium simultaneously, my hair started to grow back - dark hairs!

DOSE: 100- 200 mg daily. It is plentiful in heart, meat, kidney, and eggs, and to a lesser extent in soybeans, wheat, alfalfa, and rice bran.

8. Boron

The pivotal role of boron in bone metabolism has made it clear that it is protective against osteoporosis and therefore vital to a long and happy life, especially for women. Many more women die from complications of a fracture of the femur in the USA than of breast cancer. Researches also concluded that countries with lower boron levels in the soil had much more arthritis. It works best in conjunction with magnesium and other co-factors.

DOSE: 3 mg daily, coupled with 300- 400 mg of magnesium.

9. Alpha-Lipoic Acid

The subject of intensive current research, this may be the most important antioxidant of all in protecting the brain and neurological tissues from damage. Alpha-lipoic acid has the unique ability to pass into the brain, where is helps regeneration of other antioxidants, such as vitamin C and E and glutathione. It is also a strong chelator and may protect against Alzheimer's by removing toxic metals, which generate damaging free-radicals. It is both fat- and water-soluble, which means it is easily absorbed from the gut.

DOSE: 60- 80 mg.

10. Essential Fatty Acids

Almost the same status as vitamins, essential fatty acids are vital for tip top body and mind function. So-called omega-3s and omega-6s have different effects. You need both. Plant sources, such as borage and evening primrose, provide omega-6s and fish oils provide omega-3s. Studies show that eating lots of fish reduces inflammatory chemicals and leads to better health and more mental clarity, with less chance of Alzheimer's. Didn't your mother tell you eating fish is good for the brain?

DOSE: 500- 2,000 mg. Food sources- fish, star flower, borage, evening primrose, and flax seeds.

A final word: Although recommended doses are listed above… I advise you to meet with your health care professional before consumption. Everyone's medical history varies.

LIVE A YOUNGER LIFE

Do you want to live forever? Probably not! But most of us would be reassured to know we will feel fit, well, and active right up to the end.

It was Jonathan Swift, author of *Gulliver's Travels*, who first remarked that nobody wants to die, yet nobody wants to grow old either. Can we do anything about the unhappy paradox here?

Well, yes. The new science of anti-aging is not about living longer, though I and many doctors like me, are convinced that if you do the right things you can extend your life considerably.

It's more about increasing the quality of life. It's about feeling good, remaining active, keeping your mind alive and alert, freedom from pain and stiffness, and continuing with that most important of human feel-good activities, sex.

There's a double whammy in this. It's a great paradox of our lives, for corporate men and women such as yourselves, that during the process of striving and achievement, that just as we reach the pinnacle of our careers, the top of the corporate ladder, and socials life, biology begins to let us down. Just as we reach the dreams we always aspired to, the time and the money to fulfill them, we suddenly start to face stroke, heart disease, and cancer. It seems that maybe we ruined our health on the way up, due to lack of care and attention. But really, I put it to you that the real negative factor was just ignorance. Nobody in their right mind would deliberately shorten their life or do things can bring about ruin and demise.

But through the folly of doctors and personal doubt or confusion about the issues, we have often chosen to ignore good advice. It has been rather like ignoring a good investment and then, in later life, wishing we had bought shares in something important, for which the value has gone up and up and up over the years.

I'm talking about the value of our lives our own selves. The priceless value of good health, zest, and fulfilling sexuality.

Sex and Love

We would all like to go on finding, or I should say rediscovering, love in our partner and ourselves. Sexual vitality is important and its health benefits cannot be overestimated. And I don't mean the love of a rich old boy for a young flirt or a woman who is loaded after her husband's death suddenly finding herself surrounded by admirers. You know the sort of thing…

What I am talking about is the real honest deep-down passion for the companion who has shared your life and whom you want to continue to admire and cherish. Someone you want to hang onto and you wish they were happy and well, as you would wish it just for yourself. Or if he or she is no longer with you in life, that you can re-find yourself and live with new devotion and love that he or she would have wanted to you enjoy.

I'm not talking here about "twilight" years, so much as about the dawn of a new day!! You have to look after your health coupons!

The truth is, to have health and vitality is a choice. It is not something dished out to us at random, as many people seem to think; it has to be earned. It works like investments, as I just mentioned: a little set aside each week or month will result in fruitful rewards in later years. But far too many individuals squander their health resources and discover all too late that by a certain age the bank account is empty, all the credits used up. Zip. Zilch.

We may have a state welfare scheme but, unfortunately, the government doesn't issue health coupons. You have a full set when you are born (usually) and it is up to you to store these carefully and, if possible, get a return on the investment!

Sadly, people who don't take care of themselves are suffering from the ignorance of yesterday's science: we have always been told by the experts that aging is inevitable, there is nothing you can do, life is a lottery, it's all down to your genes, and so on. All of this has been shown in recent years to be complete nonsense. Not only is age something that can be held in check, it can be beaten. There are two counter-efforts to the aging process: firstly, that you can extend the likely years you will live, by prudent attention to diet, exercise, and lifestyle, much can be done; secondly, you can turn what years you do have in store into something far better, with more pleasure and more energy.

Actually, the two go hand in hand. When we hear the cry *"I don't want to live a long time and be an old crock,"* this is misguided and fuelled by the decrepit appearance of some old folk who have been badly let down by the medical profession and its virtual refusal to address the prevention issue. These sad wrecks are not a valid standard of what to expect; this is a measure of what shouldn't be allowed to happen!

The fact is that, for the majority of us alive today, you can say we won't live longer unless we are healthier. Adding years to your life is also a matter of adding life to your years! The few old crocks are the exception by far the majority of men and women who have lived beyond 90 are exceptionally spry and clear-headed for their age.

Take a look at the January 1973 issue of *National Geographic* magazine; there you will see men and women from Georgia, Russia (as it was), over a century old living a life full of enjoyment and vitality. One game lady whose photograph appears is between 130 and 140 years old; yet she is quite *compos mentis*; she sits with a glass of vodka in one hand and a cigarette in the other!

What does that tell us about the supposed expertise of the medical profession?

Clearly these old folk know something that so-called science doesn't. It also tells us that our human life potential is far greater than we have been duped into believing.

So where is all this leading?

As the average Western life expectancy steadily increases, more and more people are going to live beyond the age they supposed. It would be prudent to ensure that, since you will probably be one of them, you don't find yourself reaching later years with your health a broken property. All it takes is a little intelligent care now to reap the advantages later. Get rid of the bravura that "I don't care, I'll grow old gracefully." You cannot possibly know how you will feel about this in later years.

You might meet someone wonderful or start a new direction in life that would fulfill all your wildest dreams, yet your delight ends up cut short because you haven't taken care of yourself properly.

Surprisingly, there are nearly 10,000 people in the UK over the age of 100. We have become more aware of this huge group, now that the Queen Mum is one of them. If you found yourself one of them, wouldn't it be great if you could enjoy life, even then? You would want each day to be an experience to look forward to; not to wake up thinking, "Oh God, another awful day to get through!" or something equally negative.

The fact is that you may not be able to choose when you die. It would be a tragedy to have to endure a forlorn aching old age, with your body ruined; yet be unable to depart this life quietly and so have to continue to suffer it. Even if euthanasia ever become laws (unlikely), it would not be allowed for those who have simply made a mess of things and lost their enjoyment of life, due to creaking joints, fading hearing and eyesight, physical weakness, and general decrepitude.

It boils down, actually, to being intelligent. Only a fool would squander his or her future in the silly belief that nothing else exciting could happen in life. We already hear about the "Third Age" in life (retirement and beyond); those who have reached it in good shape are finding immense pleasures in life, travelling, finding new hobbies, meeting new friends and, yes, let's not be coy having a vigorous and fulfilling sex life long after the menopause or the male equivalent we've nick-named the **"andropause."**

You can control the outcome. There is a lot of up-to-the minute science to guide your footsteps into the right path. A keynote study published in the *New England Journal of Medicine* in 1990 actually showed that aging can be reversed by 10- 15 years, as judged by loss of skin wrinkles, increased strength and muscle mass, reduction in obesity, and, of course, feeling great. That's totally at variance to what is being put about, even now, a decade later, by the average medical practitioner. It's almost as if the medical profession doesn't WANT there to be any answer to aging!

Intravenous antioxidant therapy, now widely carried out in the world, can reverse the degeneration of arteries and beat free radical damage, so that more oxygen is supplied to important tissues, such as the kidneys, which excrete toxins, and, of course, the brain. We add a unique and safe substance that seems to reopen arterial pathways and gets more oxygen to the tissues.

That's always good news and the benefits in thinking processes can be immediate and obvious. Some people are finding that they don't need heart by-pass surgery after all and blood pressure and angina improve all by themselves, without drugs.

I am using an entirely new and brilliant additive to these infusions, being demonstrated by doctors in the USA to give outstanding benefits to brain functions.

People with neurological conditions, such as Alzheimer's and other dementias, parkinsonism, stroke, and multiple sclerosis are making remarkable turn-arounds in their symptoms. I believe it is good for everyone to experience these benefits and put back the appointment with old age.

There is controversy, to be sure, but that comes from people who refuse to objectively acknowledge recent progress in scientific studies. "I didn't think of it, therefore it's bunk," seems to be an all-too-pervasive sour grapes attitude in medical science these days, with everyone jostling for research grants and prize nominations.

A Note on Dying

We cannot avoid the topic of death, though I like Woody Allen's point of view:

"I don't mind dying, I just don't want to be there when it happens."

As the old saying goes, death and income tax are bad news, but everyone has to pay up! But another common misconception, circulated by ignorant doctors who don't understand the facts, is that we eventually "die of old age" we don't: not ever. We die of disease! If we take care to avoid these diseases, then we may go on living, longer and longer. This is easy to come to terms with, if you think how much Western life expectancy has gone up in the last 200 years.

The average for a male is now 74 and for a woman 79, though in some areas, the averages are another few years beyond that. This rise is solely due to the disappearance of major killers, such as smallpox, TB, cholera, and lobar pneumonia (the last was once known as the "Captain of the White Horsemen of Death," although we hardly see it today).

Logically, you can see that if we eliminate even more diseases (cancer and heart disease would be a good start), then even fewer people will be dying and the expected age span will rise even more. In theory, if ever we could eliminate all diseases, people just wouldn't die! Consider the aforementioned lady from Georgia. Sooner or later she will die, but it won't be from age but a dose of influenza, a tooth abscess that sends bacteria all over her body, a fall that leads to a fractured femur, a tumor, or whatever.

We don't NEED to die at all. So it's time to start being prudent with the health coupons we were issued with as a baby!

Cancer & Heart Disease

These two great killers account for between 80% and 90% of deaths. Yet the formula for beating these conditions is the same, really, as preventing aging. The benefit to you, as a committed anti-ager, is that you dramatically improve your chances against these two diseases. It comes as a bonus!

The truth is that it has been demonstrated over and over again that these are preventable conditions. Don't be fooled by the trigger factors, such as tobacco smoking and lung cancer. Not everyone who smokes gets cancer and not everyone who gets lung cancer has smoked; the late Roy Castle was a famous example of this.

Therefore, there are other factors at work. These other factors include nutrition, moderate lifestyle, a cleaner environment, and personal health care. Similarly, the "genes-for-everything" scientists, who keep announcing that everything from cancer to homosexuality is just a gene are being very unscientific. It will help you appreciate this is you realize that there is HUGE money in genetics and you are hearing the voice of greed, not the voice of science. Most such announcements turn out to be completely false. But this sort of propagandizing does share prices a lot of good, if not human health!

Almost all known causes of cancer and heart disease are environmental, meaning outside the body. You can control them!

Children who "inherit" from their parents also inherit bad diet and lifestyle factors, don't forget this important fact.

There is another misconception to work round - that is the widely-held fixed belief that being healthy means behaving like a freak and missing out on all the fun. This is just plain unintelligent - it is an attitude of being childish and indulgent for a few years and then advancing into chronic and not very pleasant health conditions. The same mentality would allow a family or tribe to starve, because it was too much trouble to plant next year's crops and water the seedlings. Until the 20th century that would have literally cost you your life.

It's the same sensible husbandry with your health. Take a little care now, think ahead, and you can reap the harvest of goodness for many years to come.

My own health and longevity plan is based on over 30 years of experience in advanced medical therapies. I have seen the results it produces, consistently, and have no doubt that it will benefit all human beings who want to take good care of themselves.

It is evolved from common sense and knowledge of what counts in Nature. In certain places, it might be in direct conflict to what orthodox medicine claims to be "science." Know firstly that this plan will work for you; remember also that orthodox medicine has appalling results, with worsening statistics on health in general and the appalling tendency to damage patients who come into its ambit.

When the doctors in Colombia went on strike, the death rate plummeted by 35%, only to resume its "normal" level when work resumed. When doctors in Los Angeles went on a work slow-down in 1976 to protest soaring malpractice insurance premiums, the death rate dropped by 18%. Again in Israel in 1973 when the doctors reduced their daily patient contact from 65,000 to 7,000 during a month-long strike, the death rate dropped 50% during that month. According to the Jerusalem Burial Society business for them was very bad!!

So doctors are about the LAST PEOPLE to turn to for an opinion on what counts in aging and longevity matters. Find out for yourself. Otherwise you may pay the price for ignorance. You could miss out on decades of happy vigorous life with people you love. The fact is that it doesn't matter how long you live, if you enjoy those years to the full. We like to think we are putting life into your years, as well as years into your life.

THE PLAN HAS FIVE KEY ASPECTS:
- Red-hot nutrition and diet
- Intravenous antioxidant therapy
- Direct hormone restoration
- Stress reduction
- Structural reintegration of the body

These can be explained in outline.

1. Diet and Nutrition
No, not quite the same thing. Proper nutrition is getting what you need, the right amount of macro-nutrients, such as protein, carbohydrates, and safe fats, plus micro-nutrients, including vitamins, minerals, and essential fatty acids.

I put diet in a second category because of my work in the field of food allergies. Let's use the term STRESS FOODS, so that we don't fall into the usual controversy about definitions. A stress food is something that isn't good for YOU as a person; it may be fine for others but it makes you unwell in many subtle ways. The usual result is feeling generally unwell, lacking energy, vague aches and pains, and worst of all for many intelligent people woolly brain syndrome or "brain fag," which are aptly named. My huge experience in this field, with tens of thousands of cases to report from, enables me to state categorically that the single biggest factor in anti-aging, vitality and health is AVOIDING KNOWN STRESS FOODS.

I put everything I know into my latest book *Diet Wise*; learn more at www.alternative-doctor.com/dietwise.

The results are nothing short of fantastic. Within weeks, sometimes days, the person is feeling young again, with bags of zest and a renewed attitude to life. If I had only one anti-aging tool to use in our clinics, this would be the one I would choose. It's worth can be equal to all the rest put together!

2. Chelation

Chelation means getting heavy metals out of your body. NOTHING ages us faster than poisonous heavy metals that sabotage our enzyme pathways and distort our DNA. Lead and mercury are notorious, but iron is the worst of all!

There are two ways to do it: oral and intravenous. There is much dispute, but I am now satisfied with the evidence that oral chelation works fine. It just takes longer. EDTA, the agent commonly used, is approved as a safe food additive and swallowing it is harmless. It is, after all, just four acetic acid (vinegar) molecules with a few extras (ethylene-diamine-tetraacetic-acid).

Intravenous chelation is something I did for years in my UK office. For people in big trouble with heart disease and peripheral vascular disease, it can be almost a miracle cure. We thought of it as reopening sludged arteries. I now think that is rather naive and it is probably the free-radical scavenging effect that does the most good. It works much faster than oral chelation.

Properly carried out, IV chelation is a simple, painless, and very safe procedure. It can turn back the clock on arterial aging and a growing army of people have proved it's the ideal alternative to expensive, ineffective, and very dangerous by-pass surgery. It requires you to have a weekly infusion, which lasts about three hours. I rate it as the second most powerful tool in the anti-aging armory.

3. Direct Hormone Restoration

There are many proponents of the idea that, since we lose hormones as we age, replacing the hormones will reverse aging. While it's not entirely logical to put it that way, there do seem some benefits from taking this approach.

The "big one" is human growth hormone (HGH). But that's very expensive and far from necessary. I'd put the benefits of chelation and improved diet way ahead of what you'll get injecting HGH.

You can also consider pregnenolone (the "mother hormone"), DHEA, testosterone, progesterone, and estrogen look-alikes (on no account take drug estrogens or progestogens). One of the finest anti-aging hormones comes as a surprise: melatonin. It has good anti-aging science and is even helpful against cancer, as well as putting us to sleep!

4. Stress Reduction

This is a big subject. All sorts of therapies have been invented and tried. Many are right for some and not for others.

All very interesting, but maybe not what you are looking for (if it's what you need, we'll tell you).

But I will share with you here and now the simplest and most effective stress management technique ever invented. It was tested on more than 10,000 patients over 20 years by an enlightened doctor and he found that, uniformly, those who kept it up lived significantly longer (and happier) than those who didn't bother.

It's so simple you can do it any time; in fact, you should do it all the time, every day and in all your activities. What's more, it can be described in just 14 words! What life-extension technique could be so simple and yet so very powerful?

Are you ready for it?

SAY "YES" TO THE THINGS YOU LIKE;

"NO" TO THE THINGS YOU DON'T LIKE.

That's all!

Movement and Posture

I have purposely made this a very wide category; it covers posture, movement, balance, exercise, and remedial work towards old injuries.

The benefits of exercise and how it helps us feel better and live longer is without question. Even heart attack victims do better if they get back on their feet early, instead of being told to rest, as yesterday's science used to advise!

One study, also published in the prestigious *New England Journal of Medicine*, showed that exercise created much higher levels of white cells in the peripheral blood. These defenders help us fight cancer, infections, degenerative disease, and tissue damage, so no wonder we feel better. The good news is that it does not need to be strenuous exercise.

Playing squash and riding bicycles can be overrated! In fact, hard physical exercise releases free radicals and can be damaging.

I think dance is one of the best forms of exercise imaginable, for two reasons. One, it is musical and therefore more pleasurable and less stressful than games, which are competitive (either against other people or the clock). It also does much to loosen up the FLOW of energy and it teaches you how to think and feel "I am beautiful." It isn't necessary to dance like Fred Astaire or a ballerina; neither is there much help from the spastic twitching customary on the floor of a discotheque. I am thinking simply of flowing gentle movements you can make for yourself, while listening to your favorite music in the privacy of your own home. No need to work up a sweat and therefore - ideal for many - you don't have to get into a sports strip!

If you don't get refreshing and enjoyable sensations, you are not doing this right!

Finally, you can still play squash or swim.

Posture

A healthy body isn't just about getting fit. It's also about balancing energies and posture is a very important clue to general health, as the Alexander Technique people have known for years. From chiropractic and cranial osteopathy we learn that even a tiny adjustment in the body can liberate a tremendous amount of energy that was being bottled up or suppressed.

Sometimes it is more obvious. The person stands so badly and off keel it screams at the expert that they have locked-in body problems. Unlike most anti-aging clinics, I believe that THIS aspect of health is just as important as blood efficacy, lung function and liver or kidney performance. We are living, functioning beings, so the dynamics of health are inevitably important to us. Our bodies must be supple, balanced, and integrated. Walking and standing badly can cause you to LOOK and FEEL older than you are.

Need I say more?

Finally, this is just to tell you that there are many expanding new areas of health care that have direct relevance to anti-aging and vitality. Homeopathy, for example. Modern methods have shown clearly that we can retune the body to more optimum levels. It is possible, given the right regime, to restore secretions of all-important growth hormone, which I mentioned previously. The remarkable thing is that this can be done with nothing more than trace doses of herbal and other substances. All that is taking place is that the body is being persuaded to recharge, to come back to life and continue with the markers of youth and vitality.

It all goes to prove one thing: **Nature is quite brilliant, far cleverer than doctors imagine themselves to be.** She can actually reverse the process of aging - if she is persuaded, with a little help from someone who knows what to do.

Now that's good news for us all, especially those on the slippery slope!

EXTEND YOUR LIFE WITH CARB CONTROL

Carbohydrate is the main killer in the average Western diet, *not fat*. Eskimos and other aboriginal people with very high fat levels in their diet do not suffer degenerative artery disease in the way we do in the civilized world. However, misinformation and ignorance abounds. Whatever science you read extolling the supposed benefits of carbohydrates, this will always refer to complex carbohydrates (meaning whole grains). This also overlooks the fact that many people are intolerant of grains. Despite all the propaganda, even whole grains are not "natural" foods at all. Man evolved as a hunter-gatherer and grains have only been in our diet for the last 10,000 years or so. Many people cannot digest grains but get unpleasant reactions.

Ironically, refined carbohydrates are better tolerated by these individuals than whole grains. But make no mistake, white flour, white sugar, corn syrup, white potato, and other starch-rich foods are bad for you and will shorten your life. Yet these are the ingredients commonly used by the food manufacturing industry: bread, cakes, biscuits, pasta, pastries and other confectionary items, french fries, food thickeners, coffee whiteners, white rice, and skimmed milk (milk with the fat reduced has proportionately more sugar!) - these are all stressful to your metabolism.

Sooner or later, the control mechanism that regulates the flood of such carbohydrates into your body will break down and serious, life-threatening consequences will result.

The four main resulting dangers are:

- Obesity
- Insulin resistance or hyperinsulinism
- Syndrome X or metabolic syndrome
- Diabetes

The last three items are really three progressive stages of the same condition, but all four are closely interwoven, as we shall see.

Obesity
Obesity remains close to the top of conditions that will shorten your life.

Insurance actuaries are very clear on how the percentage risk of death rises with every pound overweight; they are very exact about calculating the value of human life and the likelihood of an expensive payout. Pay attention to this cynicism!

Refined carbohydrates make you gain weight inexorably. Most people find losing weight easy when avoiding carbohydrate, without starving themselves or feeling hungry. This diet theme has been in circulation for over a century, from the original paper by William Banting, through the RAF diet, Scarsdale diet, and various other incarnations. Atkins has been probably the most famous and successful low-carb plan of all time; the acclaim is simple – it works, despite everything the critics throw at it. Now the late Doctor Atkins has spawned a whole rash of "me too" plans, such as the South Beach Diet.

Low-carb eating is gentler and more successful than low-calorie plans. World-class health author Leslie Kenton has recently reworked the theme yet again, in a fine book called *The X Factor Diet* (Vermillion 2002), and Barry Sears' *The Zone* is essentially that same life-saving information. Learn it and do it.

Insulin Resistance
Anti-aging doctors are increasingly concerned about the problem of insulin resistance as a causative factor in age degeneration. Carbohydrates of all types are digested to simple sugars, such as glucose, when they enter the gut. Eating large amounts of carb results a great deal of digestion products or a "sugar rush," which has to be dealt with safely.

One of the best-known hormones that regulate the metabolic processing of sugar is insulin (however don't forget that other hormones from the adrenal glands are also involved in this process). Basically, insulin makes cells more receptive to glucose, so they can metabolize it or turn it into glycogen, which is used as an energy store. This takes glucose out of circulation and lowers blood levels.

However, when this process has been abused for many decades, it is liable to break down. Suddenly the body ceases to adapt to glucose and, despite ever-increasing levels of insulin, glucose in the blood begins to rise. The cells can no longer utilize it properly. Cell receptors seem to have switched off and stopped listening to the signal from insulin, hence the term for this condition.

Insulin resistance is dangerous. Apart from the obvious risk of progression into the next two conditions, high insulin levels result in excess sympathetic nervous system activity, which keeps the individual tense and prone to fatigue. Sooner or later, a complete system breakdown, or advanced aging, will result.

Syndrome X

Our understanding of disordered blood glucose control advanced considerably in 1988, when Dr. Gerald Reaven of Stanford University published a paper describing what he called "Syndrome X." A syndrome in medicine means a group of symptoms that appear together as a characteristic pattern which is repeatedly encountered. In this case, the syndrome consists of five features: obesity, insulin resistance, high blood pressure, high serum triglyceride levels (bad fat), and low HDL (good cholesterol). Dr. Reaven had no idea what caused this group of symptoms to occur together, so he named it "Syndrome X."

Notice that patients with Syndrome X do not have the dangerously raised glucose levels of diabetes. But they do have insulin resistance and higher than normal levels of circulating glucose. The high level of insulin stimulates the kidneys to reabsorb sodium, which in turn results in a tendency to hypertension. Dr. Reaven believes that half of all hypertensives have insulin resistance. No one needs to be told of the dangers of high blood pressure.

Raised triglycerides, along with raised LDL (bad cholesterol), combined with lowered HDL, are disturbing. These changes in blood fats denote a major increase in the risk of arterial degenerative disease. Unfortunately, hyper-insulinism also reduces blood enzymes that prevent or dissolve blood clots. Thus, along with the undesirable changes in blood fats comes a sinister increase in the likelihood of thrombosis, making the risk of heart attack or stroke far greater than for healthy individuals.

Diabetes

The above conditions can be referred to as "pre-diabetic." Sooner or later, left untreated, the condition is going to worsen and turn into full-blown diabetes. This disease has been likened to an overview on the process of aging. Much of the degeneration in the arteries, heart, brain, and eyes seen with diabetes is the same as that attributable to aging. But it takes place much faster in a diabetic patient. The life expectancy of an individual with diabetes is therefore considerably below average.

Here we refer to type II diabetes or "late onset" diabetes. As its name suggests, this is mainly what affects older individuals. It is a direct result of collapsed carbohydrate regulation. Whereas type I diabetes is caused by the failure of the pancreas to secrete adequate insulin, in type II there is too much insulin. The two conditions are fundamentally different. In the type II condition, the body has become refractory to insulin, simply not responding to regulation as it should. Thus, despite high levels of insulin, glucose increases to unacceptable levels in the blood. Be sure you understand: untreated diabetes is a fatal disease process.

The many complications of diabetes can be summed up as follows: arteriosclerosis (leading to increased risk of heart disease, stroke and gangrene of the lower limbs), early dementia, impotence, eye damage leading to blindness, poor kidney performance, nerve damage that results in numbness and paralysis of the limbs, skin sores, carbuncles, ulcers, and poor wound healing.

Be aware then: you do not want to develop diabetes at any stage of life. Beware what you eat!

Laboratory Testing

In the old days the main test was tasting the urine to see if sugar is detectable: hence the term diabetes mellitus (sweet tasting)! Fortunately things are more scientific these days!

Doctors will insist on measuring isolated blood glucose levels, though these can be very misleading, even when fasting, and random samples are worse than useless. More helpful is the glucose tolerance test. The patient fasts overnight and then, after a loading drink of 50 grams of glucose, blood samples are taken hourly. Usually this is continued for 2 to 3 hours, but far better is to go 4 hours. The diagnostic sign is that the glucose level goes high (over 180) and stays high or is very sluggish at returning to pre-test levels. This means the cells are not utilizing the glucose properly, either through frank lack of insulin, or due to insulin resistance.

Fasting	30 minutes	1 hour	2 hours	3 hours
70-100	110-170	120-170	70-120	70-120

At least two of the recordings must be abnormal (high) to diagnose diabetes.

Hyperinsulinaemia is mainly diagnosed by sophisticated blood tests, showing abnormally high insulin levels without proportionately raised glucose levels. Blood insulin levels are difficult to measure and so not done routinely. The GTT is much more valuable if insulin is measured concurrent with the glucose levels.

The so-called insulin tolerance test means giving an injection of insulin to a fasting patient (one unit per kilogram of body weight) and taking repeated blood glucose samples every three minutes for a quarter of an hour. Insulin resistance is diagnosed if the blood glucose falls by less than 50% of the fasting level in that 15 minutes. The test is not safe to perform if the fasting glucose is less than 120 mg/dl.

Hospital doctors and internists will also measure blood hemoglobin AIC or glycosylated hemoglobin. That tells them much more accurately what long-term changes in blood levels of glucose have been like. Normal levels range up to 7%. Above 7% is bad, above 10% very bad, and above 12% is dangerous and means very poor glucose control. Experts recommend repeating this test every three to six months once diabetes has been established.

What You Can Do

By the time you have developed diabetes, you need help from a qualified and skilled doctor. But the only aim of the ordinary physician is to control the disease by keeping the blood glucose levels within normal limits. You will be offered drugs that increase insulin secretion (such as the sulphonyl ureas) or a different kind of drug, metformin, which increases the body's sensitivity to its own insulin. This simplistic approach does not go nearly far enough for you. It is far better to tackle the causes.

You can do a great deal to avoid disordered carbohydrate metabolism, or help yourself towards a recovery, if you have understood the origins of the problem. First and most obvious is to drastically curtail the amount of carbohydrate in your diet. Avoid all sugar, flour, and "white foods." What carbs you do eat, take only as whole-grain products.

Exercise and weight control are vital at all stages of life, but particularly if you are in the high-risk zone (50 plus). All knowledgeable practitioners agree that these two practices decrease insulin resistance significantly. Both also help in reducing hypertension. Do not even consider medication for blood pressure, unless all lifestyle changes fail – drugs will merely mask the problem and not eliminate the cause.

Dr. Reaven restricts carbohydrate and replaces it with mono and polyunsaturated fats, such as olive oil and fish oils. These increase insulin sensitivity and help reduce triglycerides and LDL. However, some care is required: omega-3 fats (fish and flax oil) are known to potentially impair insulin levels and increase blood glucose. This adverse effect may be avoided by adding vitamin E (400 IU daily) to the regime. The omega-6 fatty acids (evening primrose oil, star flower, borage) have insulin-like properties and they also increase sensitivity to insulin but without affecting bad blood fats.

Supplements
Top of the list is chromium, aka "glucose tolerance factor"! Take at least 400 mcg daily.

Next comes DHEA, which lowers insulin levels and also, vitally, protects organs, particularly the kidneys, against damage due to high blood glucose levels. Men need about 25 mg daily but women should not take more than 10 mg daily, or it will cause greasy spotty skin.

Next comes magnesium. A consensus panel of doctors in the America Diabetes Association agreed that magnesium deficiency may play a role in developing insulin resistance, carbohydrate intolerance and hypertension. Pay attention: it is not often that conventional doctors recommend nutrient solutions! Take 350 mg a day or more.

Vitamins B3, B6 and C are also vital. Deficiencies have shown up as insulin resistance. Take 100-1,000 mg of B3, 50- 100 mg of B6 and 2 grams of vitamin C daily, alone or as part of your health formula.

Alpha lipoic acid, a star-quality supplement steadily climbing to the top of the anti-aging league table, apart from being a powerful antioxidant has also been shown to improve insulin action. You need 200- 400 mg daily.

HUMAN GROWTH HORMONE - DO WE NEED IT?

Human Growth Hormone or HGH (also called somatotrophin) is produced by the pituitary gland. It influences the growth of cells, bones, muscles, and organs throughout the body. Production peaks at adolescence, when accelerated growth occurs. If growing children have too little, they remain dwarfs; if they have too much, they become giants. Sudden cessation of HGH can lead to drastic aging, as seen with terminal AIDS patients.

HGH is one of many endocrine hormones, like estrogen, progesterone, testosterone, and DHEA, that decline in production with age. Daily growth hormone secretion diminishes with age to the extent that a 60-year-old may secrete only 25% of the HGH secreted by a 20-year-old. The decline of growth hormone with age is sometimes referred to as somatopause, in line with menopause and the so-called andropause.

While many hormones can be replaced to deter some of the effects of aging, HGH reaches far beyond the scope of any of these hormones. Not only does it prevent biological aging, but it acts to significantly reverse a broad range of the signs and symptoms associated with the aging process, including wrinkling, grey hair, decreased energy and sexual function, increased body fat and cardiovascular disease, osteoporosis, and more.

The trouble is, it is VERY expensive. Most people would afford it, if they were SURE it would deliver that important rejuvenation effect. *The question is, does it?*

The most famous study on HGH is that published by Dr. Daniel Rudman in the *New England Journal of Medicine*[1]. Working with volunteers aged 61 to 81 at the Medical College of Wisconsin, Milwaukee, Rudman used synthetically manufactured HGH injections to replicate what is created naturally in the body's own pituitary gland. The result was quite clear: six months of injections reversed the aging process by from 10 to 15 years in patients who received the HGH, measured in terms of bone density, lean muscle mass, and reversal of fat decline. In the control group that didn't receive HGH, the normal aging process continued.

Remember, these startling findings were published in one of medicine's most conservative journals. Anti-aging science was born. Overnight, a vast Internet industry was spawned, with its own gobbledy-speak, trying to sell the gullible public HGH substitutes, taken by mouth. It looked like snake oil coming around again.

Since Dr. Rudman's initial findings, additional studies have supported the fact that HGH does not only retard aging, but it also reverses the process, as well. The consistent findings, which are proven over and over, are increase in lean muscle mass, loss of the belly fat, improved cardiovascular risk profile, more energy, and feeling good. HGH affects almost every cell in the body, helping to regenerate skin, bones, heart, lungs, liver, and kidneys to their former youthful levels. Lipid profiles are improved; the heart attack and stroke factors are diminished. Osteoporosis is blocked. That means more zest, feeling good, and enjoying life; less wrinkles, stiffness, and aches!

But, say the critics, this study was done on 70- and 80-year-olds. It isn't "valid" for anyone else. Presumably, HGH suddenly declines on your 70th birthday and to prescribe it for a 69-year-old is unethical or somehow unscientific. To me that's a bit like saying you shouldn't wear a life jacket unless you are already in the water drowning.

The "anti" brigade also points out that, although lean muscle mass is increased, studies show that contractile proteins are not affected and so strength remains unchanged. I mean, come on guys! Testosterone is what takes care of muscle tone, anybody knows that, not HGH! This is the kind of folly that non-biological medicine gets into. Our bodies are a whole system, not just an HGH machine, stuck to a muscle machine, which is stuck to a pair of testicles and so on!

Even more tellingly, the boffins urge, there is not one shred of evidence that HGH will extend your life span. True. But as I constantly point out, what our anti-aging movement is about is not so much living longer (though it counts) but feeling good, looking good, continuing to have bags of youthful energy, and avoiding those dread diseases such as cancer, diabetes, heart attacks, and strokes, that kill so many people with years still inside them. In other words, it's about staying fit and well until the very end.

Remember, though, as I also like to point out, the demographic sub-group of keen anti-agers, who follow lifestyle advice and take care of themselves, may well live significantly longer than average; nobody knows, because nobody is studying them. But their achievements would certainly be obscured by the averaging effect of the majority millions of junk-gobbling slob-out wasters who do nothing to take care of their health (though even this suicide crowd are living longer and longer and longer, as official figures show).

Consequences of HGH Deficiency

A topical briefings page, posted by the *Society of Endocrinology*, lists the following symptoms of HGH deficiency:

- Decreased energy levels
- Social isolation
- Lack of positive well-being
- Depressed mood
- Increased anxiety

They list the following clinical features:

1. Increased body fat, particularly central adiposity (a gut!)
2. Decreased muscle mass
3. Decreased bone density, associated with an increased risk of fracture
4. Increased LDL (bad) cholesterol and decreased HDL (good) cholesterol
5. Decreased cardiac muscle mass
6. Impaired cardiac function
7. Decreased insulin sensitivity (disposition to diabetes)
8. Accelerated atherogenesis (hardening of the arteries)

A review of the literature states that, overall, at least 80% of patients given growth hormone replacements demonstrate a significant improvement, especially in fat distribution, body composition, and parameters reflecting well-being and quality of life.[1]

Need I say more?

A recent study under professor S.M. Shalet, carried out here in my city of Manchester, at the world-famous Christie Hospital, aimed to study a number of pathological effects rectified by supplementing HGH but with a special wish to avoid "over-replacement." They studied 65 patients and one of the key selection criteria was poor quality of life (SRQ). Supplementation started with a very low dose, 0.8 unit/day, and aimed to normalize IGF-1 as closely as possible. The results showed that "The observed improvement in quality of life in GH deficient adults is proportionate to the degree of impairment before commencing therapy" and, furthermore, although all scales showed improvement, "that of vitality was of greatest magnitude".[2]

It all adds up to the fact that if you are deficient in growth hormone, you will benefit greatly from supplementing it. The question is: are you deficient?

Unfortunately, there are no easy tests to detect this. HGH appears in the blood at night and is present for a matter of minutes. A blood sample is very hit-and-miss. A better test is to use the marker IGF-1 (insulin-like growth factor 1). But this, too, is hardly a routine test. At least one coworker reckons that it is not such a reliable marker as we have supposed. The gold standard is called the insulin tolerance test, but it is risky and requires an in-patient basis.

I prefer to argue it this way: averages show quite clearly that we lose production of HGH as the decades pass; therefore one can safely assume that one is likely deficient. We would be far healthier with the HGH of a younger person than someone in decline. Supplementation in later decades makes sense. But why wait until you are an oldie before taking reasonable steps to put the brake on? If you were driving a car straight towards a brick wall, you would apply the brakes as soon as you knew where they were and not wait until the crash was imminent, surely.

For this reason, I think it is valid and sensible to start HGH supplementation early. But I feel strongly that it should not be taken "for life." You can snatch back some precious years but that doesn't mean you become immortal! Bearing this in mind and also invoking the Rudman study, which showed results from a six-month trial period, I think one should take HGH for no more than a year in total. Someone in their 50s would be better to stop after just three or four months. You then have another period in credit, to use later in life if you wish. The idea is to wind the clock back as far as you can while taking HGH and then let it roll forward, in the natural way.

There are plenty of steps you can take to help release HGH naturally, including weight loss, exercise, plentiful sleep, diet changes and nutritional supplements (see below).

The Regime

Patients self-administer a prescribed daily dose of HGH, starting at 0.8 unit/day . It arrives as freeze-dried powder cartridge and is easy to store. Once reconstituted however, it must be kept refrigerated and has a life of only a few weeks. A monthly supply is arranged for the patient. Dosing is easy: simply click in the right dose, touch the custom needle gun to the skin and press the trigger.

IGF-1 is monitored regularly.3 Also thyroid function, since hypothyroidism is a theoretical risk, even without growth disorder.

Side Effects

The main reported side effects are headache, visual disturbance, nausea/vomiting, carpal tunnel syndrome, and mild hypertension. However these are from high-dose growth failure cases, not anti-aging. Such side effects would be quite exceptional in the low-dose regime we use.

Oral HGH

Natural secretagogues (hormone precursors) offer a means of naturally stimulating HGH. Among the HGH-releasers recognized by holistic doctors are lysine, arginine, ornithine, and glutamine.

Arginine is an essential amino acid, meaning it is not manufactured in the body; it has to be supplied in the food we eat. Claims for arginine include an increase in fat burning and muscle building. Arginine strengthens the thymus gland, increasing its weight and activity, boosting immunity and fighting cancer. It also promotes healing of burns and wounds while generally protecting and detoxifying the body. Finally, it enhances male fertility.

The amino acid lysine boosts the effectiveness of arginine and affects growth. Ornithine can be synthesized in the body and is therefore less essential as a supplement. Similar in structure, it can be made from arginine. It definitely helps to stimulate HGH release.

Glutamine is a conditional essential amino acid but very important and cheap and easy to supplement in large doses. While one of the most abundant amino acids, it may not always be made by the body in sufficient quantities in times of stress. It is helpful to gut condition and performance and it is essential for the immune system. Without sufficiently available levels, the gut atrophies, nutrients are less well absorbed, and muscle and immunity are also lost.

GABA (gamma-aminobutyric acid), one of the most potent stimulators of HGH release from the pituitary, is a precursor to, and breakdown product of, GHB (gamma-hydroxybutyric acid), now notorious as the "date rape drug." This has put it into eclipse, though GHB is a substance that occurs naturally in every cell of the body, including the brain. The fact is that one Japanese study showed it increased HGH levels 16-fold.

Proper medical supervision by a knowledgeable physician is required in supplementing these compounds, since the glutamine-arginine-lysine stack may release insulin as well as growth hormone. We now know that raised insulin levels can be damaging and definitely SHORTEN life, so beware. Generally, when HGH levels are rising, insulin levels are falling. However, if it is possible to raise insulin levels at the same time as growth hormone; it has a very high anabolic effect. That is to say, the body builds up muscle and tissue and carries out cell repair essential to reverse aging. "You don't have to increase growth hormone very much to get a 10% to 20% rise in IGF-1 (insulin-like growth factor type 1) levels, which can have a definite effect on the body," adds Mauro Di Pasquale, MD, world-class power lifter and one of the most knowledgeable experts in the field of anabolic and HGH-releasing compounds.

References:

1. *The New England Journal of Medicine,* Volume 323, July 5, 1990 Number 1 "Effects of Human Growth Hormone in men over 60 years old." Daniel Rudman et al.
2. *Clin Endocrinology* (Oxf) 1999 Jun;50(6):749- "Dose titration and patient selection increases the efficacy of GH replacement in severely GH deficient adults." Shalet et al.
3. *Clin Endocrinol* (Oxf) 2000 May;52(5):537- "Pre-treatment IGF-1 level is the major determinant of GH dosage in adult GH deficiency." Shalet SM et al.
4. Link: www.endocrinology.org/SFE/gh.htm

OXYGEN & WHY WE NEED ANTIOXIDANTS

Despite its status as a necessary life substance for all except a few special organisms, oxygen is a highly toxic mutagenic gas [*Free Radicals in Biology and Medicine*, B Halliwell and JMC Gutteridge, OUP, Oxford 1999, p. 1). We can only survive its presence in our atmosphere because we have important antioxidant mechanisms to protect us from its damage.

Initially, the earth's atmosphere had less than 1% oxygen. But activity by blue-green algae species billions of years ago gradually increased these levels. For them, it was just a waste product of a respiration process that relied on releasing hydrogen from water. By 1.3 billion years ago, levels had risen to 1%. Around 500 million years ago, oxygen levels had reached 10%. This was sufficient to switch on the all-important ozone layer, which protects the earth's surface from blazing destructive UV radiation.

From then on, other life forms could evolve.

Oxygen may have reached 35% in the late Carboniferous age, when life was mainly plant-based. The present level of 21% was settled around 5 million years ago. As a result, oxygen is the most prevalent element in the Earth's crust (53%); rock is basically silicon dioxide, with additions

DEFINITION: Oxidation has long been taken to mean the addition of an oxygen atom to an existing chemical structure. More recently, scientists have also used this term for an exchange in which an electron is removed from a grouping. The opposite process, hydrogenation, is the addition of hydrogen; addition of an electron to a grouping is thus also hydrogenation.

About 85 to 90% of oxygen taken up in advanced animal respiration is consumed by the mitochondria. The essence of metabolic energy production in the body is that food materials are oxidized, by having electrons stripped. This releases the energy to create molecules of ATP (adenosine triphosphate), which is the body's chief energy transport mechanism. The whole process is done in a gradual step-wise fashion, involving the creation of excited forms of iron, from ferrous to ferric-haem cytochrome.

This is a very important physiological detail. It means that iron is one of the most destructive oxidative stress elements in our tissues. The removal of excess "hot" iron may be one of the principal mechanisms by which chelation with EDTA reduces or even reverses oxidative age damage.

The whole process is done under the control of a complex enzyme system called the cytochrome oxidase pathway. Cytochrome oxidase in mammals is special in that it works efficiently when there is almost no oxygen present. But xenobiotics and pollution very quickly poison this system, and so render us liable to tissue damage by oxidation.

Reactive Oxygen Species

The term "free radicals" (hence free-radical damage) was soon introduced into this debate. But, strictly speaking, a free radical is simply one capable of existing independently (hence the term "free"); they don't necessarily bite! A better term is reactive oxygen species (ROS). The chief reactive oxidation ions are O2 and OH (hydroxyl ion). The so-called superoxide radical is not, in truth, as active or damaging as the basic oxygen radical, despite its name! The quartet is made up with the peroxide ion. This is also a killer ion and is generated briefly by certain white cells to damage microbes before ingesting them. Out of place, it is potentially harmful to us.

Finally, ozone is another reactive oxygen species, which is highly destructive to living cells. However, it is little found at sea level, remaining largely in the upper atmosphere, where it shields us from harmful UV radiation. Unfortunately, urban pollution, notably with traffic emissions, in the presence of sunlight, creates dangerous levels of ozone, which we may breathe. It causes lung damage.

Antioxidants

Oxidation stress, leading to tissue damage, has now been implicated in a wide variety of disease complaints, including arthritis, heart disease, cancer, dementias, and other degenerative illnesses. Environmental pollution and overburdened lifestyles unquestionably potentiate this aging process.

Smoking and excess alcohol increase oxidative damage also. The organ most sensitive to oxidative damage is the brain.

Hardly surprising, since around 25% of the body's metabolic activity occurs in this one organ. This means real changes and loss of cognitive function - "feeling old," lethargy, confusion, and forgetfulness. There are many subtle layers and degrees of this unfortunate process, which we recognize as a loss of zest for life and a failure to think as sharply as we once did.

As we have come to understand the power and significance of oxidative tissue damage, a key process in aging, then substances which protect us from this occurrence have assumed steadily greater significance. We call these, not unnaturally, antioxidants. They can be listed as follows:

- **AMINO ACIDS** - cysteine, glutathione, methionine, taurine
- **BIOFLAVINOIDS** - anthocyanins (blue-black fruits), citrus bioflavinoids (lemon, orange, grapefruit, etc.), oligometric proanthocyanidins (OPC) in pycnogenol
- **CAROTENOIDS** - alpha and beta carotene (red, yellow and orange fruits and vegetables), lycopene (red fruits and vegetables)
- **HERBS** - Gingko, green tea, milk thistle, sage
- **MINERALS** - Copper, zinc, manganese, selenium
- **VITAMINS AND CO-FACTORS** - A, B2, C, E and coenzyme Q10, NADH (nicotinamide adenine dinucleotide)
- **ENZYMES** - catalase, glutathione peroxidase, superoxide dismutase
- **BIOCHEMICAL INTERMEDIARIES** – Glutathione

A number of proprietary "antioxidant" formulas are on sale. Typically, these include mixtures of vitamin A, beta carotene, C, E, selenium and zinc. It is advisable to eat plenty of fresh fruit and vegetables, all of which contain types of antioxidants, as you see from the list above.

Chelation therapy is now known to act primarily as an antioxidant process. Elmer Cranton, MD, one of the doyen figures of chelation therapy and author of several definitive books, thinks this is mainly by removing "pro-oxidant" ions, such as iron. It may not be all that simple. But the benefits are quite clear. I have now taken to giving glutathione IV, along with EDTA, and found startling extra benefits against aging.

Attacks on Antioxidants

In February 2007, a shocking attack on antioxidants was launched in an article published by the *Journal of the American Medical Association*.[1]

The "study" claimed beta carotene, vitamin A, and vitamin E, given singly or combined with other antioxidant supplements, "significantly increase mortality." In fact, it showed no such thing and is typical of the way in which appalling perverted science is published without question by mainstream journals, if it in any way undermines natural health and living.

Even if taking these antioxidants really was associated with a higher death rate, the "researchers" completely failed to assess or deal with the possibility that sicker people may be more desperate and more likely to try vitamins and minerals - but are also more likely to die. This would cause a bias showing antioxidant-takers died quicker. But that's a million miles from saying that antioxidants caused it!!

These hatchet jobs are often done by a "tool" called meta-analysis. That means you pool all the bad studies with those showing good outcomes, mix everything up, fudge all the figures and - hey, presto - you cancel out all the good outcomes. This review of 68 studies covered nearly a quarter of a million people and might sound impressive - if you don't know how these stories are faked.

The whole sham study tried to imply that patients were dying of vitamin supplements, when of course they were dying of heart disease, cancer, kidney failure, and so on.

Take all the antioxidants you can swallow. There are hundreds of studies showing the benefits. Natural foods are best, colored foods and... chocolate!

A *BMJ* study (December 19, 1998) showed that the more chocolate you ate, the longer you lived. Chocolate is very rich in antioxidants: the natural unprocessed variety only, I'm afraid!

Reference
1. Mortality in Randomized Trials of Antioxidant Supplements for Primary and Secondary Prevention, *JAMA*. 2007;297:842-857.

THE MOTHER HORMONE: PREGNENOLONE

You will sometimes hear DHEA described as the "mother hormone." The term would be better applied to pregnenolone, which is the basic precursor, or starting raw material, for the production of ALL the human steroid hormones, including DHEA, progesterone, estrogen, testosterone, cortisol, and aldosterone. But pregnenolone is not itself steroid hormone.

Pregnenolone has been studied extensively since the 1940s, when it was used both experimentally and medically. Pregnenolone was phased out of medical use; yet ironically pregnenolone is radically safer and more versatile than the specific steroid hormones which replaced it! Pregnenolone is safe even at 1 gram (1000mg) dosages, a claim no steroid hormone can make (20 mg or more of prednisolone, one of the main synthetic prescribed steroids, would be dangerous long-term).

One of the most important actions of pregnenolone is to counter damage caused by the natural stress hormone, released by the adrenal glands, called "cortisol" (after the adrenal cortex, where it is made). Cortisol is helpful in modest amounts, but toxic at higher levels. Amongst other things, it damages brain function and this can lead to blunting normal memory. Blocking this process may be one of the main reasons for the known memory-enhancing effect of pregnenolone. It also improved the mood and efficiency of factory workers, which may also be due to benefiting brain function, as well as enhancing mood.

Other actions of pregnenolone include limiting allergic reactions and reducing inflammatory processes, such as arthritis. It also improves energy levels by protecting our energy-producing mitochondria from environmental toxins.

Interestingly, in a study of rats subjected to spinal cord injury, administration of pregnenolone in combination with the anti-inflammatory medication indomethacin and an immune-modulating substance (bacterial lipopolysaccharide) promoted recovery of nerve function. The effect was more pronounced with combination therapy than with any one of these substances given singly or in combinations of two. We don't yet know if this works in humans the same way.

Pregnenolone enhances the activity of the cytochrome P450 detoxifying enzymes, which help our cells (especially the liver and brain) to detoxify xenobiotic poisons of all sorts.

The body's own production of pregnenolone is reduced with aging, stress, depression, hypothyroidism, and toxin exposure. The work of Ray Peat, PhD, has shown that pregnenolone may be a general "anti-stress" metabolite. However, this may not always be present in our bodies at optimal levels, precisely because it may be used up in producing all the steroid hormones, not leaving enough to fulfill its stress buffer role. Hence the need for supplementation.

Pregnenolone is generally safe and effective at doses of 50 mg to 200 mg per day. If you are self-dosing, judge it from your mood and energy levels. On no account use pregnenolone instead of medically prescribed steroids, without telling your doctor what you are doing.

NO MORE WRINKLES!

Nothing gives away our age quite so much as wrinkles, especially of the face - fine lines at the outer corner of the smile lines of the eyes (known as crow's feet). Thinning and loss of tone to the skin is one of the hallmarks of the aging process.

Can we do anything about it? *You bet.*

First, any good anti-aging measure is good for the skin and complexion. Number one among those I would put a healthy diet. It needs to be constructed on a person-by-person basis, working out the foods that suit you personally. I explain how to do this in the book, *Diet Wise*.

Botox

We all know what this is. It's a toxin (*Botulinum* toxin). It works by paralyzing the nerves to the face, those that cause expression and wrinkles.

There are several problems with this treatment:

- It can go wrong and produce deformity, even in skilled hands
- After a while it stops working. By this stage most of the facial muscles are paralyzed anyway. It is very limited.
- You will have a mask-like face. You'll wish you hadn't done it by this time but it's irreversible.

Homeopathic Botox (Better!)

This is not a homeopathic preparation of *Botulinum* toxin but a completely different formula. A preparation called MADE was developed by Massimo Debelli of Italy (hence its name) and it is quite logical. It contains all kinds of good tissue-energizing and -nourishing substances, all harmless.

MADE is intended to be injected at select acupuncture sites around the face, rather like mesotherapy.

It is normally done bi-weekly and can be continued and/or repeated as often as you like.

Homeopathic does not produce the rapid and disastrous destruction of normal facial tissue. Rather, it gently encourages regeneration and restoration of skin tissues.

Chelation

One of the more dramatic effects of EDTA chelation therapy is the diminishment of wrinkles and a return of softer, more supple looking skin.

The late Dr. Charlie Farr, from Oklahoma, performed studies that supports this happy finding. Before he began treating a group of older patients with chelation therapy, he took samples of skin from their arms. He discovered that the common stiffness and dryness they experienced with age was a result of cross-linkages of calcium. Following chelation therapy, he noticed the cross-linkages were gone and his patients were reporting softer, smoother skin.

Aging involves hard arteries and soft bones. The process of aging is what researchers and doctors call calcinosis, meaning calcium is pulled from the bones and deposited into soft tissue, settling in your arteries, joints, and skin, causing arthritis and the pale, hard, wrinkled look of aging. Calcium deposits can also cause strokes and circulation problems. What chelation therapy does is to remove calcium from the soft tissues, where it doesn't belong, and put it back into the bones, where it does belong.

In other words, **chelation can increase bone density.**

For maximum benefit, EDTA therapy should be accompanied by a carefully tailored program of vitamin and mineral supplements. This is because of the delicate balance of nutrients and the body's use of calcium. For example, those with low intakes of vitamin D have higher parathyroid function in the winter. The parathyroid glands draw on calcium reserves in the bone to keep blood levels normal. Parahormone is the hormone excreted by the parathyroid glands, which control calcium and phosphorus metabolism.

For detailed information about the device, contact Friends of Chelation Society at: 2825 Tahquitz Canyon Way, Bldg. C, Palm Springs, CA 92262. Tel: 001 (760) 4162013; Fax (760) 4162143.

For more on the fascinating, enlightening and underrated preventive and healing effects of chelation therapy, especially against aging, read the book, *Forty Something Forever* by Harold and Arlene Brecher. We're only as old as our arteries. Drink from this Fountain of Youth and be young again!

Hyaluronic Acid (HA)

HA is a special mucopolysaccharide that is the normal lubricant in human joints. When present in a joint, even one with minimal or no cartilage, it provides a cushion effect. It is also part of connective tissue and joins cells together.

Aging causes the hyaluronic acid in the skin to decrease, leaving the skin dry and wrinkled. Replenishing the HA levels in the body allow the skin to retain moisture, leaving the skin soft,

supple, and wrinkle-free. It is used in many cosmetics such as make-up and moisturizing creams.

THE ANTI-AGING VITAMIN

What Is the Anti-Aging Vitamin?

Vitamin C, we know, does some pretty cool stuff, apart from just preventing scurvy. A new study finds a link between low vitamin C in the blood and increased risk for intracerebral hemorrhage (stroke).

That's not surprising, because we know that scurvy is characterized by spontaneous bleeding, especially from the gums (if you get blood on your toothbrush, up your intake of vitamin C and don't forget the brushing with coconut oil from this issue…). Vitamin C is vital in the manufacture of collagen, which is turn helps support blood vessels and tissues.

In fact, this effect may be the real reason that fruits and veggies protect against stroke, rather than the antioxidant content (or perhaps both).

But there is an extra layer to this: **vitamin C helps reduce blood pressure significantly.** Of course, high blood pressure increases the risk of a "blowout," so it makes sense. I should explain there are two reasons for a stroke: clots, which damage brain tissue, but also bleeds, which rip up brain tissue.

So a team at Pontchaillou University Hospital, Rennes, France, decided to look into this (ah, how I love Normandy! Vivien and I were in Rennes only last year).

This was a prospective case–control study (always much stronger than retrospective studies) and included 135 participants, of which 41% had a normal vitamin C status, 45% showed some depletion, and 14% were deficient.

65 cases had had a cerebral hemorrhage episode and these were in the significantly low vitamin C patients.

The team also noticed something interesting, which is that older patients tended to have their pathology in the brain cortex or lobes, while the (relatively) younger participants had more of the deep bleeding.

Take Home

There are two clear messages I'm sharing with you here. Take lots of vitamin C, because it will help keep your vasculature in good order. But it also helps with the manufacture of collagen and we need as much collagen as possible to beat off wrinkles!

Us Boomers are fighting wrinkles and vitamin C depletion is the last thing we need. Wrinkles occur when there is too little collagen support for the skin, so it begins to sag.

For tons more good stuff on beating wrinkles, in fact beating aging and living "forever young," get my comprehensive guide: *Get Healthy For Your Next 100 Years! Visit: www.alternative-doctor.com/gethealthy*

SENILITY IS INFLAMMATION

I've been telling you for years. **Inflammation is the core of aging**. You have to quench that fire to age well.

Senility and dementia also stem directly from inflammation. Those who show signs of inflammation move earlier and quicker into cognitive dysfunction.

It was always thought that in aging our immune systems deteriorate. That's not strictly true. It changes in character. Those who stay fit in mind and body till extreme age have a vibrant immune system. But it is different from that of early life.

With age, immune cells called T-cells become more like natural killer (NK) cells, which typically target tumor cells and virus-infected cells. Now a new study that people who were most physically and cognitively resilient had a dominant pattern of stimulatory NK receptors on the T-cell surface, and that these unusual T-cells can be activated directly through these NK receptors, independently of the conventional ones.

The functionally resilient elders also show less inflammation and signs of a positive functioning immune system.

Conversely, those who aged badly had a dominant pattern of inhibitory NK receptors on their T-cells, and a cytokine profile indicating a pro-inflammatory environment.

Inhibitory NK cells, if you don't get it, means more susceptibility to disease, especially cancer.

All this was demonstrated neatly by a recent study (October 2011) from the University of Pittsburgh. The findings were published in the Public Library of Science (PLoS).

The researchers concluded that there is remodeling or adaptation of the immune system as we age that can be either protective or detrimental. It's a kind of immunological fingerprint that can identify individuals who are more likely to stay physically and cognitively well.[1]

These findings are supported by other studies, suggesting that people who take anti-inflammatories, such as ibuprofen, are less likely to get Alzheimer's, in fact 50% less likely![2]

It all adds up. Growing old and doddery is inflammation, not wear and tear, genes, telomeres, or any of that other stuff. It's fire inside.

Better get those antioxidants down fast, plenty of omega-3s (brilliant against inflammation). And cut the sugar: that's highly inflammatory.

References

1. Abbe N. Vallejo, David L. Hamel, Robert G. Mueller, Diane G. Ives, Joshua J. Michel, Robert M. Boudreau, Anne B. Newman. NK-Like T Cells and Plasma Cytokines, but Not Anti-Viral Serology, Define Immune Fingerprints of Resilience and Mild Disability in *Exceptional Aging*. *PLoS ONE*, 2011; 6 (10): e26558 DOI: 10.1371/journal.pone.0026558.
2. http://www.nia.nih.gov/NewsAndEvents/PressReleases/PR1970310AntiInflammatoryDrugs.htm.

SECTION 9

VIRTUAL MEDICINE…. WHAT I ALSO CALL MEDICINE BEYOND!

THE TRAILBLAZING ORIGIN OF VIRTUAL MEDICINE

ELECTROTHERAPY – DISCOVER THE ELECTRIC LANGUAGE OF THE BODY FOR ULTIMATE HEALING

PERSONALIZED MEDICINE WILL REVOLUTIONIZE HEALTHCARE

WHAT IS HIGH-VOLTAGE SYNDROME?

THE TRAILBLAZING ORIGIN OF VIRTUAL MEDICINE

My book *Virtual Medicine* (now *Medicine Beyond*), when it came out, broke almost all laws of medicine and showed the science (real science) behind much energy medicine and so-called "subtle energy" phenomena.

One of its critical mottoes was that "Advanced physics doesn't just say these strange energy phenomena could happen, it tells us they MUST happen." It's everyday stuff now but certainly was not in the 1990s, when I wrote it.

The first edition was published by Thorson's, an imprint of Harper Collins, one of the biggest publishing houses in the world. I wish I knew then what I know about marketing books and engaging with my audience! It would have been a blockbuster, not just a minor best-seller!

To this day, it's stolen, copied, and pirated all over the Internet. I suppose that's a kind of flattery. Anyway, I quit trying to chase abuses of copyright (but that does NOT mean I allow it into the public domain).

One of the reasons my masterwork is so popular is my hugely expanded review of DNA and how its properties affect every aspect of our health.

DNA can send out signals, which can turn chicks into ducks and revive dead seeds, which caused an elderly lady to start regrowing her teeth and allowed animals to survive a fatal dose of a poison which destroys the pancreas. In fact, they grew a new pancreas and ended up fully healthy animals.

Well, there is a lot more to come in *Medicine Beyond*. For example, expanded views of the phenomenon of death (as opposed to the experience of it), field mechanics, resonance mechanics, information theory, reverse entropy, extended mind, electrical nutrition, the Electric Universe model, how the Matrix concept applies in the real world and…as the salesman would say…much, much more!

Early readers who follow my writings will remember *Virtual Medicine* a/k/a *Medicine Beyond* all started with a conversation I had with Jacques Benveniste about an experiment in which he sent the electromagnetic "imprint" of curare thousands of miles across the Internet and killed a bunch of mice (not actual curare, just "virtual curare").

I occurred to me that we had, at that moment, entered a new age and I wanted to be part of it.

I also wanted to beat Robin Cook (author of *Coma* and *Brain*) to be the first to write a thriller about a murder in which someone switches on a computer, with a pre-programmed electronic "cyanide" message and croaks as a result!

That would be a hard crime to solve, especially in this climate of science.

If virtual substances can have a biological effect then healing remedies, too, could work in a non-material or "virtual" sense.

It was a magnificent new day dawning and my humble efforts at rounding up all the science to make it more credible, though now primitive with hindsight, at the time seemed worthy and were certainly very new.

But questions lingered. One of the most obvious ones to me was: if we can take a virtual aspirin for a headache, will we get virtual side effects?

Another was this: if a person has a real-time deficiency of magnesium, how is administering virtual nutrition going to make up the real world deficit?

It appears that what we see, feel, and touch, everything we experience, is but a concretion of consciousness into denser forms and energies. What has been considered actual reality does not even exist, never mind rule over US all.

It's only perceived to exist. From the viewpoint of consciousness it is virtual, like a dream, but from the viewpoint of experience in this very solid plane of existence seems real. Truth differs depending on whether you are viewing from a higher spiritual, soul, mental, emotional, or bodily perception.

A Word About Truth
Truth is a tricky concept at best, bright as shining gold, yet slippery as an eel's coils.

Attempts to suborn it to scientific study have proven very unsatisfactory, almost comically so. There is a method we call science. I applaud it—to look, to investigate, to speculate and theorize, then to attempt proofs or, if no proof is forthcoming, to revise the theory and continue trying, in a spirit of humble enquiry.

But the idea of science as a body of knowledge called the truth is plain laughable. As I said in the first edition of the book, our view of the world is changing fast.

A quarter of a century ago there were things that scientists were absolutely certain were true which, today, we are absolutely certain are not true…the reality is that science, as its own proponents define it, is a shifting quicksand of fashions and opinions, which regularly contradicts itself – often embarrassingly so.

Two of the grandest and most revolutionary theories of this century, Einstein's relativity and Planck's quantum mechanics, are in such disharmony that they appear mutually exclusive. Everyone knows they both throw Newton's staggeringly successful mechanical world out the window.

It is a disconcerting fact that electricity and magnetism, two of the absolutely fundamental building blocks of the universe, are so little understood that, at the deepest level, science cannot explain the nature of these energetic phenomena or how they exert their effect.

I point out these absurd contradictions in case the reader is under the illusion that science, in any meaningful sense, understands our world. It doesn't.

My greatest complaint with so-called science is not that it is sometimes wrong but that it fails to acknowledge that, whenever something cannot be shown to exist using the standard narrow approach, it is labeled "unscientific" and therefore a fake or delusion. There is never any suggestion that the problem may be the fault of science or its inadequate methodology.

Yet 100 years ago there was no way to detect radio waves. Did that mean they were an "unscientific" belief, if anyone had come up with the idea ahead of its time? Even more importantly, could it be said that because the science of the day failed to detect such a phenomenon that therefore radio waves did not exist?

This kind of thing we call "scientism," meaning an obsessive delusion with the preeminence of science.

Rupert Sheldrake, who features in the first edition of *Virtual Medicine*, has written a brilliant Philippic (almost a diatribe) on the follies of scientism in his latest book, *The Science Delusion*, called *Science Set Free* in the US (2012).

You may know that his TED talk video on this very theme was banned. Blocking a video these days is equivalent to book burning in the old days: something that the Inquisition, the Nazis and the like were fond of…but modern scientists? It's beyond shameful.

But it does mean they know they are against the ropes. A win on a technicality by Sheldrake!

Meanwhile, the forces of light and healing are at the doors of scientific despotism, hammering at the barriers to reason, love and compassion. It's the "Battle of the Karmas" (just made that up… but I like it!)

Make yourself a cup of tea and get ready to expand your mind, as I share with you the stunning findings of electrotherapy, how personalized medicine will revolutionize healthcare and more!

ELECTROTHERAPY – DISCOVER THE ELECTRIC LANGUAGE OF THE BODY FOR ULTIMATE HEALING

You will be learning more about the burgeoning specialty of Electrotherapy in times to come. I've devoted a whole chapter to it in my next book *Medicine Beyond* (which is a massive rewritten and expanded version of *Virtual Medicine*). Visit: www.alternative-doctor.com/vm

True to its ridiculous history of attacking anything they didn't think of first, medical orthodoxy has always viciously impugned any suggestion that electrical healing or electrotherapy has validity and it's been labeled charlatanism for the best part of a century.

Now they are having to eat humble pie and admit that claims, all along, had some validity, albeit in a rather hit-and-miss fashion until the advent of modern scientific trials.

We're now **learning to speak the electrical language of the body** – and using it to develop treatments for diseases from arthritis to diabetes and possibly even cancer.

It's no surprise to me, of course, nor should it be to anyone who knows of Robert O. Becker's classic book *The Body Electric*. He first wrote vividly about experiments with salamanders, in which correctly applied electrical currents could stimulate the remarkable regrowth of whole limbs.

I predicted in the first edition of *Virtual Medicine* that this is the direction healing would be going and introduced the revolutionary Russian SCENAR device, which swept the world as a result.

Cell migration and multiplication play a key role in development and healing.

Most research in this area, true to form, has been on chemical factors, totally ignoring the energy element (bioelectromagnetism). Now several studies have shown that applying electric fields can affect cell migration and division as well.

Cells and tissues essentially function as chemical batteries, with positively charged potassium ions and negatively charged chloride ions flowing across membranes. This creates electric field patterns all over the body. When tissue is wounded this disrupts the battery, effectively short-circuiting it.

Take, for example, a Scottish study, at the University of Aberdeen in Scotland, looking into repair of the cornea (in the eye).

In a healthy eye, cells pump positively charged ions into the cornea and push negatively charged ions out, creating an electrical potential of 40 millivolts.

But in damaged areas this voltage disappears, setting up an electric field between the damaged area and the surrounding corneal tissue. By enhancing or diminishing this electric field, scientists found they could speed up or slow down the rate of healing.

The conclusion: the electric field is the primary driver of the healing process. As one of the researchers stated, it's a big step forward to realize that fields play an important part in healing. They are just so far behind the pioneers in this!

Nowhere is the old adage more true than in this domain of bioelectromagnetic fields and healing (electrotherapy), that discovery goes through four stages:

    1. It's quackery and nonsense.

    2. There might be something in it

    3. There might be something in it, but where's the proof?

    4. We knew that all along!

A Little History of Electric Healing & Electrotherapy

Electrotherapy has a long history. William Gilbert, the Cambridge mathematician who later read medicine and became Queen Elizabeth's court physician in 1600, experimented with static electricity.

In 1757, John Wesley, the founder of Methodism, wrote in his diary of prescribing treatment with a specially made electrostatic machine for people *"ill of various disorders: some of whom found an immediate, some a gradual cure."*

In 1882, James Wimshurst invented the machine bearing his name.

By the end of the 19th century, the work of Faraday and many others had produced a host of convenient ways of generating electricity of various kinds: electrostatic, direct current and low-frequency and high-frequency alternating currents. Each had its advocates and to each was ascribed marvelous healing powers for every conceivable medical situation.

Magnetos proved more convenient to use than the Wimshurst and other electrostatic machines, which tended to be temperamental and intolerant of dust. Catalogues of the General Electric Company in the late 19th century had a number of such devices.

Its 1893 catalogue illustrates nine magnetos, ranging from one 20 centimeters long, boxed in pine, to the Phoenix, boxed in mahogany with a dial "to measure strength." Assorted electrodes "for foot, tooth, and ear, with plated handles" were available for the device.

Crank the handle and it generates a low-voltage alternating current. Instructions inside the lid claim that, when wound at the speed "most agreeable to the patient," this magneto will treat no fewer than 50 ailments, from weak eyes to spinal and nervous diseases, debility, fits, paralysis. and gout.

Another type of device was the induction coil, originally developed to detonate explosive charges. By 1888, GEC was offering induction coil apparatus for medical use, complete with bichromate battery, in a wooden case. By 1890 their range had grown to 10 models, with many variants, and electrodes engineered to treat particular parts of the body, from eye muscles to the spine.

Early in the 20th century so-called "hydroelectric baths" became fashionable. A wooden or porcelain bath was fitted with plate electrodes. Sometimes medicines were added to the bathwater in the belief that the patient would thereby receive whole-body treatment through the skin: cataphoresis, as it was called. Knowing what I know now, all these devices make sense and although they were not subject to modern-style scientific trials, there is little question they had benefit to some, at least equivalent to today's pharmaceutical drugs.

I was pleasantly surprised in my research to find that the famous Mayfair chemists, John Bell and Croydon, just around the corner from my former Harley Street clinic, at one time carried a range of electrotherapy devices.

They even had their own workshop, making induction coil machines tailored to what the doctor wanted for his patients in terms of output, portability and price, and the electrodes necessary to deliver the current where it was needed.

Historically, as far back as 1890, the American Electro-Therapeutic Association conducted annual conferences on the therapeutic use of electricity and electrical devices by physicians on ailing patients.

The effect of an electrical current on the body depends on its intensity. At 25 milliamps, the current, if it lasts for about 20 seconds, can stop the heart beating, so they are not inherently safe (the electric chair operates on this principle). But below 10 milliamps, whether direct current from a battery or an alternating current at ordinary mains frequencies (50 to 60 hertz), the current can create a rather pleasing tingle.

Writing in *New Scientist*, David Fishlock, an avid collector of these early devices, tells us that in the 1920s, a version of the Tesla apparatus known as Roger's Vitalator began to make its appearance in barbers' shops as a way of treating minor ailments, including bald patches and dandruff.

The barber would fit one of a number of glass tubes into an ebonite holder and switch on, whereupon sparks sizzled from the tube to scratch and tickle the pate. The maker recommended it for 127 conditions, including sexual debility, impotence, and breast development. That's barbers for you!

Fishlock asks the question: do black boxes emitting electricity or rays have a serious place in medicine? There is no doubt that the early inventions attracted the "snake-oil merchants."

As early as 1882, Silvanus Thompson, a fellow of the Royal Society and president of the Institution of Electrical Engineers, warned of the "gross impositions of the quacks and rogues who deal in the so-called magnetic appliances and disgrace alike the science of electricity and medicine while knowing nothing of either."

We shouldn't worry. Don't forget that Lord Kelvin (1824-1907), the greatest scientist of his day, declared that x-rays were a hoax!

When you consider that our entire nervous system works on electricity and electrical impulses, it's no surprise that electricity can be used to encourage faster healing times by causing cells to divide and move easily through our bodies.

I'll expand more on this fascinating field of science in *Medicine Beyond*.

Visit: www.alternative-doctor.com/vm

PERSONALIZED MEDICINE WILL REVOLUTIONIZE HEALTHCARE
Your Medical Avatar

I don't normally turn to the *Wall Street Journal* for information. But on this occasion I got it from there first, before my Medscape mailing came around.

I used to consider Medscape a lively and open-minded source for interesting news in orthodox medicine, some of it bordering on fringe. Then Eric Topol, the editor-in-chief, gave serious voice to that charlatan Paul Offit, talking about his scam book *Do You Believe in Magic? The Sense and Nonsense of Alternative Medicine*.

Throughout the text, Offit argues that healthy alternatives are not just unproven but are, in fact, proven NOT to work. To pull off this outrageous lie he had to completely and brazenly ignore the tens of thousands of papers emerging very year, showing the powerful value of nutritional supplements and the like. I'm talking about papers published in peer-reviewed journals and the quality press.

But Offit's book was "positively" received, argues Topol. Well, Nazism was positively received, wasn't it? Just not by everybody and certainly not by warm, intelligent human beings!

Anyway, the piece I'm going to talk about is not Offit but another interview with Topol; author Robin Cook.

Now let me back up a minute and mention the origins of *Virtual Medicine*. When I rang up Jacques Benveniste to talk to him about his experiments transmitting substances digitally over the Internet—and learning he had used curare to poison some mice thousands of miles away (no curare, just "digital curare")—I realized there was a book and someone must write it. I decided it would be me.

I'm talking about the book that launched the digital and cyber age of medicine and healing. The title came to mind at once: *Virtual Medicine*. Because if you can transmit "virtual" substances around the globe, everything is changed. And I wrote the book, published in 1999.

But for years afterwards I went around telling my friends I was going to beat that dude Robin Cook to the novel (Cook wrote *Coma*, which was made into a film twice). This time I would write the sensational best-seller in which someone logs on to their computer and drops dead, due to a digital cyanide signal coming through. Are you following me on this?

Of course it would be the perfect crime because:

1. There would be no cyanide

2. Every "expert" in the world would not know about virtual substances and, if told, would INSIST that such an idea was impossible!

Perfect—and if you are thinking of trying it, do not relate back to me. Please destroy this book and clean your hard drive, before doing the dirty deed! I don't want to be an accessory before the fact (do they have that charge here in the USA?)

Anyway, sad to report, I never wrote the novel; but Robin Cook did. He beat me… or at least has come close! It's just out and called *Cell* (only in hard cover to date). To commemorate the launch, Eric Topol had Cook come on his regular show and talk about it.

I soon got interested in the content. It was all about the new digitalized personal medicine: smart phone devices and diagnostic avatars the like. Wow! I predicted it all in *Virtual Medicine*, about 10 years ahead of the curve (that's what I do).

The AliveCor Heart Monitor is a hardware/app combo that turns smartphones into a portable electrocardiogram (ECG) machine. The app records and stores ECG readings on AliveCor.com, where patients and doctors can safely access the information at anytime

Welcome to the World of Personal Digital Medicine
First and foremost, the digitalization of medicine will personalize health care: Treatment will be tailored to each person as a unique individual suffering a unique illness, according to his or her genetic makeup.

Currently, therapy is based on population statistics or "averages." Patients are separated into groups defined in various ways but usually by similar symptoms or by the results of basic lab tests (like cholesterol levels). These groups are then treated with drugs that may help many people, but not all of them, and often only a fraction of them (Topol's words).

By incorporating information from an individual's DNA, the data made available through digitalization will enable clinicians to match individuals with treatments. Only patients who will benefit will get a particular drug.

This shift is huge. Giving drugs to patients who are not helped has been enormously expensive and often perverse. Particularly with anticancer drugs, it often condemns such patients to horrendous side effects for no benefit.

The Inverted Pyramid
As Cook pointed out in this interview, the whole rationale for our modern healthcare system is supposed to be to have lots of primary care doctors, a few other specialists, and a few — maybe even just one or two – super-specialists. That's supposed to be our pyramid, but our pyramid is upside down.

We have all these specialists and no primary care physicians, and it's never been solved. And suddenly, when I put all these things together, I realized that the solution to the primary care physician is going to be the smartphone, because it's not just an app to monitor your blood pressure. And it's not just an app to take a picture of your ear so that the doctor can look at it.

The cell phone can do all of these things together, and why not? **The smart phone is your primary care avatar!**

The Gutenberg Bible of Medicine
This digital revolution will democratize medicine: You will own or control the data about your own medical condition, and you will be able to analyze it instantly by your connectivity to the Web.

In many ways, the profession of medicine today is where Christianity was when the Gutenberg Bible put scriptures into the hands of the laity (1455).

But the profession is going to change, subtly and not so subtly shifting power away from the medical-industrial complex: doctors, health insurers, hospitals, medical labs and Big Pharma.

This can only be good for all of use.

The brave new world of digital medicine is coming about by the convergence of three rapidly evolving technologies: IT, or informational technology, involving wireless signaling, cloud computing and, most particularly, the spread of ever more sophisticated smartphones; medical applications of nanotechnology; and the progressively lower cost and availability of genome sequencing.

Today, all the physiological data monitored in a hospital intensive-care unit—including ECG, blood pressure, pulse, oxygenation, sugar level, breathing rate, and body temperature—can be recorded and analyzed continuously in real time on a smartphone connected to a sensor.

It can deliver information instantly to you or anyone you designate, and get this: the information rivals that collected in a physician's office or hospital setting. It can do so when you are experiencing specific symptoms—no appointment necessary—and at virtually no additional cost.

WHAT IS HIGH-VOLTAGE SYNDROME?

If you remain skeptical about electricity's central role in life forces, just wait for the publication of my new book *Medicine Beyond*! – Visit: www.alternative-doctor.com/vm

Meantime, you need to look at some genuine evidence (it's also evidence of the fact that science knows nothing, not even the limits of its own ignorance).

Consider the following intriguing and well-documented cases, that cannot be wished away by mere denial (you know, the old scientific approach: it can't be true, therefore it isn't).

One of the earliest investigated cases of an "electric person" was that of Angélique Cottin of La Perière, France. At the age of 14, a strange condition befell her in which any object she went near would retreat from her, as if pushed, like magnets repelling each other. The mere touch of her hand was enough to send heavy furniture flying away from her. No one could hold down the furniture or stop it wresting from their grasp.

A study group was appointed by the French Academy of Sciences, and a well-known physicist of the day, François Arago, published a report in *Le Journal des Débats* (February 1846). There is a lengthy translation of this report, entitled The Electrical Girl, published by *Popular Science Monthly*, Vol. 6, March 1875.

Here is an example of what they observed while studying the phenomenon.

Angélique approached a table, which was repelled as soon as it came in contact with her apron. She seated herself upon a chair with her feet resting on the floor, and the chair was thrown violently against the wall, while she was sent in another direction.

This experiment was repeated, over and over. Neither Arago, or Gougin, nor Laugier, also present, could hold the chair immovable, and M. Gougin, seating himself in one-half of it, while the girl occupied the other, was thrown upon the floor as soon as she took possession of it. The episode lasted 10 weeks before the strange manifestations finally ceased.

The Academy concluded it was all a fraud by the slight little girl; apparently she had secret muscle reflexes that allowed her to throw a 100 lb. table or chair across the room, while disguising all movement from the observers! It would have also meant she was stronger than grown men!

Of course as soon as the word "fraud" is uttered, even be it by buffoons of the day, all scientific interest ceases and the eggheads no longer have to trouble their (tiny) minds with the issue.

How Can It Happen?

Each cell in our body can generate a small charge. In his 1988 book about electric shock, Dr. Michael Shallis, an Oxford don, describes the case of Mrs. Jacqueline Priest, 22, of Sale Manchester (very close to where I had my UK headquarters).

She registered charges of static electricity more than 10 times the "normal" level. She was able to transmit miniature bolts of lightning that caused 30 vacuum cleaners and many other domestic appliances to short out or malfunction.

Gould and Pyle, in their monumental *Anomalies And Curiosities Of Medicine* (1896) mention a 6-year-old Zulu boy who gave off intense shocks and was exhibited at Edinburgh in 1882.

Foder, in his *Encyclopaedia of Psychic Science*, tells of a baby born at Saint-Urbain, France, in 1869 who badly shocked all who touched him. Luminous rays would shoot from his fingers, and when he died, just nine months old, radiance was observed around his body for several minutes.

In February of 1976, a 12-year-old boy named Vyvyan Jones from Henbury, Bristol, broke his arm. For two days after his injury, his hair stood straight up on his head and he gave terrible electric shocks to anyone around him.

The television and lights were affected by his high-voltage syndrome, flickering constantly until he left the room. Watches were also affected. Vyvyan was able to hold a light bulb in his hand and it would immediately light up. His phenomenon only lasted two days, but was unexplainable.

One of the most remarkable stories (to me) was a piece in *Electrical Experimenter* (June 1920) in which Dr. JB Ransom, chief physician at Clinton prison, New York, reported 34 convicts suffering from *botulinus* poisoning.

One had tried to throw away a piece of paper and found it stuck to his hand due to static. Soon all the afflicted inmates were on the same highly charged condition, varying in intensity with the severity of the poisoning. Compasses went wild in their vicinity and metal objects were deflected from their grasp. The effects faded as soon as they recovered.

Bioluminscence

Then there is the weird case of the "Luminous Woman of Pirano" (a tiny town in what is now Slovenia, on the Adriatic Sea). Anna Morano, aged 42, was an asthma patient. Over a period of several weeks, whenever she slept, a blue glow would be emitted from her breasts.

Dr. Protti from Padua University and a team of five other medical specialists kept a vigil at her bedside and witnessed the amazing phenomenon firsthand, taking measurements and some cine film.

Their work demonstrated that the subject doubled her heartbeat and respiratory rate during the brief minutes when the strange glow shone through her body. It was proposed that her sweating caused a luminous bacterium to glow but reports were very clear, her sweating and breathlessness came after the light.

None of the experts had any truly credible explanation for what was observed. Perhaps the best theory was that her weakened condition, due to religious zeal and fasting, increased the sulfides on her blood, which would be capable of glowing in ultraviolet light. But where did the ultraviolet light come from?

It remains a mystery. The effect disappeared after a few weeks and the woman was none the worse for her "affliction."

Harry Wood Carrington tells of a child who died of acute indigestion. As neighbors prepared the shroud they noticed the body surrounded by a blue glow and radiating heat.

The body appeared to be on fire; efforts to extinguish the luminescence failed, but eventually it faded away. Gould and Pyle in *Anomalies and Curiosities of Medicine* (1896) tell of a woman with cancer of the breast: the light from her body could illuminate the hands of a watch several feet away.

Finally (enough for now), there was a letter to the *English Mechanic*, dated Sept. 24. 1869, which described the experience of an American woman.

On going to bed, she found that a light was issuing from the upper side of the fourth toe on her right foot. Rubbing made it worse and it spread up her foot. There was a bad odor and she tried washing her foot in soap and water, but it didn't decrease the glow (thereby rendering glowing bacteria out of the question). The whole phenomenon lasted for three quarters of an hour and was witnessed by her husband.

There have been many other cases of glowing humans. Indeed, they are rather common and may extend to include the halo effect seen around holy figures or those engaged in intense spiritual activity.

Light has been seen streaming from holy priests that lit up a dark cell or whole chapel. There are simply so many of these accounts, they cannot all be dismissed. Don't forget that we all emit light from our bodies but at a level 1,000 times below the threshold of the eye.

Writing in the online journal *PLoS ONE*, researchers describe how they imaged volunteers' upper bodies using ultra-sensitive cameras over a period of several days.

Their results show that the amount of light emitted follows a 24-hour cycle, at its highest in late afternoon and lowest late at night, and that the brightest light is emitted from the cheeks, forehead and neck.

Strangely, the areas that produced the brightest light did not correspond with the brightest areas on thermal images of the volunteers' bodies.

Pathological Effect
It's very clear these strange energetic phenomena are not normal, in any sense. In fact they tend to be pathological and mainly afflict sick people. Even Angélique Cottin, the "Electrical Girl," was described as sickly and apathetic to an extraordinary degree both in body and mind. This may be the real clue we need.

In the Electric Universe model, we all live in a universe that is **flooded with highly charged electrical flows.** This current is transformed for us by our galaxy; the galactic electricity is transformed by our Sun; the Sun's violent energies are transformed Earth herself.

We still live in a sea of such unimaginable electrical energies. As I explained in *Virtual Medicine* (1999), being on Earth is like living in the heart of an immense dynamo, with its iron core rotating in the Sun's electric field.

It means that we must all be adapted to this electrical environment. But what if we fall sick; go out of kilter; un-adapt to our electrical environment? Could it not then be that for some individuals it means the electrical energy goes out of control and starts to work these strange manifestations?

I think so, and this is certainly the most plausible explanation to date. That's why I have pushed and pushed the electric universe model: there is nothing in the "universe as a cold machine" or a gravity-based physics that could possibly explain all that we have seen.

What's the number one sign of life I keep telling you?

Electricity. Not respiration, not reproduction or feeding: a cellular membrane electrical potential. Once that's gone; it's death. And in the reverse…

Mary Shelley may have had a strange prescience when she wrote her book *Frankenstein*. We all know the story, even without reading the book: mad scientist stitches together a body of sorts, using dead pieces from the morgue and from graves. What is the one missing ingredient that needed to make this monster come alive? Electricity.

Frankenstein just has to wait for the fateful lightning strike to his laboratory roof and then…

SECTION 10

THE FORGOTTEN ANTIBIOTICS THAT CAN SAVE YOUR LIFE

- THE FORGOTTEN ALTERNATIVES TO ANTIBIOTICS THAT SAVED MILLIONS OF LIVES
- THE REAL SURPRISE ANTIBIOTIC... WHAT IS IODINE?
- ALTERNATIVES TO ANTIBIOTICS - THESE FRIENDLY VIRUSES EASILY KILL DEADLY BACTERIA
- HOW PLANT OILS ARE HIGHLY EFFECTIVE AGAINST DRUG-RESISTANT BACTERIA

The golden age of antibiotics is over! Antibiotic-resistant strains of bacteria are spreading like wildfire.

But, could you survive without antibiotics?

Germs, bugs, viruses. When you were a child, all of these were lumped together. You didn't necessarily know what they were, but you knew they were bad for you. If you suffered anything from an infected cut to a severe cold, you were taken to the doctor.

You probably left with an antibiotic to take care of your troubles.

We're a little wiser these days. Now we know that all bacteria aren't bad. Many of those in your body are actually necessary for your survival. If you're a health-savvy individual, you may have a few containers of pro-biotic yogurt in your refrigerator at all times for better digestion – made possible by "good" gut flora.

Victims of the Cure

Some viruses are being manipulated by science to battle diseases such as HIV. Scientific cases of the attacker being used to fight itself. Not all the news is good news.

Unfortunately, many of the antibiotics prescribed for decades are no longer effective because the bacteria they were used to combat are now immune. We're becoming victims of the cure.

Penicillin was discovered in 1928. At the time, it was a miracle cure. Before the discovery of the first antibiotic, anything from syphilis to splinters could and often did lead to death. Once an infection entered the body, it spread rapidly.

With the dawn of antibiotics, science believed it had finally conquered infection. The general opinion was that humans could not survive without antibiotics. That prediction held true for 33 years.

The Evolution of the Superbug

In 1961, the first case of what would become known as methicillin-resistant *Staphylococcus aureus* (MRSA) was diagnosed in the United Kingdom. MRSA, as its name suggests, is a staph infection that's immune to methicillin, a potent antibiotic.

The dangerous truth is that MRSA isn't the only "superbug" out there. Looking to ESKAPE? Don't go to your nearest hospital. ESKAPE is an acronym for *Enterococcus*, *Staphylococcus*, *Klebsiella*, *Acinetobacter*, *Pseudomonas*, and *Enterobacter*.

These are the most common organisms found in the standard hospital environment.

Hospital-acquired infections kill at least 100,000 people every year. That is three times more than the number of people who die annually from HIV. With the passage of time and the overuse of prescribed antibiotics, many organisms have developed an immunity to treatment.

The same is true with old diseases such as gonorrhea, chlamydia, and syphilis. One night's indiscretion once meant an embarrassing visit to the doctor and an injection. Now, once again, it can mean a death sentence.

Even tuberculosis is reappearing on the medical horizon. Resistant strains are popping up in various areas of the world. Once curable, nearly 1.5 million people die from this ancient disease every year. More than 500,000 of those infected suffer from a strain that is resistant to treatment.

Doctors are being more selective about antibiotics these days. No longer does every frantic parent who brings in a child with a runny nose leave with an antibiotic prescription. Regrettably, it may be too little, too late.

There is another source of antibiotic resistance. It has only recently become a topic of serious discussion. You may be surprised to learn that much of the fault lies on your dinner table.

Antibiotics and Our Food Supply
Were you planning to enjoy a steak tonight? Perhaps some ham or chicken instead? If the meat you purchased was not organic, then you may be unknowingly ingesting mass quantities of antibiotics.

Today, more than 80% of antibiotics distributed in the United States are not given to humans. Instead, they are being force-fed to healthy animals. The logic is that antibiotics promote growth and creates healthier food.

One small side effect is that it is increasing the cases of drug-resistant *E. coli* and salmonella.

Science Will Save Us!
We can look to the medical and scientific communities for answers. Right? They've done it before and they can do it again.

You may not like the answer to that question.

When Jonas Salk cured polio in 1955, he made the compassionate choice to give it away for the benefit of humanity as a whole. His selfless decision has improved the lives of millions.

Only five major pharmaceutical companies are currently researching new antibiotics. As of 2008, only 15 of the 167 drugs under development have the potential to treat organisms with multi-drug resistance. None of them has been released to the marketplace.

Why isn't more effort being devoted to something that is a major catastrophe waiting to happen?

Sadly, the answer is money. For example, it is far more lucrative for the pharmaceutical giants to focus their resources on a new diabetic drug that a patient has to take once a day for the rest of his or her life. An antibiotic that is a one-dose cure all isn't going to put profits in their pockets.

We have options. Can you survive without antibiotics? Yes, you can. There are dietary choices you can make such as buying foods labeled organic or antibiotic free whenever possible.

You will also be shocked to discover that there are many safe and effective ancient remedies that worked **better** than traditional antibiotics…but they were buried.

Keep reading to discover these for yourself…

THE FORGOTTEN ALTERNATIVES TO ANTIBIOTICS THAT SAVED MILLIONS OF LIVES

These antibiotics can't be patented, are cheap and plentiful, and are Nature's blessed gifts to us. You can access them anywhere, except perhaps the darkest polar nights.

Can you guess what they are?

Fresh air and sunshine.

You probably think I'm joking. But fresh air and sunlight are among the oldest concepts in medicine. Florence Nightingale famously promoted them. What's more, they were effective.

She slashed hospital death rates with a host of hygiene improvements – including throwing open the windows. *"It is necessary to renew the air round a sick person frequently, to carry off morbid effluvia from the lungs and skin,"* she wrote.

But less well known is the fact that **"Nightingale wards,"** as they became known, had their long sides south-facing to let in plentiful sunlight.

Soon the health benefits of sunshine became more widely recognized, particularly for people with tuberculosis, which in Victorian times caused around one in five deaths in our crowded cities.

Sunlight not only kills airborne bacteria and those on the skin, but also seems to kill TB microbes inside the body, probably by boosting production of vitamin D, which has powerful effects on the immune system.

By the turn of the 19th century, "solar clinics" were in vogue, utilizing fresh air and sunlight as part of TB treatment. Hospital beds were wheeled on to balconies or conservatories with special glazing that allowed ultraviolet light to pass through.

What Does Science Say?

Actually, there's a very interesting report in *New Scientist*, about two experimenters at the Porton-Down defense facility in the UK (for those of you living outside the UK, this is a well-known bio-warfare site).

Microbiologists Henry Druett and K. R. May had speculated about what would happen if deadly pathogens were exploded over a major city: how long would the microbes remain viable?

To find out, they exposed *E. coli* to fresh air and were astonished that all viable microbes were dead within two hours, while controls kept in boxes at identical temperature and humidity largely survived.

So Florence Nightingale was right! Open windows not only diluted pathogens but actually destroyed them. The term *"fresh air factor"* was so named; it's the newest-oldest antibiotic!

The sunlight is no mystery either. As I said, we know it **boosts vitamin D levels and that will favor the immune system over invaders.**

Trouble is, these cheap and effective remedies fell out of favor, due to the rise of antibiotics and their manifest success in conquering infections.

Moreover, in the 1970s, energy conservation became a big issue. Open windows and circulating air are the kiss of death to economical heating. Everything was sealed up.

We entered the era of *"sick building syndrome"* (tight building syndrome in the USA).

Filtered air, it emerges, is deadly because it circulates pathogens to an unnatural and dangerous degree. As we get more and more crowded together in our cities and buildings, the dangers increase.

For instance, US soldiers stationed in the Saudi Arabian desert during the first Gulf war got more coughs and colds if they slept in air-conditioned barracks than if they bedded down in tents and warehouses.

Another study looking at Chinese college students found that 35 percent of those who slept in poorly ventilated dorm rooms got an infection over the course of a year, compared with 5 percent in rooms that were better ventilated.

That's a seven-fold decrease in pathogenic activity. It's time to go back to the old ways.

They DID work, as I have explained.

Is There a Fresh Air Factor?

The answer is *hydroxyl radicals*. These short-lived molecules are constantly produced in the atmosphere through reactions between ozone and water, catalyzed by airborne organic chemicals from plants. They kill bacteria but are (relatively) harmless to humans.

But it's also possible to produce them synthetically and I expect devices of this type will be widely available commercially, as the obvious failure of antibiotics looms larger and larger.

The Sunlight Factor

Science has the answer here too. We know that UV light is antiseptic. But it is also supposedly dangerous.

Drenching kids with UV light to boost their vitamin D levels was fashionable when I was a kid but soon went out of favor, as it was realized that UVB damages skin. Now we even worry about UVA.

But it has been found that the most useful wavelength is 207 nm. At this wavelength, the UV is absorbed by protein molecules and therefore penetrates only a short way into human cells; it does not reach the DNA to cause mutations.

Microbes, on the other hand, are so much smaller than human cells that they completely absorb the light and are zapped.

Now a lamp has been developed that emits only UV at 207 nm. Studies on cells grown in the lab have shown that this narrow band does not harm human skin tissue cultures, yet it kills bacteria, including MRSA.

I've written about the use of UV technology (and plain blue light) in my block-buster compendium of alternative antibiotics. You need to get it and read it. No use waiting till somebody is deadly ill. There are countless cases of people feeling a little ill at breakfast time and being dead before bedtime. That's how fast bacteria multiply and do their deadly work.

The Bacteria Social Network
Also, in my book *How To Survive In A World Without Antibiotics*, (visit: www.alternative-doctor.com/wwa) I explained what we call quorum sensing in bacteria. It's like microbial Facebook!

When enough bacteria are present and "texting" each other, they reach a critical trigger point and suddenly explode as pathogens.

In the pipeline now are "quorum-blocking" drugs, which, rather than killing bacteria, merely stop them from mounting such an attack; it's like shutting down their Facebook accounts. Importantly, such drugs are probably less likely to trigger resistance than conventional antibiotics.

Another option is phage therapies, using viruses genetically engineered to destroy bacteria. Here the *New Scientist* journalist and editor got it wrong. According to them, such a strategy is some years away from reaching the clinic.

In fact, as I explain in my book, phage therapy is alive and well in the Eastern bloc. Russia has a long and successful track record of using this kind of approach to microbes.

The drawback, as I explained, is that there is only one killer virus "phage" for any given pathogen. It will kill and eat its target bacteria all right, but there is no general phage to kill all or most pathogens, like penicillin does.

The Future
In the meantime, I think it pays to learn from the heroes of the past. Florence Nightingale slashed the death rate in the hospitals of the Crimean War. Until she came along, soldiers were more likely to die of "hospital" than they were to die of wounds on the battlefield!

It's like today, when patients are very likely to catch a dangerous infection when they go to hospital. In the UK, 9% emerge with an infection they wouldn't have caught elsewhere. In the USA, 100,000 a year die from such hospital infections.

That's three times the number that died of HIV.

The World Health Organization has published a report urging all healthcare settings to use natural ventilation as far as possible, even referencing Florence Nightingale.

In Mumbai, India, an old-style sanatorium is being refitted as a clinic for people with drug-resistant TB, making use of an open-air regime. It has high ceilings and open balconies. We seem to have come full circle in hospital design. Don't miss out on the wealth of antibiotic alternatives available today.

THE REAL SURPRISE ANTIBIOTIC…WHAT IS IODINE?

What, iodine? *Well, why not?* You probably remember when Mom used to spread it on a skin wound (you might have thought she did it to hurt you on purpose!).

Sure, it stings. But it's also very effective. Maybe you don't know but surgeons (at least in my day) swabbed the patient's skin with iodine, before throwing the sterile drapes over the patient, leaving just a teeny window in the fabric to work through.

Truth is, iodine is a very good antiseptic **(kills germs dead on contact).**

It is also a very good antibiotic. Its use as an antibiotic/antiviral/anti-fungal has been completely ignored by modern medicine. But iodine works against microbes in two ways:

1. It kills germs, as I said, though when taken internally, you have to adjust the dose, of course, to avoid hurting the patient.
2. It also boosts the immune system and makes it much more dynamic at removing predatory pathogens.

I'll explain these two aspects as we go along.

Meantime, don't forget that iodine has other very important roles to play…

Fertility
Take fertility, for example. In the old days, in some inland areas such as the high Andes, seafood, fish eggs, and seaweed were highly valued, because the iodine content of these foods kept women fertile.

Without that supplemental iodine, women experienced many stillbirths and miscarriages. Infant mortality is highest in areas known for iodine deficiency.

Generally speaking, the further inland (further from the ocean), a person is living, the lower the iodine content of food and crops grown there. Iodine is certainly the **"ocean nutrient"**!

Thyroid Function
Iodine is food for the thyroid gland, which simply can't function unless it is present in adequate amounts. Iodine deficiency can lead to swelling of the thyroid gland (goiter), as it tries to cope. Ultimately, lack of iodine can lead to hypothyroid states and all that that entails: low energy, weight gain, poor hair and nails, heavy periods (women), loss of libido (back to babies again!), and slowed, thickened speech.

This is textbook stuff, I don't need to give you references.

Immune System

I came across the power of the thyroid to support, or damage, immune function when I started using electronic acupuncture diagnostic machines in the 1980s.

Time and again, thyroid would be the underlying cause (i.e., further upstream) than cancer or infectious diseases.

That again makes iodine very important to immunity and this goes far beyond the mere antiseptic effect. This is via immune modulation.

Brain Development

Iodine is quite crucial to proper brain and neurological growth. Children from very low-iodine regions were historically likely to be severely mentally retarded; a condition we used to call cretinism. Nowadays we don't use the term, since it has insulting overtones. But remember the word: it will help you understand the sad plight of iodine deficiency in growing infants.

Today we call it untreated *congenital hypothyroidism* (with or without a goiter). But its very existence shows you the power and important of this not-so-humble nutrient.

Brain development is absolutely dependent on normal thyroid hormone levels. A progressive intellectual deterioration occurs with each passing week in the absence of appropriate thyroxine replacement.

Severe developmental and physical delays occur by six months of age. Treatment in infancy will reverse the physical changes, but sadly not the neurological damage.[1]

Iodized Salt

All this was thought to be fixed by the supplemental addition of iodine to our diets. That was done in a cute way (too cute, because it backfired): iodine was added to table salt.

Spot the problem? Right, the medical profession has been advocating low-salt diets for nearly 50 years, without even considering it as a "low-iodine diet." Plus, with the modern food industry practices of adding bromine to bread and fluoride to our water (both of which compete with iodine), we are suddenly back to the iodine deficiency of old.

It's a problem. You definitely need to supplement iodine. I'll tell you what and how much shortly.

Antibiotic Effect

Back to where we started: iodine as an antibiotic.

As early as June 1, 1905, an article was printed in the *New York Times* about the successful use of iodine for consumption/tuberculosis.

In 1945, J.D. Stone and Sir McFarland Burnet (who later went on to win a Nobel Prize for his clonal selection theory) exposed mice to lethal effects of influenza viral mists. But deaths were prevented by first putting iodine solution in mice snouts just prior to placing them in chambers containing influenza viruses.

Iodine exhibits activity against bacteria, molds, yeasts, protozoa, and many viruses. Most bacteria are killed within 15 to 30 seconds of contact. It's probably superior and way less toxic than the chlorine dioxide protocol (MMS of Jim Humble).

Please note that iodine and chlorine are both similar; they are elements called halogens. Iodine penetrates bacterial cell walls, and although its precise killing mechanism is uncertain, it's likely related to retardation of bacterial protein synthesis, disruption of electron transport, DNA denaturation and/or membrane destabilization.

Are There Any Dangers?

What is being missed by armchair proponents of iodine is the possibility that iodine, too, may have dangerous side effects (nutty holistic "health researchers" seem to believe everything orthodox is toxic at any dilution and that "natural" substances can do no harm at any concentration).

Well, aren't opium and hemlock natural? Too much of them and your heart will stop beating permanently!

Anything that impairs electron transport in the cell or has the potential to denature DNA should be viewed with caution.

Plus, I found a 1926 correspondence series in the *JAMA*, raising the very real possibility that ingested iodine in therapeutic quantities could cause the break down and release of old tuberculosis.

Tests on guinea pigs certainly give pause for thought: the iodine-treated guinea pigs died rapidly, with rampant and widely disseminated TB at autopsy.[2]

I am compelled therefore to suggest that iodine is far from the **"best antibiotic"** we have, as Dr. David Derry believes, and I advise caution, certainly where there is a history or possibility of TB (that would include me, since all my farming uncles and aunts and other relatives were at very high risk of TB and we drank plenty of raw milk).

Remember that TB never really goes away or gets cured; it simply goes into deep hibernation, waiting for the immune system to take a week off work!

Homeopaths have even suggested the emergence of a TB miasm!

Administration and Doses

So, if you want to take iodine, what should you do? First, let me state that you have to have it. Even with a history of TB, you need to supplement iodine. Thyroid, remember, is your master metabolism gland (see my own newsletter "Engine Speed" here).

Forget the iodized table salt. It's not enough. Seafood of all kinds is better.

But you should take, at least from time to time, full-on supplements of iodine, whether you are hypo-, hyper- or normal thyroid. It is especially important for the next few years to take sufficient iodine to lock out the bad stuff: radioactive iodine 131, stemming from Fukushima and still, don't forget, Chernobyl. The 1986 disaster was worse than Fukushima and we're still here![3]

Once ingested, radioactive iodine concentrates almost exclusively in the thyroid gland, where the radiation can cause either destruction of the gland, or lead to the development of thyroid cancer.

Individuals who experienced Fukushima radiation were found to quickly develop unnatural thyroid nodules.

Young children and fetuses, who have fast-growing thyroid glands, are the most susceptible to exposure to radioactive iodine, and the effects of exposure also tend to show up more quickly in children compared to adults.

Note that milk is a potent source of contamination: when cows eat grass contaminated with radioactive iodine, the iodine concentrates heavily in milk (another very good reason not to eat milk, raw or pasteurized).

The best way to take it, in my view, is Lugol's iodine (5% organic iodine, 10% potassium iodide and 85% water).

You can also get tincture of iodine. As I have said elsewhere, try to get your supply from old stocks and old shelves, to avoid contamination with radioactive iodine. The only way to do that is to ask your supplier.

The best dose is 10 mg to 12 mg daily. You can go up to 50 mg daily for loading purposes but not for long.

But rather than act in a hurry, recognize that it will take more than half a year to correct a major iodine deficiency.

Be patient! I'm giving doses in milligrams, because there are many different strengths of iodine preparations; classical Lugol's, for example, comes in 1%, 2%, and 5%, as well as the original 10% strength.

For those who object to the alcohol content of tinctures on religious grounds, you can get iodine kosher certified alcohol-free from Cedar Bear Naturales.

You can also get Iodoral tablets and Iodizyme-HP tablets, available at 12.5mg strength.

Meanwhile, don't be daft and make sure to avoid goitrogens in your diet for a while, as they hinder iodine utilization. Such foods included kale, cabbage, peanuts, soy, Brussels sprouts, cauliflower, broccoli, kohlrabi, and turnips.

If you are confident that your iodine levels are adequate, you could turn this around and say to eat them, to prevent the ingress of radioactive iodine (not really recommended)!

Selenium

Don't forget selenium. That's another very cancer-protective element and probably vital in the post-Fukushima era.

Selenium works intimately with iodine as precursors to thyroid hormones. The selenium content of the thyroid is higher than that of any other body part. It's crucial to the conversion of T4 hormone to the more active T3 form.

During times of selenium deficiency, the body will use any available selenium for the thyroid. Even the brain and neurotransmitters "take a back seat" to the functioning of the thyroid in regards to selenium status within the body.

So don't just supplement with iodine but be sure to add in 100 mcg or, better still 200 mcg of selenium. The higher dose is highly cancer protective (and also, incidentally, locks out toxic mercury).[4]

References
1. *Paediatrics Child Health*. 2003 February; 8(2): 105-106. PMCID: PMC2791432 Cretinism: The past, present and future of diagnosis and cure.
2. Scott R. Edwards, M.D., Iodine In Tuberculosis, *JAMA*. 1926;87(7):509-510. doi:10.1001/jama.1926.02680070055027
3. http//content.hks.harvard.edu/journalistsresource/pa/society/health/thyroid-cancers-in-ukraine-related-to-the-chernobyl-accident/
4. Naithani R. Organoselenium compounds in cancer chemoprevention. *Mini Rev Med Chem*. 2008 Jun;8(7):657-68.

ALTERNATIVES TO ANTIBIOTICS - THESE FRIENDLY VIRUSES EASILY KILL DEADLY BACTERIA

The technical word is *bacteriophage* (which means "eater of bacteria"), or often just phage for short. Special viruses have this useful skill. We may harness them for deliberate use, pumping phages into a person challenged with a bacterial infection. We call this "phage therapy."

It's a viable alternative to antibiotics. I gave it some coverage in my blockbuster book of alternatives to antibiotics: *How to Survive in a World Without Antibiotics*.

The idea has been around since the 1920s and was kept alive in Russia and Eastern Bloc countries, where phage therapies are used regularly. There was even some interest in the West, but after the discovery of antibiotics in the 1930s and 1940s, doctors and scientists lost interest (as with the Rife machine and other antibiotic "alternatives").

Today, with the collapse of antibiotics and the emergence of worldwide, dangerous, and drug-resistant bacteria, phage therapy suddenly starts to look attractive again and is being re-introduced here.

There may come a time when you have to trust your life to a bunch of invisible marauders, let loose in your body! Phage therapy has many potential applications in human medicine as well as dentistry, veterinary science, and agriculture.

People need to get over their natural revulsion at a virus infection. There are good guys out there! We have even developed "oncolytic" viruses, meaning they destroy cancer cells.

History of Phages

Phages (I'll use the shorter term from now on) were first identified by English microbiologist Frederick Twort in 1915 and again in 1917 by French Canadian microbiologist Felix d'Herelle.

Not long after his discovery, d'Herelle used phages to treat dysentery, in what was probably the first attempt to use bacteriophages therapeutically. The studies were conducted at the Hôpital des Enfants-Malades in Paris in 1919, under the clinical supervision of Professor Victor-Henri Hutinel, the hospital's Chief of Pediatrics.

The phage preparation was ingested by d'Herelle, Hutinel, and several hospital interns, in order to confirm its safety before administering it the next day to a 12-year-old boy with severe dysentery.

The patient's symptoms ceased after a single administration of d'Herelle's antidysentery phage, and the boy fully recovered within a few days. This experiment was never officially published.

The efficacy of the phage preparation was "confirmed" shortly afterwards, when three additional patients having bacterial dysentery and treated with one dose of the preparation started to recover within 24 hours of treatment.

The first study to enter the medical press came in 1921, when Richard Bruynoghe and Joseph Maisin used bacteriophages to treat staphylococcal skin disease.

They injected bacteriophages into and around surgically opened lesions, and the authors reported regression of the infections within 24 to 48 hours. Several similarly promising studies followed and, encouraged by these early results, d'Herelle and others continued studies of the therapeutic use of phages.

For example d'Herelle used various phage preparations to treat successfully thousands of people having cholera and/or bubonic plague in India.

Specificity

Bacteriophages are much more specific than antibiotics, meaning one phage will only attack and "eat" one particular bacteria and no other. Each infection requires a particular phage to treat it. Consequently phage mixtures are often applied to improve the chances of success, or samples can be taken and an appropriate phage identified and grown.

On the plus side, phages can hypothetically be chosen to be indirectly harmless not only to the host organism (human, animal, or plant), but also to other beneficial bacteria, such as gut flora, thus reducing the chances of opportunistic infections.

They have a high safety factor, that is, phage therapy would be expected to give rise to few side effects.

Another big advantage is that, since phages replicate inside the patient, a smaller effective dose can be used. In fact a repeat dose may not even be necessary.

Phages are currently being used therapeutically to treat bacterial infections that do not respond to conventional antibiotics, particularly in Russia and Georgia.

Phages are especially promising for biofilms, bacteria which secrete themselves a protective polysaccharide layer, which antibiotics typically cannot penetrate.

Cold War Medicine

Isolated from Western advances in antibiotic production in the 1940s, Russian scientists continued to develop already successful phage therapy to treat the wounds of soldiers in field hospitals.

In WW2, phages were also used to treat many soldiers infected with various bacterial diseases, e.g., dysentery and gangrene.

Russian researchers continued to develop and to refine their treatments and to publish their research and results.

However, due to the scientific barriers of the Cold War, this knowledge was not translated and did not proliferate across the world.

A summary of these publications was published in English in 2009 in *A Literature Review of the Practical Application of Bacteriophage Research,* and my subscribers who are practitioners may want to pursue this reference.

There is an extensive library and research center at the George Eliava Institute in Tbilisi, Georgia. Phage therapy today is a widespread form of treatment in that region and, so far as I can determine, testing for phage strains for use in the United States has to be done via labs in Tsibilisi.

Acne Cure?

Phages could even open up a line of advance against that dread affliction of teenagers: acne. It turns out that those who don't get acne have a phage-type virus on their facial skin.

It's probably why the causal bacterium, *Propionibacterium acnes*, does not flourish and cause zits.

Scientists have used genetic sequencing to identify 11 new viruses with the potential to kill the *P. acnes* bacteria that leads to intense breakouts. Other promising present-day research is pointed at bed sores, leprosy, and drug-resistant staph infections.

What About Resistance to Phages?

Good question. It's possible. But phages are live too and so they can fight back!

Just as bacteria can evolve resistance, viruses can evolve to overcome resistance (however, the ability to evolve raises certain safety questions).

The body might also mount its own attack on phage viruses. I found one study from Poland in which that happened to 2 out of 44 cases. It's always a theoretical complication.

A few research groups in the West are engineering a broader-spectrum phage, and also a variety of forms of MRSA treatments, including impregnated wound dressings, preventative treatment for burn victims, and phage-impregnated sutures.

My own interest in this topic was refreshed last week, when I met a Russian MD well-versed in phage therapy. I had a friend in the same city who had been successfully treated for an MRSA infection, using phage therapy. This got me thinking…

I am pursuing more of this line of therapy and will keep you posted on future developments, including where to get supplies.

HOW PLANT OILS ARE HIGHLY EFFECTIVE AGAINST DRUG-RESISTANT BACTERIA

If you have read my book *How To Survive In A World Without Antibiotics,* you'll know I have described the **powerful antibacterial effects of everyday plants and their essential oils.** Even culinary herbs and spices, such as thyme and cinnamon, have antibiotic effects.

White tea extract actually outperforms two major antibiotics: *tetracycline* and *vancomycin*, for heaven's sake!

New research, reported last week at the Society for General Microbiology meeting in Edinburgh, Scotland, has repeated everything I discovered and reported.

The study took place at the Technological Educational Institute of Ionian Islands in Greece. Researchers investigated the effects of plant oils against multi-drug-resistant *Staphylococcus aureus*, or MRSA, a bacterium that causes hospital-acquired infections and is dangerous because it frequently does not respond to a whole range of antibiotics.

Recently a strain of MRSA has emerged that is five times more deadly than before; it kills 50% of infected cases.

Professor Effemia Eriotou, who was in charge of the research, said:

"We didn't know that essential oils were going to have that great an anti-microbial activity. And it's really amazing that they are killing all these bacteria and yeasts as well.

That's great news for *Candida* and yeast sufferers!

Essential oils from eight plants were tested, including thyme, basil, peppermint, and cinnamon. They all had significant anti-bacterial activity, but essential oil from thyme, a spice frequently used in Mediterranean cooking, killed almost all of the bacteria in a Petri dish within an hour. Almost as effective was cinnamon oil.

Scientists had noticed that cheeses mixed with herbs had no bacteria, which were present when there were no herbs. So Eriotou started investigating.

You need more information like this. It will save your life some day. Antibiotics are failing now BIG time. It's getting truly dangerous again, like it was 60- 70 years ago.

I came across this article about antibiotic-resistant bacteria and couldn't wait to tell you about it!

Fox News reported a class of fast-growing killer bacteria classified as an urgent public-health threat.

According to a new report by the U.S. Centers for Disease Control and Prevention (CDC), at least 2 million people in the United States develop serious bacterial infections that are resistant to one or more types of antibiotics each year, and at least 23,000 die from the infections.[1]

Modern antibiotics are not just failing big time; they are DANGEROUS.

We are seeing a steady increase in resistance rates and one reason for that is the over-prescription of antibiotics, which causes the pathogens the opportunity to outwit the drugs that are ultimately used to treat them.

This diarrhea-causing superbug that is antibiotic-resistant is not only raising alarms in the US…

Last March the chief medical officer for England said antibiotic resistance poses a "catastrophic health threat." That followed a report last year from the World Health Organization that found a "superbug" strain of gonorrhea had spread to several European countries.[2]

Threats of these superbugs that are drug-resistant are ranked into three categories – but they are also based on health impact factors such as the total number of cases, the ease by which they were transmitted, and whether there are effective antibiotics available for treatment.

Over the last decade there has been a huge increase in "urgent" cases and even the strongest antibiotics are not effective against it.

My Thoughts…

I've been saying for several years now that The Golden Age Of Antibiotics Is Over.

We are all at risk now. However, there are many great natural antibiotics that got eclipsed in the 1940s and 1950s. But they worked then and will work now and maybe one day could save your life…

It's one of my pet sayings that the commonest cause of death is ignorance.

This is a topic on which you can't afford to remain uneducated.

References
1. Fox News Health http://www.foxnews.com/health/2013/09/16/drug-resistant-superbugs-deemed-urgent-threats-cdc-says/print, published Sept. 16, 2013.
2. *Loc. cit.*

Antibiotics Kill – So Take Control of Your Health Today…

Lots of antibiotics kill. In my view, it is unethical to prescribe them and you wouldn't get any from me, unless the situation was already life-threatening. Even then, if it was me or my own family, I would rather rely on IV mega-doses of vitamin C than any antibiotic. 50- 100 gr of vitamin C is much more certain and quicker (works in an hour to two!) against antibiotic-resistant bacteria.

The bottom line is nobody should be thinking "antibiotics." We should be thinking of "alternatives." And here's the joker: there are thousands of viable alternatives. Hundreds of them work as well as antibiotics.

As I have mentioned, the Golden Age of Antibiotics is over. Bacteria have won the war, hands down, and that's the truth.

Well, not quite. There are, as I said, hundreds of healthy, safe and EFFECTIVE alternative modalities of treatment. You need to learn about them and learn NOW, not when somebody is in bed with life-threatening pneumonia (non-hospital pneumonia, which is the fourth commonest cause of death in the UK and sixth commonest in the USA).

I suspect those of you who haven't yet bought my eBook *How to Survive in a World Without Antibiotics* are still living in a dream world, thinking you are OK.

Infectious diseases can strike anywhere and move terrifyingly fast. We are going back to the old days, when bacterial infections can kill within hours.

Get the knowledge you need to stay safe and take care of your loved ones. Go here to learn what you need to know to SURVIVE IN A WORLD WITHOUT ANTIBIOTICS.

Visit: www.alternative-doctor.com/wwa

SECTION 11

VITAMINS, ANTIOXIDANTS & SUPERFOODS

- VITAMIN C CAN HALVE YOUR CHANCE OF A HEART ATTACK
- VITAMIN D HAS MORE AMAZING PROPERTIES
- COCOA IN CHOCOLATE IS GOOD FOR THE HEART
- DID YOU EAT YOUR SULFUR TODAY?
- FLAX SEED OIL - AMAZING!
- HERBS CAN REALLY WORK FOR PAIN
- THE NUMBER ONE ANTIOXIDANT
- WHAT IS CHIA? DOES IT WORK FOR WEIGHT LOSS?
- VITAMIN E TRIUMPHS AGAIN
- WHO LIKES ARTICHOKES?
- VITAMIN B1 MEGA DOSES REVERSE EARLY-STAGE KIDNEY DISEASE
- SOMETHING NEW FOR ALLERGIES?
- WHY NUTRITION IS NOT VITAMIN ACCOUNTABILITY

One of my pet *bitches* (is that a sexist remark?) is the idea that nutrition comes down to so-many milligrams of this and so many units of that and so many teaspoonfuls of the other…

This mistake is found across the board, from certified nutritionists and dieticians, through MDs, to alternative health writers who ought to know better.

I fought back with a lecture I gave in Malaysia some time ago. I still have the PowerPoint; I called it "Nutrition Bullets." It's probably time to serve it up for the Web. I'll do that as soon as I get some spare time.

There were several key points – in other words bullet points – that have little or nothing to do with measured quantities. They have everything to do with dynamics, function, and biochemical individuality.

My main point is that losing focus by concentrating on isolated technical information and spurious quantitative measurements does not lead to a workable science of nutrition.

We need a bigger picture; the Interstate freeways map, not the hikers' side paths and byways!

I don't believe that the creation, repair, and maintenance of healthy body tissues can be reduced to itemized lists of figures, like a supermarket shopping list. This kind of "nutrient accountancy" shows a deplorable lack of understanding of the way Nature works and the meaning of holistic integration of health.

The picture today is very complex, with traditional foods all but gone and, as farming methods change, the value of foods changes. You'd never think that to read the nonsense published as official "nutrition."

In fact, Pandit Professor Dr. Med Sir Anton Jayasuriya and I were trying to debate a suitable word for this bigger view of things just before he passed away. The best we could come up with was nutritionology, which is obviously not going to fly!

Any suggestions, anybody?

The adding numbers view violates all the laws of accountancy, in that there is no balance to the balance sheet!

So what are the key issues?

These are 10 basic simple nutrition rules:
This is not just the first, but my #1 nutrition rule (the only one that matters):

Rule #1 - No one will cure anything to last, no matter how brilliant you are, or what your healing paradigm or belief system is, if the patient is in a negative nutritional balance.

Think about this: Nothing in the body is fixed. It ALL changes over, every few months. Therefore nutrition is a vital renewal, healing, and construction factor. Without it you can't repair joints, even if the guru laid his hand on you and the pain went away!

This is my rule #2 and another biggie - What you are eating that you shouldn't is of far more importance than what you not eating that you should. I learned this in decades of pioneering work in the food allergy field. Almost ANYTHING was curable, from cancer to muscular dystrophy, from schizophrenia to arthritis, if you took away negative hurtful foods. And the bandit foods were different for everybody. Adding things in (supplements) is trivial next to expert food elimination.

Rule #3 (so far, they are in order of priority) - Every individual is different and varies in nutritional requirements from time to time and different individuals have highly disparate nutritional requirements at any one time. Isn't that obvious; we are all different? Well, not according to the textbooks!

Rule #4 - RDAs (daily values) take no account of different rates of absorption, individual biological variation, stress demands, or that the minimum requirement to avoid fatal avitaminosis is a totally different concept than the amount required for optimum health. Yet research shows that our requirements for B vitamins go up over a hundredfold when we are under severe stress!

Rule #5 - Natural foods in their natural state manifest energetic properties that bear no relation to their biochemical composition. The whole is more than the part! This makes a nonsense of ORAC values, "active ingredients," and all the other humbug surrounding the supplement industry. You only have to look at Kirlian photographs of "live" foods and cornflakes from a packet to tell the two are universes apart.

Rule #6 - Another HUGELY important factor that changes EVERYTHING, as soon as you incorporate it into your thinking: What is swallowed does not equate to nutrition. Malabsorption and dysbiosis are rampant. Digestive unwellness is the norm.

So much of what is swallowed never enters the metabolic stream! Stories abound of portable toilets having tablets and capsules that are so undigested you can still read the manufacturer's name on them!

Rule #7 - No nutrients act alone, they are all interdependent. All studies that purport to examine the effects of certain vitamins and minerals in isolation are likely to be misleading. Duh! Why don't scientific trials and studies use this obvious fact?

Rule #8 - Nutrition for detoxication is a life-saving factor in the modern world. We cannot have functioning enzymes to keep our bodies healthy and poison-free if essential nutrients are lacking. Enzymes are the life force driving an organism's metabolism. Now we need a whole new science of keeping our body mechanisms working, in the face of severe oxidative stress that simply did not exist when we were hunter-gatherers. The whole topic goes way beyond the avoidance of "deficiency diseases," like scurvy and beri-beri. [Incidentally, beri-beri is a local Sri Lankan word meaning *very weak*.]

Rule #9 - Foodstuffs, notably plants, contain pharmacologically active substances. The effect of these drugs can rightly be seen as a sub-function of nutrition (a complex, vast subject!). Caffeine isn't just a brain stimulant; it affects your blood pressure, heart rate, kidney function, and numerous other less investigated functions. Some plants, as you know, have hormone-like and anti-hormone effects. Isn't this part of nutrition too, if we eat them? I think so.

Rule #10 - This is an odd ball, but you need it! What goes in doesn't necessarily come out! (Nutritional implosion?) You can see evidence from colonics of food residues from many years earlier. Ignore the pseudo-science of most colonics people. They claim the bentonite residues are bowel content; they are not (just bentonite strings).

But I have confirmed stories with my patients on many occasions of the individual seeing a detox stool that contained some identifiable food eaten years before.

The record known to me was a patient of mine who had some showers of green cake decorations in her stool which she had not eaten for over 40 years. They were still green, for heaven's sake!

As I write, it is clear there is so much to this topic, that's why I am sharing this valuable information with you. *You won't find it anywhere else.*

VITAMIN C CAN HALVE YOUR CHANCE OF A HEART ATTACK

Vitamin C - you know it's good for you. Linus Pauling famously showed that 2 grams a day protects from viruses and cancer.

But did you know that vitamin C can actually reverse artery plaque and reduce arteriosclerosis as we age? You read that right: it is not just protective, but it can also REVERSE the age damage of arteries.

Dr. James Enstrom from the University of California studied the vitamin intake of over 11,000 people for 10 years. He found that 300mg of vitamin C a day reduced risk of heart disease by 50% in men and 40% in women. The test also revealed that a higher intake of vitamin C boosted life expectancy by 6 years.1

We know that lack of vitamin C leads to deterioration in collagen elasticity. In fact, skin won't heal; small blood vessels damage easily, leading to bruising, and teeth drop out. Blood vessels also deteriorate and that may lead to the scarring that we call "plaque" (thick plates inside the blood vessel walls).

Vitamin C is essential for the prevention of dangerous plaque buildup. Dr. Matthias Rath divided a group of guinea pigs into two groups. One group received only the equivalent of 60 mg of vitamin C a day in humans (the recommended daily allowance or RDA). The other group got the equivalent of 5,000 mg of vitamin C per day. In all other respects their diets were identical.

In just vie weeks, the guinea pigs who received 60 mg of vitamin C per day developed significant plaque deposits – especially in areas around the heart. The arteries of those who received 5,000mg of vitamin C per day were strong and clear without plaque.[2]

Why do we need these high doses of vitamin C?

Because we can't make our own. Most animals can manufacture their own vitamin C, which is why you don't see cows, dogs, and cats running around with flu and colds! Guinea pigs are like humans and can't make on-board vitamin C, which is why Dr. Rath used them.

References:
1. Enstrom J. *Epidemiology*.1992; 3:3, pp 194-202.
2. Rath M. *Why Animals Don't Get Heart Attacks... But People Do!* 2003. MR Publishing, Inc.

VITAMIN D HAS MORE AMAZING PROPERTIES

You really CANNOT afford to go short of vitamin D. Remember, it's silly cheap, so there is no need to skimp. You can get 5,000 IU (plenty for an adult), 240 caps, for under $8 if you Google it!

Take only D3, by the way, not the very inferior form of D2. Vitamin D2 was the first synthetic form of vitamin D. Vegans use it. D2 can be used to fortify foods, it's in some vitamin D supplements, and is the type put in all vitamin prescriptions. Therefore, don't bother your doctor for a script. You'll get junk nutrition.

Vitamin D insufficiency has been associated with a variety of clinical disorders and chronic diseases, including impaired balance, decreased muscle strength, mood and cognitive dysfunction, autoimmune disorders such as multiple sclerosis and diabetes (types 1 and 2), and certain forms of cancer. Woa!

This goes way beyond preventing rickets! It even goes beyond vitamin D as an immune stimulator.

Now, evidence is linking it to Parkinson's disease, but remember that's not quite the same as saying it causes the disease (correlation is not causation, as the saying goes). For example, lack of mobility, which is naturally a result of Parkinson's, may result in plummeting vitamin D levels.

In this new study, the researchers looked at 157 people with early, untreated Parkinson's disease and found that 69.4% had some lack of vitamin D, and 26.1% had vitamin D deficiency at the start of the study.

That's pretty bad in itself. But by the end of the study period, these levels had dropped to an appalling 51.6% and 7%, respectively. Bear in mind this means 7% of RDA, which is ridiculously low anyway.

Oh, and did I mention that vitamin D is associated with Alzheimer's, too?

Yes, a British study, presented at the Alzheimer's Association's International Conference in Honolulu (July 2010), showed that older men and women with low levels of vitamin D are nearly four times as likely to have problems with their memory, attention and logic.

Researchers have begun to think vitamin D is important to brain health by protecting the blood supply to the brain. It may also help to clear toxins from the brain, helping to break down amyloid-beta protein, the substance that is thought to play a role in causing Alzheimer's disease.

A related report, also published in July 2010 by some of the same researchers in the *Archives of Internal Medicine*, had similar results. It reported that older men and women with low levels of vitamin D don't do as well on tests of reasoning, learning, and memory as those with higher levels.

Participants completed interviews about their health history, had medical examinations, provided blood samples, and took tests measuring thinking skills at the start of the study and again after three years and six years.

The analysis reveals, that compared with participants who had sufficient vitamin D levels, those who were severely deficient experienced a substantial decline in thinking and in executive function - the ability to organize thoughts, make decisions and plan ahead.

And in case you are wondering: the authors say that the link between vitamin D deficiency and cognitive decline persisted even after adjusting for diet, health, and other factors!

Better get some and start taking it, before you forget why you should!

He he!

Another Reason Why Vitamin D Is One of the Most Amazing Natural Substances for Human Health

Deficiency of this vital substance is a possible risk factor for a host of other diseases, including multiple cancers, arthritis, diabetes, multiple sclerosis, and even tuberculosis.

Now, it seems, vitamin D has been found to lower blood pressure. Meaning that the Western deficiency in vitamin D (partly caused by government's stupid low recommendation of only 200 units) is one of the likely reasons we are seeing an epidemic of hypertension just now.

A recent study showed that a vitamin D deficiency before age 45 was associated with a threefold increased risk for hypertension in midlife. By the end of the trial, when the average age of the women was 53, about one in four had developed high blood pressure.

There are two important health messages I can discern. One is obvious: get plenty of vitamin D (these researchers suggested 10 times the RDA, or about 4,000 units!).

Many foods, including milk, yogurt, breads, and cereals, are fortified with vitamin D, but is very difficult to get adequate levels of the vitamin from food sources alone.

The other message is that whatever you do when you are kids has a very powerful impact on health in later life. Kids who are gaming couch potatoes, obese, and fed on junk are going to grow up sick and die young.

Get them outdoors in the sunshine. If you live in northern grey climes, then supplement. It's dirt cheap, considering its benefits; less than $10 for a month's supply of 2,000 unit capsules.

[SOURCES: American Heart Association 63rd High Blood Pressure Research Conference, Chicago, Sept. 24, 2009. *JAMA*/Archives journals, news release, March 14, 2011.]

COCOA IN CHOCOLATE IS GOOD FOR THE HEART

Spanish researchers put 42 men and women on a diet that included 40 grams of unsweetened cocoa powder (about 1.4 ounces) mixed with skim milk daily, or plain skim milk. During the study, participants didn't take additional vitamins or supplements, and the only cocoa-containing products they consumed were those provided by researchers.

After one month, those who drank the cocoa-flavored milk had **lower levels of inflammatory markers** associated with heart disease than those drinking the milk alone!

That result was critical because the participants, whose average age was about 70, were at high risk of cardiovascular disease because they had diabetes and three or more risk factors for heart disease, including smoking, high blood pressure, high levels of LDL "bad" cholesterol (more than 160 milligrams per deciliter), low levels of HDL "good" cholesterol (below 35 milligrams per deciliter), obesity, or a family history of early coronary heart disease.

Cocoa **increased** HDL (good) cholesterol, and **lowered** levels of LDL (bad) cholesterol. Cocoa was shown to have anti-inflammatory, antioxidant properties. The study is published in the November 2009 issue of the *American Journal of Clinical Nutrition*.

The secret is polyphenols; these are major antioxidants that protect your heart. Of course diehard idiots will tell you to eat more green veggies instead of "unhealthy" chocolate.

Do you know what? A 2-oz bar of untreated (natural) chocolate contains more antioxidants than a whole lousy plate of raw broccoli. I'm not kidding!

This is recent research, but I have been on the chocolate story for years, because of my fabulous "Doctor's Chocolate" and the care I took to make sure it conformed to all that we know of heart-healthy and anti-inflammatory science.

DID YOU EAT YOUR SULFUR TODAY?

Sulfur is a superfood, if ever there was one. We need plenty of it.

Sulfur is part of our detox mechanisms; what we call Phase II detox is moderated mainly by glutathione and consists mainly of conjugating toxic molecules with things like a sulfate radical. That renders the toxin relatively harmless and it can be excreted, via urine, bile, or skin.

The precursors of glutathione, such as N-acetyl-cysteine (NAC) and s-adenosyl-methionine (SAMe) are, essentially, just sulfur donors. Sulfur is present in certain foods, such as the crucifers; break open some raw broccoli and sniff it. You'll see what I mean.

(Wherever you get stinky smells, sulfur is the reason. Garlic is rich in sulfur, which is why it smells, and it is a great detoxer! The repellant smell of rotten eggs is hydrogen sulfide, a simple compound of hydrogen and sulfur).

Sulfur is a nutrient probably more important to health than magnesium, zinc, iron, copper, sodium, iodine - and, for that matter, many vitamins. It accounts for about 1% of our body weight, for heaven's sake!

You'll have heard of MSM (methylsulphonylmethane) for joints and ligaments.

Sulfur-containing crucifers (cabbage and broccoli family) are known to help fend off cancer. The active agent is indol-3-carbinol and that too is rich in sulfur.

Is this beginning to add up for you?

Sulfur is so essential for life that you would die without it, yet it is hardly ever mentioned in books on nutrition.

But the old folks kinda knew about it. They used to dose kids on brimstone and treacle; remember? Brimstone and treacle is prepared by mixing an ounce and a half of sulfur, and half an ounce of cream of tartar, with eight ounces of treacle; and, according to the age of the child, giving from a small teaspoonful to a dessertspoonful, early in the morning, two or three times a week.

Not surprisingly, it made kids pretty sick and probably worked by stopping the child from voicing their suffering so they didn't get the "cure"! But the sulfur does kill most parasites, so this was a good worming mix.

Interestingly, sulfur has been a common ingredient in homeopathic remedies, developed in the 19th century and still popular today as over-the-counter remedies.

Now researchers understand that sulfur forms part of the matrix of bone joints in the form of chondroitin sulfate and glucosamine sulfate.

Yessir, we need plenty of that! Don't forget.

FLAX SEED OIL – SIMPLY AMAZING!

Sometimes thought of as the "new" craze, flaxseed has a l-o-n-g history!

Flaxseed was cultivated in Babylon as early as 3000 BC. By the 8th century, King Charlemagne believed so strongly in the health benefits of flaxseed that he passed laws requiring his subjects to consume it.

Now it's enjoying a renaissance (literally: new birth) and flaxseed is found in all kinds of foods, from crackers to frozen waffles to oatmeal. Scores of new products are flooding the market that list flax or flaxseed as an ingredient. It's not only being supplied to humans but flaxseed is also fed to the doughty chickens who are charged with producing for us all those eggs that are "higher in omega-3 fatty acids."

It's a natural foodstuff; that's good. It's reputation is centered mainly on the omega-3 content. But flaxseed also contain **lignans**; in fact 75 to 800 times more lignans than other plant foods. Lignans in flaxseed have been shown to reduce atherosclerotic plaque buildup by up to 75%. So great for the heart.

Lignans also have certain estrogenic properties. A 2007 study reported that 2 tablespoons of ground flaxseed (taken twice each day) cut a menopausal women's hot flashes in half. And the intensity of their hot flashes dropped by 57%. That's pretty significant. And it was quick: the women noticed a difference after talking the daily flaxseed for just one week, and achieved the maximum benefit within two weeks.

Flaxseed also reduces bad cholesterol, improves blood sugar in diabetics, and lowers inflammation in any tissue.

Finally, flaxseed has great anti-cancer properties. You may have read in my publications that Joanna Budwig built one of the most successful cancer treatments around this humble seed. I explained in detail how this harnesses the special electrons (pi electrons) released from the Sun, which have the magic equivalent of oxygen when they reach the tissues.

The best way to take it is cold-pressed flaxseed oil (otherwise it is worthless).

You can grind your own flaxseed, to make oil (more like a paste really). Don't forget to do this. Remember how Oprah was embarrassed on the air on one of her programs when she was told you have to grind it first! She hadn't been doing it right and was just passing poop full of undigested flax seeds!

Don't grind it till the moment you need it. Air turns fresh oils rancid very quickly. Add fresh ground flaxseed to your oatmeal, smoothies, soup, or yogurt. You can use it in baking. Substitute ground flaxseed for part of the flour in recipes for quick breads, muffins, rolls, bread, bagels, pancakes, and waffles. Try replacing ¼ to ½ cup of the flour with ground flaxseed if the recipe calls for 2 or more cups of flour.

Keep it refrigerated at all times. Pour it cold onto salads too!

HERBS CAN REALLY WORK FOR PAIN

An herb called **Brazilian mint** (*Hyptis crenata*) treats pain as effectively as a synthetic aspirin-style drug called Indomethacin, according to researchers at Newcastle University (England).

Hyptis crenata has long been used in Brazil to treat a range of painful health problems, such as headaches and stomach pain. This study is the first to scientifically prove the pain-relieving properties of Brazilian mint.

The study was presented Nov. 24, 2009, at a conference in India, in advance of publication in an upcoming issue of the journal *Acta Horticulturae*.

"What we have done is to take a plant that is widely used to safely treat pain and scientifically proven that it works as well as some synthetic drugs. Now the next step is to find out how and why the plant works," Study leader Graciela Rocha said in a university news release.

Brazilian mint is traditionally taken as a tea infusion.

[SOURCE: Newcastle University, news release, Nov. 24, 2009.]

THE NUMBER ONE ANTIOXIDANT

Forget noni juice, acai berry and all the ORAC lies and hype: the master antioxidant, and the original star, has always been **superoxide dismutase (SOD).** It has been called the *"master guardian."* Compared to vitamin C, this nutrient is 3,500 times stronger.[1]

In aging studies, researchers discovered that mammals that produce the highest levels of SOD have the longest life spans. And, according to Cutler, when they genetically engineered fruit flies to have double the amount of this nutrient, the fruit flies lived twice as long.[2]

SOD is so vital that production starts when you're in the womb. In one study, genetically engineered mice whose bodies couldn't make their own SOD died in just days from massive free radical damage.[3]

That's how important antioxidants are!

Unfortunately, levels drop off as we age, leading to a buildup of free radicals.[4]

Moreover, native levels of SOD vary by as much as 50% from person to person, depending on genetic and other factors.[5]

That may be why some people age quickly and why others live to a ripe old age without any problems.

You should be concerned about how much SOD is in your body. It would be great if we could supplement it but haven't been able to. Till now…

A patent has been passed which claims to have solved the problem of getting SOD absorbed by the oral route, without being destroyed by the digestive process (US Patent 6 04 5809).

The new process wraps SOD in a protective coating, which enables it to pass through your digestive tract without being damaged.

The new patented, absorbable form of SOD is available in Dr. Al Sear's antioxidant formula RES-3, along with two other well-recognized antioxidants that make it pretty formidable protection.

References
1. Colman J. "Life Span-Increasing Effects of Super Oxide Dismutase (SOD)." *LEM*. Winter 2005/2006.
2. Cutler RG. "Antioxidants and longevity of mammalian species." Basic Life Sci. 1985;35:15-73. And Cutler RG. "Antioxidants and aging." *Am J Clin Nutr.* 1991 Jan;53(1 Suppl):373S-9S.
3. Li, et al. "Cardiomyopathy and neonatal lethality in mutant mice lacking manganese superoxide dismutase," *Nature Genetics*. 1995. 11:376-381.
4. Lishnevskaia VL. "The role of free radical oxidation in aging." *Adv Gerontol*. 2004;13:52-7.
5. Ueda K, et al. "Levels of SOD in Japanese people." *Acta Med Okayama*. 1978 Dec;(6):393-7.

WHAT IS CHIA? DOES IT WORK FOR WEIGHT LOSS?

I'd never heard of chia till I got an advisory from WebMD. Apparently, it's being sold as a weight loss aid. Probably the reason I have never heard of it is that it doesn't work!

Chia is an edible seed that comes from the desert plant *Salvia hispanica*, grown in Mexico dating back to Mayan and Aztec cultures. "Chia" means strength, and folklore has it that these cultures used the tiny black and white seeds as an energy booster.

Chia seeds are a concentrated food containing healthy omega-3 fatty acids, carbohydrates, protein, fiber, antioxidants, and calcium.

Chia seeds are an unprocessed, whole-grain food that can be absorbed by the body as seeds (unlike flaxseeds, which have to be ground to be digestible). One ounce (about 2 tablespoons) contains 139 calories, 4 grams protein, 9 grams fat, 12 grams carbohydrates, and 11 grams of fiber, plus vitamins and minerals.

The mild, nutty flavor of chia seeds makes them easy to add to foods and beverages. They are most often sprinkled on cereal, sauces, vegetables, rice dishes, or yogurt, or mixed into drinks and baked goods. They can also be mixed with water and made into a gel.

So far, so good, right?

But does chia work for weight loss? Nah...

David Nieman, a professor at Appalachian State University in North Carolina, **found no reduction in body weight, body fat and no improvement in traditional cardiovascular markers from 50 grams of chia per day**, despite the claims.

It's the *Hoodia* and hydroxycort story all over again.

For weight loss then, a resounding NO.

VITAMIN E TRIUMPHS AGAIN

Really, the torrent of positives is just boring!

There are really two parts to this latest story: this study strikes at the continuing oft-quoted nonsense that antioxidants, especially vitamins C and E and beta carotenes, are bad for you, and also points out that nutrients have a major impact on Alzheimer's disease (something the drug-run Alzheimer's Association consistently denies, while pushing its useless drug recommendations).

Alpha-tocopherol, one of the more common forms of vitamin E, has been widely studied for potential protective effects against the onset of Alzheimer's disease.

Whenever people equate alpha-tocopherol with "vitamin E," you can know they are getting it wrong. Really WRONG.

Alpha-tocopherol is a synthetic manufactured substance. It contains none of the many variants found in the natural vitamin E. Vitamin E is really a family of eight substances, with different prefixes (gamma-tocopherol etc.).

And when you read the vitamin E has "no benefit" on heart disease, or that it may even be dangerous, know that it's not vitamin E, just the synthetic stuff.

However, not everyone is a phony or a fool. Dr. Francesca Mangialasche, from the Karolinska Institute in Stockholm (Sweden), and colleagues knew what they were doing. They studied a group of 232 men and women, ages 80 years and older, who were dementia-free at the study's start. The researchers follows the subjects for six years, tracking the onset of Alzheimer's disease and measuring blood levels of all eight natural vitamin E components.

What they found was pretty telling: those patients who had higher blood levels of all the vitamin E family forms were at a markedly reduced risk of developing Alzheimer's Disease, as compared to subjects with lower levels. In fact a 45-54% lower risk, depending on the vitamin E component.

The researchers conclude that:

The neuroprotective effect of vitamin E seems to be related to the combination of different forms, rather than to alpha-tocopherol alone. High plasma levels of vitamin E forms and reduced Alzheimer's disease risk in advanced age.[1]

References:
1. Francesca Mangialasche, Miia Kivipelto, Patrizia Mecocci, Debora Rizzuto, Katie Palmer, Bengt Winblad, Laura Fratiglioni. *Journal of Alzheimer's Disease*, Vol. 20 No. 4, Pages 1029-1037, 5 July 2010; DOI: 10.3233/JAD-2010-091450.

WHO LIKES ARTICHOKES?

*If you like a*rtichokes, you are in luck.

As I wrote in my book: **Love Your Liver**, globe artichoke (*Cynoma scolymus*) is a really good liver support plant, right up there with milk thistle and schisandra! In fact, globe artichoke is a kind of thistle. Don't mix this up with the jerusalem artichoke, which is the tuber of a sunflower-type plant.

European doctors have been using artichokes to treat jaundice and other liver complaints since as far back as the 18th century. Artichokes protect the liver from damage and even help it regenerate.

It was not until the 1930s that German and French researchers began to study artichokes in their laboratories. Later, Italian researchers joined them to produce a substantial amount of research. It is reported to stimulate bile secretion and to act as a diuretic, antidyspeptic, lipid-lowering agent, and antioxidant in human studies.

Cynarin, luteolin, cynardoside (luteolin-7-O-glycoside), scolymoside, and chlorogenic acid are believed to be artichoke's active constituents. The most studied component, cynarin, is concentrated in the leaves.

In one study, dozens of Polish workers who were exposed to the toxic chemical fumes of carbon disulfide were given an artichoke extract for two years, which protected them from damage, according to their blood work. The results of this study were presented in 1960 at the Symposium on Drugs Affecting Lipid Metabolism in Milan, Italy.

I found a study on PubMed that said the same thing.

In this toxic world, it's nice to know there are vegetables that specifically protect our beleaguered livers. You can find out other ways to help your liver help you by getting this eBook: *Love Your Liver*. Visit: www.alternative-doctor.com/liver

I don't have recipes for globe artichoke, unfortunately. All we do in our house is cook 'em in water and serve with butter and sea salt! Too bad they are so fiddly to eat.

Artichoke hearts are probably easier to serve. Check out this comprehensive artichoke salad from the BBC.

VITAMIN B1 MEGA-DOSES REVERSE EARLY-STAGE KIDNEY DISEASE

You may not know that diabetes is a sure path to kidney damage. As I said, diabetes is fast-aging.

I just came across an interesting study showing that *thiamine*, vitamin B1, can protect the kidneys from damage, at least in the early stages.

What surprised me was the very large doses used by the researchers. These were even beyond what we used to call *"megavitamin therapy"* doses (not recommended).

The research came from the Warwick Medical School, UK, in collaboration with researchers at the University of Punjab and Sheik Zaid Hospital, Lahore, Pakistan (beautiful old castle in Warwick, by the way. Richard de Beauchamp, 13th Earl of Warwick, was the man who supervised Joan of Arc's trial and execution).

Back to kidneys! Kidney disease, or diabetic nephropathy, develops progressively in patients with type 2 diabetes. Early development of kidney disease is assessed by a high excretion rate of the protein called albumin in the urine.

The Warwick team discovered that taking high oral doses of thiamine (300 mg) can dramatically decrease the excretion of albumin and reverse early stage kidney disease in type 2 diabetes patients. In fact the albumin excretion rate was decreased by 41%.

The Warwick research group has already conclusively proven that type 2 diabetes patients have a thiamine deficiency, which could also be the key to a range of vascular problems for diabetes patients.

[SOURCE: Rabbani et al. High-dose thiamine therapy for patients with type 2 diabetes and microalbuminuria: a randomized, double-blind placebo-controlled pilot study. *Diabetologia*, 2008; DOI: 10.1007/s00125-008-1224-4.]

SOMETHING NEW FOR ALLERGIES?

Our old friend vitamin D again.

We know that vitamin D is great. It does far more than just protect us from rickets!

It turns out to be an immune super-booster too; its presence in adequate amounts reduces the risk of cancer and infections.

Not so surprising then, that it **helps reduce allergies**. In a study published in the *Journal of Clinical Investigation*, researchers report finding that vitamin D not only substantially reduced the production of the protein driving an allergic response, but it also increased production of the proteins that promote tolerance.

Mold allergies, especially to common mould (*Aspergillus fumigatus*), can often cause severe complications for asthma sufferers - but not all.

The study was designed to find why only a certain sub-set of patients with asthma suffered from the mold allergy. They discovered an association between vitamin D and a bandit protein (called OX40L), which was critical in driving the allergic response to the mold.

Patients with low levels of vitamin D had more of the trouble protein and less of the protective ones. When vitamin D was supplemented, that reversed.

So again the way is open to a good treatment of asthma, without using the usual dangerous asthma drugs (which probably kill as many people as the disease does).

Just take lots of vitamin D: 4,000- 5,000 IU is fine. Plus it's one of the cheapest vitamins in town!

"Our study provides further evidence that vitamin D appears to be broadly associated with human health," said the chief researcher.

A bit of an understatement, I think!

Interestingly, Dr. Carl Reich MD in Canada was treating asthma kids with vitamin D; thousands of kids in fact. They pulled his license; but not for vitamin D use. For claiming that coral calcium was the cure for cancer (silly man!)

[SOURCE: *Journal of Clinical Investigation*, published online ahead of print, doi:10.1172/JCI42388. "Immune Tolerance to *Aspergillus fumigatus* versus Allergic Bronchopulmonary Aspergillosis: roles of OX40L and vitamin D in humans and mice." Authors: J.L. Kreindler, C. Steele, N. Nguyen, Y.R. Chan , et al.]

SOME OF MY WEBSITES YOU MIGHT LIKE TO VISIT

Alternative Doctor
www.alternative-doctor.com
Discover alternative health articles, videos, inspiration, and quotes directly from my years of research. You'll find I dig deep beyond traditional health care and conventionally accepted wisdom to help you live a longer life!

Diet Wise
www.alternative-doctor.com/dietwise
Food is what really matters…and eating the *wrong foods* can create allergies and suppresses your immune system. By eating the wrong kinds of food you actually weaken your immune system and could spark a chain reaction that creates the perfect environment for cancer cells to attack and thrive. Check out my amazing world-class food regime, that's been proven to be the best immunity and cancer fighting diet, for the last 32 years.

Cancer Research Secrets
www.www.alternative-doctor.com/stopcancer
I'll share with you how diet, emotions, and your environment are at the root cause of cancer and yet there is always a cause. "Cancer Research Secrets" is your GPS to the heart of the problem, a user-friendly map to find your way around and get to the cure you or a loved one so desperately need.

How to Survive In A World Without Antibiotics
www.alternative-doctor.com/wwa
Antibiotics have been terribly overused. Find out how to survive antibiotic resistant bacteria and how these natural alternatives are better than drugs!

Get Healthy For Your Next 100 Years
www.alternative-doctor.com/gethealthy
Don't kid yourself with the "short life but a happy one" baloney. Get it right and you have a whole second life to come, full of fun and vigor. Get it wrong and you'll live mainly in regrets, limitations and discomfort. *Get the inside story on why yesterday's science is wrong.*

Fire In The Belly
www.alternative-doctor.com/firebelly
Did you know…the secret to better health lies in your gut? Find out the surprising cause of most diseases, states of mind and aging processes… it's the biggest medical breakthrough ever!

Ultimate Guide to Natural Pain Relief
www.alternative-doctor.com/nopain
When pain comes calling…be ready! The most up-to-date compilation book filled with natural pain relief solutions for headaches, migraine, back pain, arthritis, cancer pain, sports injuries and much more!

Alternative Doctor Newsletter
www.alternative-doctor.com/newsletter
This is where I chat intimately with my subscribers: on anything from mind, body, and spirit to the latest science discoveries, medical studies, current events, fun tidbits, and more…